Early Intervention in Psychiatry

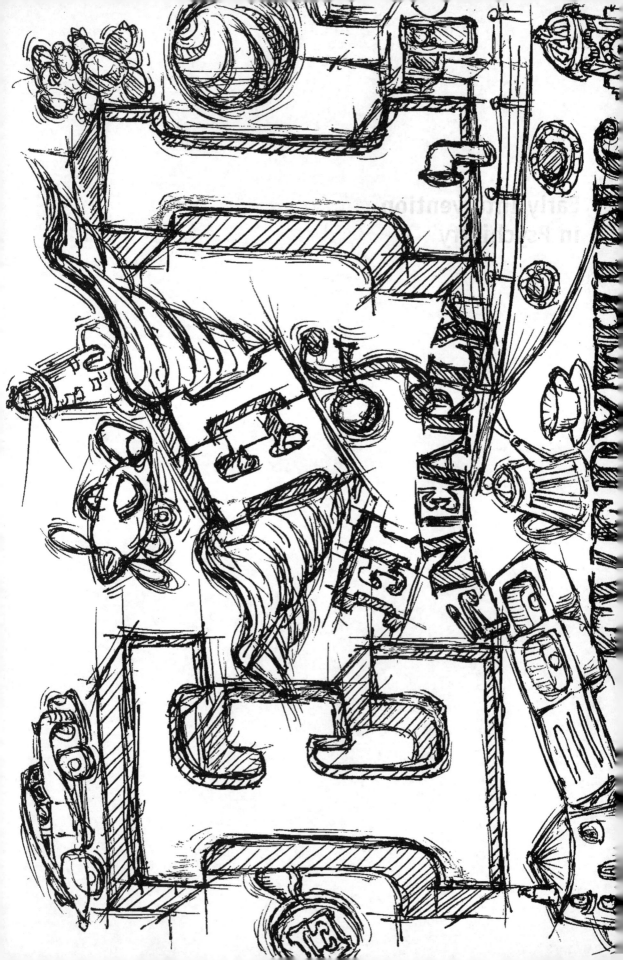

Early Intervention in Psychiatry

EI of nearly everything for better mental health

Edited by

Peter Byrne

Homerton University Hospital, London; Royal College of Psychiatrists, UK

Alan Rosen

School of Public Health, University of Wollongong
Brain and Mind Research Institute, University of Sydney
Mental Health Commission of New South Wales, Australia

WILEY Blackwell

This edition first published 2014 © 2014 by John Wiley & Sons, Ltd

Registered office: John Wiley & Sons Ltd, The Atrium, Southern Gate, Chichester, West Sussex, PO19 8SQ, UK

Editorial offices: 9600 Garsington Road, Oxford, OX4 2DQ, UK
The Atrium, Southern Gate, Chichester, West Sussex, PO19 8SQ, UK
111 River Street, Hoboken, NJ 07030-5774, USA

For details of our global editorial offices, for customer services and for information about how to apply for permission to reuse the copyright material in this book please see our website at www.wiley.com/wiley-blackwell.

Library of Congress Cataloging-in-Publication Data

Early intervention in psychiatry (Byrne)
 Early intervention in psychiatry : EI of nearly everything for better mental health / edited by Peter Byrne, Alan Rosen.
  p. ; cm.
 Includes bibliographical references and index.
 ISBN 978-0-470-68342-2 (cloth : alk. paper)
 I. Byrne, Peter, 1964- editor.   II. Rosen, Alan, 1946 January 3- editor.   III. Title.
 [DNLM: 1. Mental Disorders–prevention & control.   2. Early Medical Intervention–methods.   3. Mental Health Services–organization & administration. WM 400]
 RC454.4
 616.89–dc23

2014014775

A catalogue record for this book is available from the British Library.

Wiley also publishes its books in a variety of electronic formats. Some content that appears in print may not be available in electronic books.

Set in 10/12.5pt Times Ten by Aptara Inc., New Delhi, India
Printed in Singapore by C.O.S. Printers Pte Ltd

1   2014

Dedication

This book is dedicated to one of our Early Intervention of Nearly Everything *book co-authors, Professor Helen Lester, who died on this journey at the height of her academic and practical achievements, many of them concerning early intervention in primary care settings. She left a young family behind her. We also pay tribute to all the contributing authors in this book, from whom we have learned so much of value relevant to early prevention and intervention in a wider world. We acknowledge too all the people with lived experience of mental illnesses and their families, and the many dedicated service providers and researchers from whom we have learned about the immense value of earlier intervention approaches to many mental health conditions. Finally, we sincerely thank our families for their unflinching support for this, at least initially, quixotic dash into uncharted territory, and forbearance in living with our cognitive absences from them at times, due to our intermittent preoccupation with this most absorbing project.*

Contents

Part V   Conclusions

List of Contributors

Marco Armando Child and Adolescence Neuropsychiatry Unit, Department of Neuroscience, Children Hospital Bambino Gesù, Rome, Italy; School of Psychology, University of Birmingham, Edgbaston, Birmingham, UK

Iyas Assalman Newham Centre for Mental Health, London and East London Foundation NHS Trust

Jane Barlow Mental Health & Wellbeing, Warwick Medical School, University of Warwick, UK

Arvin Bhana School of Applied Human Sciences, Howard College, University of KwaZulu-Natal, Durban, South Africa

Maximilian Birchwood YouthSpace; University of Warwick, UK

Sophie Bridger Mental Health Foundation, UK

Helen Bruce University College London, Institute of Child Health, London, UK; East London NHS Foundation Trust, London, UK; Barts and the London School of Medicine and Dentistry, London, UK

Peter Byrne Homerton University Hospital, London; Royal College of Psychiatrists, UK

Tom Callaly Barwon Health, Geelong, Victoria, Australia; School of Medicine, Deakin University, Geelong, Victoria, Australia

Andrew M. Chanen Orygen Youth Health Research Centre & Centre for Youth Mental Health, The University of Melbourne, Melbourne, Australia; Orygen Youth Health Clinical Program, Northwestern Mental Health, Melbourne, Australia

Philippe Conus Treatment and early Intervention in Psychosis Program (TIPP), Service of General Psychiatry, Department of Psychiatry CHUV, Lausanne University, Switzerland

Jayne Cooper Centre for Suicide Prevention, Centre for Mental Health and Risk, University of Manchester, Manchester, UK

Patrick Corrigan　Illinois Institute of Technology, Chicago

Walter Cullen　Department of General Practice, University of Limerick Medical School, Limerick, Ireland

Franco De Crescenzo　Child and Adolescence Neuropsychiatry Unit, Department of Neuroscience, Children Hospital Bambino Gesù, Rome, Italy

Mark Deady　National Drug and Alcohol Research Centre, University of New South Wales, Sydney, Australia

Linda Dowdney　University College London, Institute of Child Health, London, UK

Gráinne Fadden　Meriden Family Programme, Birmingham and Solihull Mental Health NHS Foundation Trust, Birmingham, UK; University of Birmingham, Birmingham, UK

Rick Fraser　Early Intervention in Psychosis Service, Sussex Partnership NHS Foundation Trust, Sussex, UK

Isabella Goldie　Mental Health Foundation, UK

Helen Herrman　Collaborating Centre for Mental Health, University of Melbourne, Parkville, Melbourne, Victoria, Australia

Rajeev Jairam　Gna Ka Lun Adolescent Mental Health Unit, South West Sydney Local Health District, Campbelltown, New South Wales, Australia; School of Medicine, University of New South Wales and University of Western Sydney

Nav Kapur　Centre for Suicide Prevention, Centre for Mental Health and Risk, University of Manchester, Manchester, UK

Tony Kendrick　Hull York Medical School, University of York, York, UK

Martin Knapp　Centre for the Economics of Mental and Physical Health, Health Service and Population Research Department, Institute of Psychiatry, King's College London, UK; Personal Social Services Research Unit, London School of Economics and Political Science, UK

Kristin Kosyluk　Illinois Institute of Technology, Chicago

Brian Lawlor　Mercer's Institute for Research on Ageing; Trinity College Dublin; St Patrick's and St James's Hospitals, Dublin, Ireland

Helen Lester　Primary Care, School of Health and Population Sciences, University of Birmingham, UK

Crick Lund Department of Psychiatry and Mental Health, University of Cape Town, Rondebosch, Cape Town, South Africa

Craig Macneil Treatment and early Intervention in Psychosis Program (TIPP), Service of General Psychiatry, Department of Psychiatry CHUV, Lausanne University, Switzerland

Karl Marlowe East London NHS Foundation Trust, London, England, UK

Paul McCrone Centre for the Economics of Mental and Physical Health, Health Service and Population Research Department, Institute of Psychiatry, King's College London, UK

Andrew McCulloch Mental Health Foundation, UK

Louise McCutcheon Orygen Youth Health Research Centre & Centre for Youth Mental Health, The University of Melbourne, Melbourne, Australia; Orygen Youth Health Clinical Program, Northwestern Mental Health, Melbourne, Australia

Patrick McGorry Orygen Youth Health Research Centre, University of Melbourne, Melbourne, Australia

David Meagher Department of Psychiatry, University of Limerick Medical School, Limerick, Ireland

Nick Meinhold Monash University, Victoria, Australia; University of Queensland, Brisbane, St Lucia, Queensland, Australia; Community Healthfulness Cooperative, Melbourne, Victoria, Australia

Irwin Nazareth Department of Primary Care & Population Health, London, UK

Celia O'Hare The Irish Longitudinal Study on Ageing (TILDA), Department of Medical Gerontology, Trinity College Dublin, Ireland

Nicola C. Newton National Drug and Alcohol Research Centre, University of New South Wales, Sydney, Australia

Inge Petersen School of Applied Human Sciences, Howard College, University of KwaZulu-Natal, Durban, South Africa

Leora Pinhas Eating Disorders Program, The Hospital for Sick Children, Toronto, Ontario; Department of Psychiatry, University of Toronto, Toronto, Ontario

Paddy Power Treatment and early Intervention in Psychosis Program (TIPP), Service of General Psychiatry, Department of Psychiatry CHUV, Lausanne University, Switzerland

Rosemary Purcell Centre for Forensic Behavioural Science, Swinburne University of Technology, Melbourne, Victoria, Australia

Alan Rosen School of Public Health, University of Wollongong; Brain and Mind Research Institute, University of Sydney; Mental Health Commission of New South Wales, Australia

Hannah Schwartz St. Mary's Hospital Center, McGill University, Montreal, Canada

Jan Scott Newcastle University & Centre for Affective Disorders, Institute of Psychiatry, UK

David Shiers National Early Intervention Programme, England; Leek, North Staffordshire, UK; National Mental Health Development Unit, London, UK

Jo Smith National Early Intervention Programme, England; Worcestershire Health and Care NHS Trust, Worcester, UK; University of Worcester, Worcester, UK

Martin St-André Sainte-Justine University Health Center, Université de Montréal, Montreal, Canada

Sarah Steeg Centre for Suicide Prevention, Centre for Mental Health and Risk, University of Manchester, Manchester, UK

Danny Sullivan Centre for Forensic Behavioural Science, Swinburne University of Technology, Melbourne, Victoria, Australia; Victorian Institute of Forensic Mental Health, Clifton Hill, Victoria, Australia

Maree Teesson National Drug and Alcohol Research Centre, University of New South Wales, Sydney, Australia

Garry Walter Discipline of Psychiatry, University of Sydney; Child and Adolescent Mental Health Services, Northern Sydney Local Health District, New South Wales, Australia

Amy C. Watson Jane Addams College of Social Work, University of Illinois at Chicago, Chicago

Jennifer Wong Eating Disorders Program, The Hospital for Sick Children, Toronto, Ontario

D. Blake Woodside Department of Psychiatry, University of Toronto, Toronto, Ontario; University Health Network, Toronto, Ontario

Keiko Yoshida Department of Child Psychiatry, Kyushu University Hospital, Fukuoka City, Japan

Foreword

Prevention of mental illness can take many forms and should be at the heart of mental health services. Traditionally, prevention has been classified into primary, secondary and tertiary. Virtually all psychiatric clinical practice is about secondary and tertiary prevention by treating the symptoms when they have developed and require intervention. In many cases, the development of these symptoms and the accompanying distress will determine where help is sought from and who is approached for intervention. The recognition of early distress has to be achieved carefully, as there is a serious danger that normal responses to stress or distress themselves may be pathologised and medicalised.

Early intervention can be seen at multiple levels – as an intervention at an appropriate stage before symptoms become resistant to intervention or as early recognition of the need to intervene. There are clearly ethical dilemmas which need to be resolved. Primary prevention is not only about mental health promotion and reduction in precipitating factors, but also about improving resilience. Early intervention is about treating people who are at risk of developing disorders as well as intervening at an early stage to improve the possibility of recovery. Clinicians as well as stakeholders need to be aware of the possibilities that early intervention in many conditions may help. We know that children with conduct disorders are more likely to develop personality disorders when they grow up. This development if averted may contribute to huge savings in the long run. One of the major challenges is for health to work with education, the criminal justice system and other departments to achieve this reduction. Another major challenge is where early interventions are based and placed – whether this is in primary care or secondary care. In either case, should they have strict boundaries? In which case, it is inevitable that further fragmentation and exclusion criteria come into play. The advantages of early intervention are many – through early and better engagement of the individuals and their carers and families – such approaches may reduce stigma and enable carers to learn about the illnesses and their consequences. For some psychiatric conditions, early intervention will take place in adolescence, whereas for others it will be in older age. These interventions need to be comprehensive, evidence based and interdisciplinary, no matter where they are placed.

Those individuals and families who may be at risk need to be educated and engaged in understanding what may precipitate certain illnesses, what the predisposing and perpetuating factors may be and how the individual, their families and society at large cope and manage these.

Interventions at antenatal stages, especially maternal support and abstinence from alcohol, smoking and drugs, can help. Postnatal support and educating about maternal and parenting skills will enable the development of better attachment patterns in infants and children. Education about bullying and other factors at school will enable children to manage better in facing these and future adversities. Better physical health, physical exercise and employment all provide strategies for coping with stress and distress. There is compelling evidence that social inequalities, poor public transport, lack of green spaces can contribute to mental ill health.

It is heartening to note that there appears to be an increasing interest in prevention of mental ill health and mental health promotion. It is vital that these issues are taken up at both undergraduate and postgraduate levels. The present volume, with its array of topics and authors, will provide a further platform for ongoing discussion and debate but, more importantly, will contribute to practical advice which mental health professionals across disciplines will find helpful.

Dinesh Bhugra CBEPhD FRCPsych
Professor of Mental Health and Cultural Diversity
Health Service and Population Research Department
Institute of Psychiatry, King's College London
London, UK

I

The Rationale for Early Intervention in Nearly Everything

1
Introduction

Peter Byrne[1,2] and Alan Rosen[3,4,5]
[1] *Homerton University Hospital, London*
[2] *Royal College of Psychiatrists, UK*
[3] *School of Public Health, University of Wollongong*
[4] *Brain and Mind Research Institute, University of Sydney*
[5] *Mental Health Commission of New South Wales, Australia*

Early intervention (EI) is arguably the single most important advance in mental health care of the past decade. In terms of all-time advances in mental health care delivery, EI is up there with the consumer, family, recovery, and human rights for psychiatric disability movements, person-centred and holistic integrated services, effective psychotropic medications and psychotherapeutic interventions, evidence-based psychosocial interventions and mobile assertive community-centred service delivery systems. EI represents a key shift in both theoretical standpoint and service delivery, and marks an end to the first era of community psychiatry – where we set up 'accessible' clinical structures by locality, and patients were expected to adapt to these. With EI, practitioners reconfigure how they work to engage, negotiate and agree interventions support and care with their service users. From a general practitioner (GP) perspective, some modern community mental health teams (CMHTs) have 'raised the bar' to focus only on those with severe mental illness (SMI), now implicitly or formally defined as established psychotic disorders. Many CMHTs decline people in crisis or in the early stages of illness: by the time their referral is accepted later on, engagement is harder and many interventions have a reduced efficacy. Like all useful ideas, EI is a simple one and has instant appeal to people in early stages of illness (crucially often *before* insight is lost) and to their families. Key clinicians, notably GPs and mental health professionals also have a strong self-interest in designing and supporting efficient EI services. It is both self-evident to them, and increasingly evident from emerging studies, that such timely approaches could save much harder and longer clinical endeavour further down the track. We list the key pioneers later (Chapter 27), many of whom have contributed to this book. Their work, along with impressive citations at the

Early Intervention in Psychiatry: EI of nearly everything for better mental health, First Edition.
Edited by Peter Byrne and Alan Rosen.
© 2014 John Wiley & Sons, Ltd. Published 2014 by John Wiley & Sons, Ltd.

end of each chapter, should persuade readers new to EI that this will be a key component of the twenty-first century mental health care. This book's main aim is to affirm for every clinician, every purchaser of services and other interested parties the high value of EI in most care settings from cradle to grave.

Prevention

Caplan's three levels of prevention are well described [1, 2]. Primary prevention prevents the disorder from occurring in the first place, secondary restores health from an existing disorder, while tertiary attempts to claw back better function from persistent or long-term disorders. In mental health service delivery, most effort and money are devoted to tertiary prevention/maintenance treatment, where the quality of rehabilitation may be so variable that the term 'rehabilitation' may sometimes be a euphemism for habitual low-grade custodial care. Secondary prevention is the early recognition and treatment of psychiatric disorders: to date, the best evidence and best practice has been implemented in EI for psychosis in young people (see Chapters 7, 9, 15 and 21). This book will inform interventions in people from all age groups, building on the core components of excellent services: engaging, low (negative) impact practices that are culture- and age-sensitive with robust crisis interventions, assertive case management, flexible home visiting, family consultations and in and out of hours, active response services. EI teams should have a low threshold to identify individuals warranting assessment, monitoring and sometimes treatment, reduce stigma in patients and their local community, engage individuals with emerging symptoms and their family carers in low-key pre-emptive services even if formal treatment is not indicated, not wanted or not available, locally or anywhere. Their primary aim is to treat vigorously the first signs of the disorder in the first 3 years ('the critical period'). In managing a complex mix of possible noncases and cases, medication is only one option and part of phase-specific organic and psychosocial interventions: comprehensive therapeutic assessment, crisis intervention, education, family work, cognitive behavioural therapy, assertive community treatment, substance misuse and vocational interventions, to name but eight.

Overview: structure of this book

EI principles also support service users and carers in their individual recovery models, and dare to aim for full remission or generate hope that their symptoms do not develop into lifelong disability. A large part of primary care, child psychiatry and consultation–liaison (general hospital) psychiatry works as secondary prevention, but within large caseloads across secondary services including CMHTs, there are many opportunities for EI. This book's approach will be:

- Across the age spans, identifying the best EI practices in specific groups.

- Comprehensive: most common psychiatric disorders will be addressed – that is the 'nearly everything' of our subtitle. Because most psychiatric subspecialities have developed in isolation, they may be unaware of hard-won lessons from other colleagues in engaging and managing people from different demographic groups and cultures. Whether your patient is 8 or 80, there is much to be gained from an EI ethos.

- Evidence based, with an emphasis on **outcomes** (e.g. improvements in symptoms, social functioning, concordance, quality of life, service satisfaction) and **outputs** (e.g. interventions, contacts with services, clear care pathways that encourage referrals). Where these are available and reliable, screening instruments will be discussed.

- International, with authors and promising studies and experiences recounted from Asia, Australasia, Europe and North America.

- Practical: though it is challenging to cross different cultures and diverse health care provision, authors will try to answer readers' questions about how excellent EI service configurations might look (Section III), and which clinicians are best placed to intervene.

- Interdisciplinary and collaborative: this book was written for all interdisciplinary team members, our mental health and primary care colleagues (nurses, social workers, psychologists, occupational therapists, vocational rehabilitation and supported housing specialists, peer workers etc.), doctors (psychiatrists, GPs, public health doctors, paediatricians, adolescent specialists, physicians, geriatricians and more), managers, purchasers/commissioners and other health care providers. The book will also be useful to trainees in these disciplines, postgraduate students and commentators and to service user and family groups.

- Flexible and holistic: one of the key lessons from EI Psychosis Teams internationally has been NOT to send young people elsewhere (to another service) to address their substance misuse problems, or to separate organisations to deal with educational/training, housing, relationship problems. Although we did not brief authors about physical health care, this was raised frequently by the individual authors, and new approaches are set out later.

- Pragmatic: for clinicians with scarce resources, prioritising early identification (precursor symptoms and prodromes) to reduce current long durations of untreated illness and to set out core interventions that reduce psychological morbidity.

- Future proof: where evidence appears relatively sparse (e.g. eating disorders, learning disability, bipolar disorder) or where research continues apace (e.g. psychosis, dementia, delirium), expert clinicians will summarise the advances and predict where best practice will lie in the future. Though it may be attractive to researchers, the book is aimed primarily at clinicians, service planners and providers.

We begin with contributions from two key groups, whose interests mostly overlap – service users (consumers) and carers (families) – before hearing the economic arguments in the fourth chapter. The next six chapters have artificially divided the life span into five stages. Our needs change as we attach, individuate, enter adolescence then adulthood, before biology and our environment act upon us in middle age through to later life. We also include a key chapter on transition – from children's services to general adult psychiatry as Chapter 8. As health care providers this is an inevitable transition that should herald an orderly handover of care. Certainly in Europe, and we believe elsewhere, clinicians have not managed this well, and there are lessons to learn. Although artificial, we have laid out settings and levels of prevention in the next five chapters. We accept the same patients are attending GPs (Chapter 13) as are admitted to general hospitals (Chapter 14), and every one of them benefits from primary prevention (Chapter 11) and voluntary sector activities (Chapter 12). Though this might seem theoretical, we think the principles that drive the evidence might be similar but the different settings require different strategies to deliver EI. Not least, each setting has a different story to tell about the institutional and other obstacles to EI.

Inevitably, we expect busy clinicians and students to go straight to the third section and Chapter 16 (the common mental disorders of depression and anxiety) and thence to the following eight chapters that are disorder specific. EI sceptics, and there are many, might need to explore the challenges from their comfort zones by looking at familiar diagnostic categories. We could have picked up to 10 additional, discrete disorders for this section but we think the material covered lends itself to the treatment of the 'nearly everything' our title boasts. Chapter 15 summarised the gains of EI Psychosis Teams across the world, but we felt strongly that bipolar disorder, still with the longest time to definitive diagnosis of any psychiatric condition, merited a separate space as Chapter 21.

In addition to Patrick McGorry's Afterword, we have three concluding chapters. Without the social movement described (and indeed led) by Shiers and Smith, allied to evidence-based stigma-reduction strategies (pioneered by Pat Corrigan and colleagues), EI would crash and burn. If our only arguments were short-term gains, especially financial, then the passion that drives EI would continue to shine brightly but would then move on to other challenges. The final concluding chapter contains a challenge to adapt our 'headsets' as Americans might say, to a public health oriented, preventionist and early interventionist approach to all substantial mental health disorders. It summarizes the strengths and benefits of this approach. It also contains cautions and caveats which urge us not to overclaim for this territory, and not to disband specific EI in psychosis teams or merge them with generic teams, on the perhaps illusionary rationale that such CMHTs could do a bit of EI of everything, as well as everything else they must do, and end up being nothing much to anybody.

What do we mean by prevention?

In primary prevention, it is easier to reduce precipitating factors (especially those proximal to illness onset) than predisposing factors, but some (coping style, social supports, resilience and other protective factors) are also amenable to interventions. Secondary prevention will remain mostly synonymous in this book with EI, and tertiary prevention, beyond the scope of this book, is the treatment and rehabilitation of established disorders. By this late stage, illness (disability) is long term: the person has developed recurrent severe depression, 'chronic' schizophrenia, or the medical complications of alcoholism/eating disorder, and the health professional's role is to 'pick up the pieces' in an attempt to reduce distress and restore a modest proportion of previous social functioning. EI has the dual objectives of treating previously undiagnosed disorders and treating patients in the early stages of an illness where they have the highest chance of recovery. Ethical concerns (e.g. overdiagnosis – treating people who do not have, and will not develop, the disorder) will be covered in individual chapters and the concluding chapter. They also focus on many of the initial benefits of EI (improvements in engagement, therapeutic alliances, less stigma and greater self-knowledge of relevant mental health disorders) and the prevention of collateral damage (comorbidities, losses of educational, employment and housing opportunities, disrupted relationships, widening health inequalities) which can both give a 'head-start' or provide a reserve of functionality and resilience to augment the effective management in patients who progress towards longer-term disability.

The how of prevention

Preconception advice and interventions, for example genetic counselling, are examples of primary preventative measures [3]. Similar measures are set out in individual chapters. Before a person becomes ill, and in the *lead in* time after someone develops symptoms ('biological disadvantage') but does not seek or achieve healthcare advice, most post industrial societies resource *universal measures* of prevention [1]. These are designed to help everyone: restrictions on alcohol sales and minimum pricing of alcohol to reduce general consumption and thereby alcohol consumption by people who are misusing alcohol, improved social capital, combating stigma through media campaigns. There are also *specific measures* [1] aimed at known, vulnerable groups: children from disadvantaged backgrounds, or people with chronic medical illnesses. Universally applied preventive measures are to be preferred for their greater potential to make a large positive effect on a population, and their less stigmatising impact on individuals. For this we need national initiatives, driven by research, where we end the artificial separation of the psychological from the physical [4].

Evidence

As we commissioned each chapter, we were aware that the practical gold standard for EI currently is the international effort to provide EI for young people with psychosis [5–7]. It is common, in EI psychosis services for example, to start secondary prevention for one disorder (typically anxiety, but frequently depression), in the context of simultaneous/parallel primary prevention for another (psychosis or comorbid substance misuse). The point here is that EI services (in any age group, any given disorder) need to understand and practice both primary and secondary prevention. While we can speak of general principles of EI, there is no assumption that these work in every (age) group, in every setting, at every stage of a (particular) disorder. To explore just one disorder, there are multiple differences in the detection and management of depression when this occurs in older people [8], women in the postpartum period [9], and in adolescents where classic presentation symptoms are the exception not the rule [10]. We have therefore encouraged the chapter authors to find the best evidence that should lead the best practice in their area, mindful that none of us, even in the developed world, have unlimited access to the resources necessary to run high quality mental health services. You will read about these age groups (Section II), settings (Section III) and disorders (Section IV) with no claim that 'one size fits all' in EI. As general psychiatrists, we were frequently pleasantly surprised to see impressive successful trials of treatments to challenge therapeutic nihilism in conditions like alcohol misuse [11] and eating disorders [12].

Parallels with medicine

At the time of writing, the Royal College of Psychiatrists (UK) in collaboration with service user groups has successfully lobbied the UK Government to sign up to *Parity of Esteem*. Parity of esteem (http://www.rcpsych.ac.uk/pdf/OP88.pdf) means that, when compared with physical health care, mental health care is characterised by:

- equal access to the most effective and safest care and treatment

- equal efforts to improve the quality of care

- the allocation of time, effort and resources on a basis commensurate with need

- equal status within health care education and practice

- equally high aspirations for service users and

- equal status in the measurement of health outcomes.

With this in mind, it would be unthinkable to deny or delay EI in cancer, myocardial infarction, stroke, or ANY serious physical illness. The consequences of late intervention in mental disorders mean more suffering for people with treatable disorders, and for their families. Because other bad things happen to people with severe mental illness (SMI), late intervention also means that our friends and family with SMI die between 10 and 20 years earlier than they would have if they never had a mental health problem (http://www.rethink.org/media/810988/Rethink%20Mental%20Illness%20-%20Lethal%20Discrimination.pdf). At time of submission, the Royal College of Psychiatrists' General Adult Faculty has set out 25 ideas to improve the poor physical health of people with mental illness as their first Faculty Report (https://www.rcpsych.ac.uk/pdf/FR%20GAP%2001-%20final2013.pdf). Appropriately, the first of these measures is the Lester Cardiometabolic Health Resource (www.rcpsych.ac.uk/quality.aspx) developed by Professor Helen Lester, who was third Editor on this volume, until illness prevented her from continuing with this project.

There is a second parallel with EI in medicine – the main down side of EI, overdiagnosis. Here, there are concerns that people (who by rights should not be just thought of as 'patients') are being 'overdosed, overtreated and overdiagnosed' [13]. Overdiagnosis, where asymptomatic people are 'diagnosed' with a disease that will not lead to symptoms or early death, is said to waste in excess of £128 billion in the US Healthcare system each year. Much debate prevails about disease mongering, overmedicalisation, mission (diagnosis) creep, and shifting thresholds to label people 'ill' and providing treatment that wastes their time and scarce resources [13]. Mental disorders fare relatively well in this critical review [13], with only attention deficit disorder getting a dishonourable mention. This is a complex condition, plagued by comorbidities, covered in Chapters 18 and 24. There is, however, no room for complacency in mental health: we will not medicalise behaviours (e.g. sex 'addiction') and do not advocate any potentially harmful treatments (by definition, medications) unless there is a safe, scientific prediction that individuals have or will go on to develop a treatable psychiatric condition. We now have highly reliable evidence that psychological and family interventions (but not necessarily anti-psychosis medication, except supplements like omega-3 fatty acids or fish oil) will prevent transition to psychosis in people with at-risk mental states [14].

And finally

We boast innovation in this book: we asked authors to write about their area of expertise on a blank page – with tips on how to deal with, overcome or effectively bypass the obstacles of 'unfit for purpose', ill-designed services, professional intransigence, the inertia of habitual practices and conventional wisdom. And to achieve change in the context of limited resources. The advantage of this endeavour has been to gather the best available evidence in one book – to enable busy clinicians and health care providers, among others – to make the arguments locally to get the effective services that individuals and families living with mental disorders deserve. Right now, they need ready access to the best services, as early as possible in the courses of their conditions. The unique purpose of this book is to gather the best available evidence of EI of many disorders and in many clinical systems, in one place. We anticipate that some will find gaps in the breath of coverage here, and expect that research will drive the evidence even further forward. At the very least, we hope to provoke and inspire.

References

1. Paykel ES and Jenkins R (eds). (1994). *Prevention in Psychiatry*. Gaskell.
2. Jenkins R and Ustun TB (eds). (1998). *Preventing Mental Illness: Mental Health Promotion in Primary Care*. Proceedings of a UN conference. John Wiley & Sons, Ltd.
3. Mario M, Juan JL, Norman S, et al. (eds). (2005). *Early Detection and Management of Mental Disorders*. Proceedings of a WPA conference. John Wiley & Sons, Ltd.
4. Jorm A and Reavley N. (2013). Preventing mental disorders: the time is right. *Medical Journal of Australia* **199**: 527.
5. Birchwood M, Fowler D and Jackson C. (2001). *Early Intervention in Psychosis*. John Wiley.
6. McGorry P and Jackson H. (1999). *The Recognition and Management of Early Psychosis: A Preventive Approach*. Cambridge University Press.
7. McGorry P (ed.) (journal) *Early Intervention in Psychiatry*. http://onlinelibrary.wiley.com/journal/10.1111/(ISSN)1751-7893/issues.
8. Sirey JA, Bruce ML and Alexopoulos G. (2005). The treatment initiation program: an intervention to improve depression outcomes in older adults. *American Journal of Psychiatry* **162**: 184–188.
9. Murray L, Wilson A and Romaniuk H. (2003). Controlled trial of the short- and long-term effect of psychological treatment of post-partum depression. *British Journal of Psychiatry* **182**: 420–427.
10. Babor TE, Ritson B and Hodgson RJ. (1986). Alcohol-related problems in primary health care settings: a review of early intervention strategies. *British Journal of Addiction* **81**: 23–46.
11. Thapar A, Collishaw S and Potter R. (2010). Managing and preventing depression in adolescents. *British Medical Journal* **340**: 245–258.
12. Shoemaker C. (1998). Does early intervention improve the prognosis in anorexia nervosa? A systematic review of the treatment-outcome literature. *International Journal of Eating Disorders* **21**: 1–15.
13. Moynihan R, Doust J and Henry D. (2010). Preventing overdiagnosis: how to stop harming the healthy. *British Medical Journal* **344**: 19–23.
14. Stafford MR, Jackson H, Mayo-wilson E, et al. (2013). Early interventions to prevent psychosis: systematic review and meta-analysis. *British Medical Journal* **346**: 12.

2

How Early Intervention Can Turn Things Upside Down and Turn a Patient Into a Psychiatrist

Nick Meinhold

Monash University, Victoria, Australia
University of Queensland, Brisbane, St Lucia, Queensland, Australia
Community Healthfulness Cooperative, Melbourne, Victoria, Australia

Introduction

When I became unwell I was placed in a system of early intervention and given 18 months of high quality care, encouragement and support. I have been given different diagnoses at various times and it is difficult to classify the symptoms I have experienced into a single mental health disorder. It is my opinion that early intervention is an effective system that is independent of a particular illness and beneficial for people experiencing mental ill health across the board.

The lead up to psychosis

Growing up can be a painful experience, and I was never one to do things the easy way. Plenty of excuses come to mind and I admit I tried on a few. My family went through some rough times and I lost things that I felt were very important. For much of my early adolescence I was focused on a career in basketball and this goal was well on track after state selection and a tour around America. Then multiple sports injuries requiring surgery forced me to take stock and finally I gave up my dream. There were also issues in my family, which broke apart when I was fifteen, but when I look back now it seems that

Early Intervention in Psychiatry: EI of nearly everything for better mental health, First Edition.
Edited by Peter Byrne and Alan Rosen.

there was nothing entirely out of the ordinary to justify my anger at the world. Nothing that was not true for a lot of other people anyway.

I was angry and I made bad choices. Perhaps I lacked the foresight of age or the insight of maturity but I know in my heart that I had an urge to be destructive and I wanted to hurt myself. Maybe I just needed the world to see my pain.

Whatever the reason, my teenage years were an ever increasing cycle of self-destruction. Drugs and alcohol played a part but they were just the most readily available implements for the work of wreaking havoc on self. If no drugs had been available, I am sure I would have found something else. Whether it was relationships gone wrong, physical injury, legal consequences or horrible come downs, the results of bad choices were all fairly similar. They just bloody hurt.

You might wonder why someone would enter such a cycle. Why not just stop? I would like to be able to answer that question but I do not have an answer now just as I did not have then. Perhaps too many of the choices we make are on a level we do not have access to. Maybe we are subconsciously influenced by our relationship with ourselves, or maybe we just create situations that reflect the way we feel. I doubt I will ever really know. I have read a lot of theories on why people become self-destructive and how a negative self-image comes about. I wish we understood it in a way that we could discard unhelpful attitudes and stop creating unflattering and inaccurate ideas about ourselves. Personally I think that the issue of self-image is crucial, and where a constructive change can be most effective. A path that leads to pain, anguish and ill health has to begin somewhere.

As I destroyed my life I saw a lot of my friends take similar paths and I saw a reflection of my own anger and desire for self-destruction in their choices. The similarities drew us together and we pushed each other to ever-greater levels of chaos. We would consume any drugs we could find, get into fights and wreck whatever was in our way. Nothing justifies such terrible behaviour but perhaps we were trying to break the world in which we felt imprisoned. We were united by a desire to push until something shattered. Some of my friends are still at it and some are no longer around. Some found relationships and family or committed to jobs and careers. For me, I pushed until something shifted, but it was not the world that broke, it was my perceptions and reasoning and ultimately, my mind.

Amongst friends that often argued, trust was a fragile commodity. A slew of bad choices culminated in some major losses and I entered a downward spiral. Escalating levels of drug use and emotional turmoil felt like a weight dragging me down. I stopped doing anything that was remotely healthy. Eventually I even stopped eating and sleeping.

Psychosis and mania

Pushing a brain and body beyond their limits can only end badly. My thinking became focused around ideas of the future and I felt that I was able to perceive things I had not previously been aware of.

I was living at one of the colleges of Melbourne University, by nature a very competitive environment. As I gradually became unwell, my declining rationalisation fabricated conspiracies involving the college community and I managed to enrol some of my friends and a few members of the staff into my agenda. One such conspiracy that I remember centred on one of the staff, who also happened to be the father of a friend. I came to believe that he was controlling the other staff by blackmailing them with secrets of terrible acts he had forced them to carry out. The delusions of an unwell mind can be incredibly elaborate in design and complex in detail. I am sure all of the people whom I believed I had convinced, in truth remained doubtful, but it is difficult to entirely disregard a passionate declaration of genuine conviction, no matter how bizarre the content. Of course at first, the theories I communicated were more unusual than inherently sinister, grandiose rather than conspiratorial, and we all love to be inspired.

The first stage of mania was an incredible feeling, like reaching the very pinnacle of joy and staying there, riding a wave. The incredible feeling eventually became an inflated sense of my own abilities and place in the world. Initially it was all very exciting but over time grandiose ideas became conspiratorial suspicions and my mind created elaborate stories with bizarre and complex causal relationships. In retrospect, there was a strong theme of control in my delusions and I became convinced that someone at my friend's work was controlling everyone with some kind of supernatural force, because particular words had been used in conversations. I do not remember the particular words or why I believed they had a particular meaning. I think this is part of the illness, to make connections that no rational mind would make and to take them on as truth.

Most of my memories of that time are very blurry but I have flashes of extreme emotional turmoil and psychological pain. Perhaps my mind created an alternative reality to escape into. I was certainly at the centre of the delusions I created, frightening and bizarre as they were. It seems counterintuitive to construct an illusion that creates so much misery but mental illness never seems to make much sense.

Involuntary treatment

My friends put up with my strange ideas and behaviour for as long as they could but eventually they agreed that the situation was more than they could deal with and contacted the local hospital.

I was couch surfing and moving around a bit but I had been spending a fair bit of time at one particular place. A friend owned a house in Melbourne and had seen other people become unwell with psychosis. He rang around and sorted out a Crisis Assessment Team (CAT) that included a psychiatric nurse and an occupational therapist. They came over and introduced themselves. I was in a very open state and told them everything they wanted to know. Perhaps it is contradictory but despite being unwell and delusional, on the whole I maintained a very truthful and candid manner throughout. Interestingly, I have found this to be true of many people I met who were struggling with their mental health.

I agreed to go for a ride and meet some new people. I am sure the CAT team had become very adept at using language that would create intrigue rather than suspicion and I do not see deception in the variation. I remember sitting in the back seat, feeling surrounded by nervous people. At one point I made a joke about the level of tension, which I did not understand and mistook as something others might have seen as fun, like we were playing a game and I had not been told the rules. The laughter was loud and sudden, like a release after a long period of suspense. I did not mean anyone any harm but I was aware that I no longer had any fear, which made people uncomfortable. We rode the rest of the way in silence and I watched the world slide by out of the window, no doubt in my mind that everything was as it should be.

Arriving at EPPIC

The Early Psychosis Prevention and Intervention Centre (EPPIC) was described to my friends as a lovely facility overlooking the Melbourne Zoo. There was indeed a view. Through the bars of the cage that surrounded the balcony we were allowed to smoke on, you could see the external fence of the zoo in the distance. I am sure this exaggeration of the facts was a part of the overall strategy of getting someone who was very unwell into a facility where they could be appropriately treated and I harbour no ill will towards the staff who created the small deception. In all of my experiences in the treatment of psychosis, the ideal situation seemed very far from the reality, but the people involved have always been well intentioned. Psychosis is a horrific experience for everyone involved and I believe we make the best of a very difficult situation.

On arrival, I was interviewed by a psychiatrist with a group of people in tow. I do not remember much of the conversation but I remember being excited about the idea of living at EPPIC, which was described as a wonderful place full of interesting people. The latter part of the statement proved to be quite accurate. I was taken up to my room and then left to my own devices.

I can of course only relay what remains of my memory of the events and there may well be interactions and situations that I have simply forgotten.

Meeting my housemates

The inhabitants of my new home were as disparate in appearance and character as any group I have ever encountered. The dynamics were complex but a clear hierarchy emerged. A giant Turkish guy who claimed he had killed and been to prison was the obvious leader. A young Maori kid was even bigger and they often clashed, with destructive results. When violence threatened to flare up, we all got out of the way and waited for the security guards to sort it out. Unfortunately the security guards were not always around and the ward at times felt like a dangerous place.

With so many extremely unwell young people thrown together in a relatively confined space, you had to stay alert. Delusions by definition were not based on evidence, often shifted quickly and seemed completely random. I had the sense that we were all trying to work out the meaning behind everyone else and decide how they all fit into our own constructed worlds.

Everyone was unpredictable, but there was a special kind of unpredictability in psychosis that came from abusing speed and ice. Most of the patients I spoke to had been using drugs of some kind and strangely, different kinds of illness seemed to spring from the various groups of drugs, though this may just have been my perception.

Living at EPPIC

Despite the potential danger, the facilities were wonderful, and the grounds quite beautiful. We also had plenty of activities to keep us occupied, everything from music sessions, where everyone ended up indiscriminately thumping their randomly assigned instruments, to art therapy where we created similar chaos with paint and craft supplies. Many found an outlet and diversion in activities they had never previously had the opportunity to experience.

We were fed well despite meal times being a trial for the staff. Getting all of the inpatients together always had the potential for disaster. Being confined created a level of tension that could erupt in altercations in an instant and many delusions seemed to involve the food we were given. Apparently I stopped eating for some time as I became convinced there was a conspiracy to poison us. With so little control over our situation many took the opportunity to rebel by refusing their food or arguing over its contents. We were called in individually to a private room to take our medication and this also became a focus for many delusions, including my own.

Many of the delusions were very dark with themes of violence, conspiracy and sex being common. They often had a disruptive effect, to greater and lesser degrees. For example at one point, I offended the noses of my fellow patients for several days when I stopped showering, as I had become convinced I was going to be killed in the shower. Unfortunately it was not always just the sense of smell that was assaulted. Backing people into a corner, even if it is only in their minds, will of course produce varying results. Sometimes I was surprised that the staff could manage to keep everyone safe.

Maintaining control

As social animals, it seems isolation is the worst kind of punishment we can endure. At EPPIC there was an area I heard people call the ICA, where a patient could be viewed at all times from an adjacent office and any violent or unsafe behaviour could be immediately addressed. Most of the time I was there it was empty and the threat of being sent there and effectively isolated was a very potent form of control.

We were a group of agitated, often aggressive, unpredictable and extremely emotional young people. Most were naturally very angry at being detained and were eager to disrupt the control of their perceived captors. The measures that the staff employed to maintain that control were strict at times but never draconian. The security guards could be rough but if you did as you were told they left you alone. In an extremely tough situation I think that, on the whole, the staff did an incredible job of treating us with dignity and respect.

In fact, we were given the sense that we had control over our circumstances and ultimately our destiny, although I did not realize that at the time. When this occurred to me, I was recalling the balcony enclosed with prison style bars where everyone smoked profusely. One day, on exploring the extent of my detention I chanced upon the rubbish dump beneath the balcony that was a foot deep sea of cigarette butts. The sight disturbed me and I became determined to convert the butt wasteland into a clean environment. I imagine the futility of my task was not lost on the staff, but despite this, I was assisted with provision of the appropriate tools and encouraged to take charge of making a change that I felt was important.

Time to go

After roughly 2 weeks it was decided I could go home. Apparently I was still quite unwell but had passed a critical point. Someone suggested to my parents that they were unsure just how many of my responses were truthful, as I had demonstrated an ability to tell the psychiatrists what they wanted to hear. They also told my parents that staying at the psychiatric unit was actually making me worse. I do not know why the final choice was made to send me home but I imagine it is always a complex decision and having parents that were able to alternate taking time off meant I would be cared for.

Unfortunately I went back to old habits and smoking weed put me back where I had started after just a few months. I went back into EPPIC for another 2-week period. My memories of the two admissions are probably mingled and each was fairly similar. After the second admission, I knew that if I ever wanted to have any kind of freedom, I had to accept that my old life was over and start making difficult choices that would lead to a more positive result.

Life as an outpatient

In the 18 months following my admissions that I spent as an outpatient of EPPIC, I was diagnosed with bipolar and schizoaffective disorder. I did not fully accept those labels but I did continue to experience mood swings and paranoid delusions of life-threatening intensity.

Having regular appointments to talk to someone was really helpful. My case manager was a constant source of positive energy and inspiration and created a familiar link between busy psychiatrists and overwhelmed family and friends.

We met weekly to begin with, then less frequently as I became more able to cope. It was an incredible balancing act by my case manager; giving me the support I needed while always encouraging me to take charge of my own life. I knew when things got tough I could organize a chat over the phone or move forward an appointment, and sometimes that was all I needed to find the strength to keep going.

My time as an outpatient was a buffer that separated acute care and the challenge of finding my feet in everyday life. People from the outpatient program acted as a vital lifeline in times of need and for my family, feeling we were part of a community that was equipped to deal with the situation was invaluable.

The following 5 years

After a long run of manic energy, depression inevitably struck. It was a dark depression, so deep I believed I would never come out of it. I struggled to get out of bed for over a year, and I was still living with ongoing symptoms of psychosis. There were many times I really considered ending the struggle and I cannot express the agony of that time but my intention is not to elicit sympathy. Part of the reason I was there was a string of bad choices, part was bad luck and I am sure other influences played their part. The experience was as close to hell as anything I could imagine but being surrounded by strong support and people who believed in my recovery, I never gave up and every now and then I noticed that things had gotten a little easier.

Over the next 5 or so years I fought my own mind every second of every day and slowly climbed out of the dark place in which I had suddenly found myself. There was never a time where I suddenly felt as though I had shaken off my illness. Intermittently I would notice that the last few months had been less of a trial and I was expending less energy, keeping the darkness at bay.

I read everything I could get my hands on that might offer some advice on finding a way out and I tried every kind of healing modality, fitness regime, herbal remedy and psychological method I could find. I think regular, intensive exercise is the best treatment I have experienced and there is mounting evidence for this [1]. Certain aspects of eastern philosophy, particularly those summarised in Acceptance and Commitment Therapy [2] were also helpful. Researching my options was never a simple task as I often struggled to find the stillness to sit and read. Terrible thoughts and emotions had a way of sneaking up and overwhelming me. I slowly pieced together some tools that worked but it was as though my mind was bouncing around a prison of my own making and just as I thought I may have found a way out I would bounce somewhere else and lose sight of it.

And then the next 5 years

I had to rebuild, or create new ways to find, many things I had always taken for granted. I lost many of my memories. One loss that I particularly noticed was the ability to do simple mathematics. It was a loss I felt I could not accept, so in an attempt to regain what I had lost I began reading primary school mathematics textbooks. Each day for as long as I could manage, I would sit and work my way through simple addition and subtraction, then later through fractions and long division. I believe I found solace in the structure and felt a sense of progress. Whilst only small goals, I was regularly achieving something and in a life that often appeared to be going nowhere, even a slow progression was infinitely better than stagnating in the one place.

In fact, relishing the sense of achievement that came from a structured curriculum, I enrolled in a private computing course. Making the journey to the classroom environment was challenging and being around teachers and students could be an ordeal, but they allowed the subjects to be taken at your own pace and I gradually made my way through the course. I even found a job with the qualification I received but despite having several years of recovery behind me, I was still quite unwell and the anxiety of a real job with responsibilities and consequences was more than I could cope with. My confidence had taken a hit so I decided to stick with what I knew and continue with more formal education. I did increase the challenge though, by enrolling in a university degree.

I was older than most of my classmates, and my social abilities were another casualty of my waning but continuing illness. Nevertheless, the structure and support were there and after a few years I even managed to achieve high grades. I always tried to take on further challenges though. A habit had formed from the time when incrementally challenging myself was all I could do to stay alive; I took on teaching mathematics, I got involved in clubs and social activities. I even took an acting class at one point.

I was at the wheel of my journey of recovery, but without the incredible support of some amazing people I probably would not be here today. My parents put up with so much but somehow were always willing to take more. The few friends who could handle my strange ideas would come and visit, helping to break the monotony. Support and advice from health professionals was important, although I was never an easy patient. I spent most of my time during those years thinking about what was going on and contemplating how I could find my way out. I am not sure how conscious it was but I always pushed myself to do a little more than I found comfortable.

Now

Somewhere around 10 years after I first became unwell I found that, more often than not, I was confident and at ease with myself. My life had become an undertaking that overall was an incredibly enjoyable experience. After my initial two admissions, I never again became psychotic and the unstable peaks and troughs of mania and depression had gradually become the ups and downs of everyday life.

The illness I went through was the worst kind of prison I could ever imagine. Each of the tools that I learned in my recovery I continue to use and I keep growing all the time, in my health and as a person. Having found my freedom I am now determined to help others do the same. I took on the challenge of studying medicine with the intention of becoming a psychiatrist. My goal is to obtain the knowledge and tools that our society has built over a long period of time in order to understand psychosis from a different angle. As I walk with people on a part of their journey, I hope a widened perspective will allow me to discover truths that may have previously gone unnoticed.

There are many things I owe to the interventions I received, and the system and the people that made them possible. In a sense I have come full circle and, in collaboration with others who have a personal understanding of mental ill health, we are building a new model of mental health recovery, born of experience and aimed at maximising the healing potential of the journey of recovery.

The future

I now believe that there are several things that can make a difference and give people the greatest chance of recovering from mental illness. First, by giving the body everything it needs to be healthy, including a nutritious diet, daily exercise and the removal of toxins and poisons. Emotional and spiritual health is also important and activities such as meditation, yoga and nature walks give a sense of ease and peace that is conducive to health and recovery. Finding a creative outlet like acting, music or art, through local groups, courses or personal practice, can help lift us free of old pain and negativity. We also benefit greatly from having the sense of belonging that comes from working in a team and contributing to the community in a meaningful manner. This builds self-esteem and self-worth and gives the confidence that is necessary to take on the challenge and the responsibility of taking control of your life. I believe a person needs to take responsibility for the choices they make in response to their set of circumstances in order to become free from their mental illness. Towards this end, giving people gradually increasing levels of challenge and responsibility gives them the greatest chance of recovery.

Having identified these requirements, I tried to envisage a facility that could provide all of these components and after discussing my ideas with many people over a long period of time, we began the establishment of a non-profit health retreat business, the Community Healthfulness Co-operative in the Yarra Valley, Victoria, Australia [3], which is primarily staffed by people recovering from or dealing with mental illness.

I have since searched out other alternative health care models that provide support and encourage recovery. As part of my studies I moved to Brisbane and came across Stepping Stone Club House, an organisation where members help to run the service. Amongst the different aspects of the services, they offer assistance with housing and employment, as well as affordable food and social recreation. It is a truly wonderful place, staff are friendly and supportive and everyone makes an effort to ensure you feel welcome. By being encouraged to contribute to running the place, members are given an important sense of purpose. I joined the Clubhouse and every time I was there I felt empowered and connected to people.

Having a role and responsibility in a group, and the sense of connection we gain from that, seems to be a vital element to all people's mental health. While it is essential to have a system where a person who becomes unwell is provided for, on all levels in the short term, as that person recovers they need to be challenged in a way that is appropriate to their ability to cope with that challenge at that time.

In my experience, it is a lack of control over our emotions that leads to maladaptive coping strategies and learning to deal with ongoing external challenges gives us the generalised ability to cope with situations we cannot control. We take for granted the ability to influence our world that comes from practicing, over and over, the process of facing challenges and making decisions that have a lasting impact. As people recover from mental ill health, they often lose the chance to practice managing their lives and making decisions that affect others.

Creating the community healthfulness cooperative

When I first started discussing my ideas for a place where people could support each other to intensify and strengthen the recovery process, we decided to create a cooperative so that everyone would have the sense of control over their situation. A cooperative is a business owned and controlled by the people who use its services and the model removes the separation between the service provider and the people in need of the service. By working together, a cooperative can reach an objective unattainable by individuals acting alone and by each member having equal ownership, we empower individuals to practice managing the challenges of a real-life situation.

There are obviously serious challenges to a cooperative model and recovering from mental ill health is a vulnerable time. In order to ensure the safety of everyone involved, we continue to consult with experts and seek feedback on every aspect of the model we are creating. Australian of the Year, Professor Patrick McGorry, has agreed to act as our patron and we continue to engage professionals and people involved in highly accountable and responsible walks of life, so that at all times the important challenge of responsibility is balanced with the crucial protection of safety and well-being.

In the cooperative I describe, people recovering from acute mental illness are given the opportunity to live on a property in exchange for working as part of a team, helping to provide a health retreat service for themselves and others. Working in a group of people united by a shared goal, we have secured land, built a driveway entrance and planted a large orchard and vegetable crops.

The project aims to provide respite and true asylum, a space where people will have the chance to rest and recuperate, as well as being given the opportunity to begin rebuilding their lives and creating their future. Using practices of sustainability and a holistic approach to mental health, the cooperative will be aided by a paradigm where the health of the individual is viewed as a singular aspect of the health of the entire environment. By maintaining a sustainable environment, people recovering from mental illness will gain skills in balancing the many aspects of a healthy environment and learn to apply these skills in managing their own health.

As a product of early intervention, I will continue contributing to the health of my peers and I hope I can demonstrate the power of giving people the appropriate assistance at the proper time.

Conclusion

As I work towards my goal of becoming a psychiatrist and work with others to create a community-driven mental health service, I hope people see the benefit of an early intervention system, not only in giving someone the best chance to recover from a devastating illness, but also in the benefit to society that comes from life beyond recovery.

Those of us struck down by mental ill health have an incredible amount of potential to share with the world. If we focus on giving people everything they need in the early stages of illness, we offer them the greatest chance of a life that benefits us all. I hope my story can act as an example of why this is true.

References

1. Ratey J and Hagerman E. (2008). *Spark: the Revolutionary New Science of Exercise and the Brain.* Little, Brown and Company.
2. http://www.actmindfully.com.au/ (accessed on 26 April 2014).
3. Grey F. (2010). Introducing…Community Healthfulness Co-operative in the Yarra Valley, by Nick Meinhold. OurConsumerPlace Newsletter.

3

Involving the Family in Early Interventions

Gráinne Fadden

Meriden Family Programme, Birmingham and Solihull Mental Health NHS Foundation Trust, Birmingham, UK; University of Birmingham, Birmingham, UK

Introduction

The involvement of family, social networks and those who are important in the life of the person presenting with difficulties is core in early interventions. When intervening early, it is much more likely that the individual will be functioning at a level where they are still engaged with families and relatives. The extent of involvement will vary depending on where the person is on the continuum of lifespan development. Clearly, there is recognition that for children with difficulties, the family must be involved, and this also applies at the other end of the age spectrum where older people are often dependent on family for support and care. It makes sense from several perspectives to support people in using those resources that are naturally there in their lives, particularly where this results in the avoidance of dependency on expensive secondary and tertiary services.

The evidence presented in this chapter confirms that people are willing to engage in family-based approaches, with a high rate of treatment retention when families are involved. The involvement of those who are significant in the person's life fits with models of recovery, and clearly, if an individual is deprived of this support, they are missing a key resource that could aid their recovery. Fostering competencies that can be incorporated into everyday environments and activities in both the individual and those who are close to them makes it more likely that gains will be maintained. Family-centred approaches tend to have a number of core values such as a non-blaming attitude towards families, collaborative working relationships between family members and professionals, the empowerment of families by emphasising concepts of choice and control, an emphasis on strengths

---

Early Intervention in Psychiatry: EI of nearly everything for better mental health, First Edition.
Edited by Peter Byrne and Alan Rosen.

rather than deficits and a goal of enhancing functioning. Family interventions are usually individually tailored and phase-specific.

Reviewing family involvement and family interventions can be complex as there are a variety of ways in which family approaches are delivered. These can include working with whole families, parents or other relatives on their own, the individual with difficulties and significant family members, subgroups of families, for example supporting siblings, working with several families together including the person experiencing problems as occurs in multifamily groups, or without the affected person as happens in carers' support groups. This chapter will attempt to summarise what is currently good practice in relation to the role that families can play in early intervention. A range of disorders will be referred to, and early psychosis will be used to illustrate what can be achieved by offering tailored family interventions and what the main issues are. A broad definition of family referring not just to immediate or blood relatives, but to those who are important in the lives of the individual, for example extended, reconstituted or proxy families will be employed.

Family interventions across the lifespan

The benefits of the early involvement of the family have been described across the lifespan from birth to later life, and in the context of a range of diverse disorders.

Childhood developmental disorders

In a review of services for children with special health care needs, Bruder [1] traces the development of the concept of family-centred care from the 1960s when it was first described through to the integral involvement of families in early intervention by family empowerment [2] into a philosophy of care and a set of principles to guide service delivery. The rationale for family intervention is clear: experiences in the family context are critical to the child's development [3]; the caregiving family is constant in the child's life; the caregiver has the most time and greatest opportunity to influence the child's development and competence, even where professional input is available [4]. Parental attitudes and beliefs have a powerful influence on the child [1], and if their resources are utilised to the full, costs to communities and schools are decreased because children arrive at school ready to learn [5].

Dunst [6] outlined the features of family-centred early intervention programmes as practices that: regard families with dignity and respect; share information so that families can make informed decisions and choices about intervention options; use practices that are individualised, flexible and responsive; encourage collaboration and partnerships between professionals and families; provide the support needed by families to help them to care for their children and result in the best outcomes for all. Ingber and Dromi have added the attitude of treating parents as experts regarding their family's needs [7], and Brotherson et al. highlight the importance of home visiting in meeting emotional needs [8]. Where progammes adopt these features, for example with families of children with hearing loss, engagement and satisfaction with services are better [9]. A study by Moeller [10] highlights the benefits of family-based early intervention. High levels of family involvement correlated with positive language outcomes, and conversely, limited family involvement was associated with significant child language delays at 5 years, especially when enrollment in intervention was late. Significantly better language scores were associated with early enrollment in intervention. In spite of the obvious benefits of this type of approach, there are difficulties translating these principles into everyday practice worldwide [5, 9, 11].

Adolescent problems

Moving across the developmental lifespan, the value of involving the family in terms of preventative work in reducing health-risk behaviours and promoting social adaption in early adolescence has been examined. Family-centred intervention has been used to attempt to reduce antisocial behaviour and substance use with successful outcomes: young people in families who engaged in the intervention based on contact between professionals, school and families, and using principles of motivational interviewing exhibited lower rates of antisocial behaviour and substance misuse compared with matched controls [12].

In a review of family-based treatments for serious antisocial behaviour including conduct disorders, delinquency, substance abuse and criminal behaviour in adolescents, Henggeler and Sheidow [13] describe the benefits of a range of family models including multisystemic therapy, functional family therapy, multidimensional treatment, foster care and brief strategic family therapy. They note that these therapies are characterised by being flexible, strengths focussed, pragmatic and individualised. Particular issues they highlight include the need for more evaluation of these approaches with different cultural groups, and also issues linked with implementation, with many of these programmes being provided through purveyor organisations rather than through traditional mental health systems. This raises issues for those areas that cannot afford to import them, or have trained practitioners to deliver them. Other reviews in this area confirm that there is now clear evidence that family therapy is an efficacious treatment approach for adolescent substance misuse, although the authors once again highlight the need for further research in the area of 'implementation science', given the lack of widespread use of family-based approaches in routine clinical practice settings [14].

For an extensive review of family work for child and adolescent disorders, Kaslow et al. cover a wide range of disorders including mood, anxiety, attention-deficit disorder, hyperactivity, disruptive behaviour and developmental disorders including autism spectrum and eating disorders [15]. These are summarised in Table 3.1, indicating the extensive range of approaches to working with families that have been developed. The authors point out that the term 'family interventions' is a rubric, and that for most disorders, multiple family-based interventions appear to be of value. They highlight implementation issues linked with the resource-intensive nature of family programmes and draw attention to the way in which practitioners often use conceptualisations and techniques from multiple approaches, referred to as a 'common factors' approach rather than adhering to a single evidence-based approach with fidelity.

Eating disorders

One of the areas where the role of the family seems to be central and the interplay between family involvement and early intervention is clear is in relation to the management of eating disorders, in particular, anorexia nervosa. A significant study carried out at the

Table 3.1 Summary of family-based interventions for child and adolescent disorders based on review by Kasow et al. (2012) [15]

Disorders	Randomised controlled trials	Considerations	Promising interventions: non RCTs
Depression	• Stress-busters with parent component – school-based, CBT and family intervention • Coping with depression (for adolescents and including parent group) • Attachment-based family therapy • Penn Resiliency Program • Family psychoeducation • Multifamily psychoeducational groups	The addition of parenting elements seems to enhance most of the approaches	• ACTION programme for depressed girls with gender-sensitive material • Depression Experience Journal – computer-based psychoeducational intervention for families using a narrative approach
Bipolar disorder	• Family-focussed treatment • Multifamily psychoeducational groups • Individual family psychoeducation	Some studies show that benefits are mediated by parents beliefs about treatment	• Child and family focussed group intervention based on CBT framework
Anxiety disorders	• Family cognitive behaviour therapy • Combined CBT and attachment-based family therapy	Need trials with larger sample size and younger children	• Multidimensional family therapy • Behavioural consultation in schools • Narrative family therapy • Parenting techniques/parent education
Attention-deficit hyperactivity disorder	• Parent–child interaction therapy • Triple P Positive Parenting Program • Incredible Years (Multiple levels with parent, teacher, child)	More RCTs needed with broader age range	• A range of different family approaches including mediation
Oppositional defiant disorder	• Parent–child interaction therapy • Triple P Positive Parenting Program • Incredible years (IY) (Multiple levels with parent, teacher and child)	Parent programs need to be adapted for older youth	• Combination of IY with program to assist youth with literacy problems • General paucity of new family-based interventions

(continued)

Table 3.1   (*Continued*)

Disorders	Randomised controlled trials	Considerations	Promising interventions: non RCTs
Autistic spectrum disorders	• Limited empirical examination of family-based interventions • Results from parent-managed intervention programs not as good as for centres specialising in ASD	Problems because of complexity of study designs	• Parent education or parent-managed intervention • Relationship-focussed interventions
Eating disorders	• Maudsley approach for Anorexia Nervosa	Research needed for family-based approaches for Bulimia Nervosa	• Attachment-based perspective incorporated into systemic therapy • Family-orientated preventative interventions

Maudsley Hospital in London comparing individual therapy with family therapy, and which followed people up for 5 years demonstrated that outcomes, in particular, weight gain, were better in those offered family therapy early in the course of the disorder [16]. Where there was a long duration of illness, both treatment modalities were associated with a poor outcome. Lock [17] highlighted the need for prevention and early intervention for those at risk of anorexia nervosa, given the evidence that symptoms develop long before the full syndrome becomes apparent. Highlighting further the benefits of family therapy, Lock noted that family therapy appeared to produce positive effects more quickly than individual therapy, prevent dropout and play a significant role in reducing the need for more expensive inpatient and residential treatments [18]. He also pointed out that treatments needed to be phase-specific. For example, for younger teenagers, the key issues may be early socialisation and identity, whereas for older adolescents issues related to dating, leaving home or making decisions about further education may be more pertinent. This is a theme that is referred to in much of the literature around the topics that are addressed in family work involving young people across a range of disorders.

A series of further studies continues to confirm the positive benefits of working with the family when a young person has an eating disorder. It is clear that this type of approach is both effective and acceptable to both the young person with the problem and the family and can be delivered in different formats such as manualised family-based treatment [19]. In this study, participants reported a range of positive outcomes including increased closeness, communication, openness, honesty, problem-solving skills, parental understanding, awareness of feelings, family support, patience, cooperation, appreciation and overall happiness, with decreases in arguing and criticism. The mechanism whereby positive results are achieved has been shown to be linked with the development of a strong therapeutic alliance with parents [20].

This is achieved through having a collaborative therapeutic stance, a non-blaming attitude where parents are absolved of responsibility for causing the disorder, where parental guilt is reduced and where there is a focus on symptoms rather than aetiology. The principle of externalisation is used whereby everyone is battling against the symptoms rather than against the child. Results demonstrated that a strong early alliance with the family prevented dropout [20]. This central role played by the family was again demonstrated in a study by Lock et al. where a decline in problematic family behaviours was one of the key factors that increased the young person's chance of remission [21]. A further randomised controlled trial comparing individual treatment with family-based treatment demonstrated the greater effectiveness of the family treatment at both follow-up points indicating that the involvement of the family results in sustained change and improvement [22]. These long-term benefits were again highlighted in a review by Treasure and Russell [23] who point out the superior effects of family therapy at 5 year follow-up and conclude that effective family-based treatment applied early in the course of the illness can shape the outcome for at least 5 years.

Older adults

Another area where there is increasing interest in early detection and intervention and the role of family caregivers is at the other end of the lifespan spectrum in relation to older people with dementia and memory difficulties. This is to a large extent driven by the changing demographics worldwide with increasing life expectancy. Dementia has a major impact on carers in terms of stress and reduced quality of life, and the key role played by family members in the care of those with dementia is well documented. Studies to assess the benefits of both the impact of early intervention and psychosocial support targeted at families have been ongoing for some time. Moniz-Cook et al. examined the impact of early family counselling at the time of diagnosis with dementia [24]. The focus was psychoeducational, concentrating on those abilities that were still preserved, on crisis prevention and coping strengths, and on emotional issues, particularly feelings of loss linked with anticipated increasing disability. The intervention also offered active training in memory management which was home-based and involved the carer. Improvements were found in memory scores in the group where the family approach had been employed, and carer wellbeing was better. In the control group where there was no family intervention apart from written information, there was an increased likelihood of breakdown of home care.

The benefits of early diagnosis in dementia have been described by other researchers – the person and their family carers can plan for their futures and avail themselves of a range of help, support and treatments [25]. The current literature clearly points to the value of early diagnosis and intervention involving psychosocial approaches for caregivers in delaying or preventing transitions into care homes thus resulting in huge cost savings [25, 26, 27]. There appear to be clear benefits therefore for early intervention for those referred to services prior to assessment and diagnosis: this helps shape positive attitudes, encourages the maintenance of pleasures and relationships, allows the provision of information that addresses fears and can be delivered in many cases by primary care staff [28]. Intervening early seems to improve feelings of self-efficacy, and communications skills training has been identified as a key component of successful interventions [29]. Caregivers report communication difficulties with their relative even in the initial stages of the disorder, and these escalate unless the caregivers are offered communications training. The authors conclude that as caregiving responsibilities are of long duration in dementia, it is imperative that home-based care models that are responsive to caregiver needs are offered right from the point of contact with services [29].

Family intervention in early psychosis

An area that has received much attention in recent years is the development of early intervention for people with psychosis, with services developing in several countries [30]. Central to all of these services is the concept of involving the family of the young person and those who are important in their social networks[31, 32, 33]. The rationale for family engagement is clear:

- Young people are often living with their family [34], and by working in this way, the young person is understood in their social context

- Families often initiate and sustain engagement with services [35, 36, 37, 38], although families may face obstacles when trying to engage [39]

- It facilitates the establishment of collaborative relationships between the individual, family and services, and supports the family's understanding, relationships and adjustment to change [40]

- Young people highly value the involvement of family and find the family environment supportive [41]

- Family interventions have been found to be one of the key elements of effective intervention in early psychosis [42], and the reductions in relapse and hospitalisations evidenced in dedicated early psychosis services result from the delivery of family interventions [43]

- Reduces the level of distress that carers experience and assists them in their role in supporting the young person towards recovery [44], thus minimizing the risk of problems developing in individuals or in the family as a whole

- Families can experience a range of difficulties including stigma [45, 46], regret, grief and loss reactions [47, 48, 49], and a range of concerns about the young person including worries about their self-esteem and identity, social behavior and substance abuse [50]. They report emotional demands, and describe sacrifices they have to make as a result of their caring roles [48]. Working with the whole family ensures that these issues are addressed

- Addresses the needs of all family members, including siblings who experience a range of difficulties connected with their brother or sister with psychosis [51, 52]

- The cost savings that result from early psychosis services have been well evaluated and documented [53], and family interventions play a major part in this because of the reductions in relapse rates and hospitalisations.

Key elements of effective family intervention in early psychosis

Family interventions in early psychosis have been delivered in a number of formats including individual family approaches [54], brief psychoeducational styles with a limited number of sessions [55], carers education groups [56, 57], combinations of group and individual components [58] and multi-family groups [59, 60]. The number of randomised trials is still limited, and many of the studies are small and not well controlled. Results have been variable, and as many of the studies evaluated family work as part of an integrated early psychosis service, it has been difficult to separate out the role played by the family intervention *per se* in influencing outcomes [61]. Some have reported positive outcomes in terms of lower hospitalisations and higher level of functioning [58], and others in relation to positive outcomes for family members in terms of reduced isolation, improved understanding and relationships [56]. Brief educational approaches that are not individually tailored may not be as acceptable to families [55], and it is not clear whether multifamily groups produce positive outcomes. The study by Rossberg et al. [60] demonstrated that although there were fewer drop outs in the group attending multifamily groups, these participants showed less improvement than those in the control group and had significantly longer duration of psychotic symptoms during the follow-up period [60]. The meta-analysis by Bird et al. [43] clearly demonstrates that family interventions in early psychosis reduce relapse and readmission rates significantly. There is an acceptance, however, that more research is necessary to determine what are the necessary components of effective family interventions at this early stage, and in what format or combination of formats these should be delivered [62, 63]. There is also research currently underway to assess the potential benefits of family interventions in the prodromal stage of psychosis [64].

Currently there is sufficient information from existing studies to have a reasonable idea of the main elements that family interventions in early psychosis should consist of, and these are listed in Table 3.2. The clearest descriptions of these come from the sites where pioneering early intervention services were established such as Birmingham, United Kingdom; Melbourne, Australia and Calgary, Canada. Common features of the interventions

Table 3.2 Early psychosis – features of effective family interventions

- Detailed assessment of the family's knowledge, strengths and coping resources and areas of difficulty [40, 65]
- Family, individual and clinicians reaching a shared understanding around the disorder and substance misuse [40]
- Information on how to access, understand or negotiate services that are unfamiliar, including transitions between services [39, 45]
- Information sharing and increasing understanding [31, 65]
- Relapse prevention strategies and 'staying well' plans, although these can be difficult to introduce as the individual and family may find the possibility of relapse difficult [40, 57, 66]
- Problem-solving about day to day issues [40, 65]
- A focus on communication [40, 65]
- Counselling about grief and loss, and adjustment to changed expectations [47, 49, 57]
- Different types of family input at different points in time – phase specific [31, 65]
- Attention to individual differences between and within families [31, 68]
- Culturally sensitive content [65, 67]

include assessment, sharing of information, relapse prevention strategies and a focus on communication and problem-solving [40, 65, 66]. Any approaches to helping the family need to be sensitive to the cultural norms and beliefs in individual families [67].

There is also a detailed information available about how these approaches can be delivered in practice [40, 68], and also in supporting siblings within the family [69, 70]. The other area where family work is being shown to have beneficial effects is in families of young people with bipolar disorder. Young people offered family-focussed treatment showed significant improvements in depression, hypomania and psychosocial functioning [71]. Macneil et al. describe how work with families of young people with bipolar disorder helps them to differentiate 'normal' adolescent behaviours from symptoms of a mood disorder and helps them to respond appropriately to the young person during the first episode [72].

Conclusion

Lucksted et al. describe a clear rationale for the early involvement of families – dysfunctional family patterns are commonly the result of illness and disorder, so intervening early will prevent this from happening [73]. Others highlight the fact that family interventions enhance the chances of a favourable outcome [74]. Family approaches are clearly acceptable to families, provided they are culturally sensitive [67, 75].

References

1. Bruder B. (2000). Family-centred early intervention: clarifying our values for the new millennium. *Topics in Early Childhood Special Education* **20**(2): 105–115.
2. Dunst C, Trivette C and Deal A. (1998). *Enabling and Empowering Families: Principles and Guidelines for Practice*. Cambridge, MA: Brookline Books.
3. Guralnick MJ. (1999). Family and child influences on the peer-related social competence of young children with developmental delays. *Mental Retardation and Developmental Disabilities Research Reviews* **5**: 21–29.
4. Kochanek TT and Buka SL. (1998). Patterns of service utilization: child, maternal and service provider factors. *Journal of Early Intervention* **21**(3): 217–231.
5. Bruder MB. (2010). Early childhood intervention: a promise to children and families for their future. The Free Library, www.thefreelibrary.com (accessed 9 April 2014).
6. Dunst CJ. (2002). Family-centered practices: birth through high school. *Journal of Special Education* **36**: 139–147.
7. Ingber S and Dromi E. (2009). Demographics affecting parental expectations from early deaf intervention. *Deafness & Education International* **11**: 83–111.
8. Brotherson MJ, Summers JA, Naig LA, et al. (2010). Partnership patterns: addressing emotional needs in early intervention. *Topics in Early Childhood Special Education* **30**(1): 32–45.
9. Ingber S and Dromi E. (2010). Actual versus desired family-centered practice in early intervention for children with hearing loss. *Journal of Deaf Studies and Deaf Education* **15**(1): 59–71.
10. Moeller MP. (2000). Early intervention and language development in children who are deaf and hard of hearing. *Pediatrics* **106**: 43–52.
11. Tang HN, Chong WH, Goh W, et al. (2011). Evaluation of family-centred practices in the early intervention programmes for infants and young children in Singapore with measure of processes of care for service providers and measure of beliefs about participation in family-centred service. *Child: Care, Health and Development* **38**: 54–60.

12. Stormshak EA, Connell AM, Véronneau MH, et al. (2011). An ecological approach to promoting early adolescent mental health and social adaptation: family-centered intervention in public middle schools. *Child Development* **82**(1): 209–225.
13. Henggeler SW and Sheidow AJ. (2012). Empirically supported family-based treatments for conduct disorder and delinquency in adolescents. *Journal of Marital and Family Therapy* **38**(1): 30–58.
14. Hogue A and Liddle HA. (2009). Family-based treatment for adolescent substance abuse: controlled trials and new horizons in services research. *Journal of Family Therapy* **31**: 126–154.
15. Kaslow NJ, Broth MR, Smith CO, et al. (2012). Family-based interventions for child and adolescent disorders. *Journal of Marital and Family Therapy* **38**(1): 82–100.
16. Eisler I, Dara C, Russell GF, et al. (1997). Family and individual therapy in anorexia nervosa: A 5-year follow-up. *Archives of General Psychiatry* **54**: 1025–1030.
17. Lock J. (2003). A health service perspective on anorexia nervosa. *Eating Disorders* **11**: 197–207.
18. Lock J. (2004). Empowering the family as a resource for recovery: an example of family-based treatment for anorexia nervosa. In: H Steiner (ed.), *Handbook of mental health interventions in children and adolescents: An integrated developmental approach*, pp. 758–781. San Francisco, CA: Jossey-Bass.
19. Krautter T and Lock J (2004). Is manualized family-based treatment for adolescent anorexia nervosa acceptable to patients? Patient satisfaction at the end of treatment. *Journal of Family Therapy* **26**: 66–82.
20. Pereira T, Lock J, Oggins J. (2006). Role of therapeutic alliance in family therapy for adolescent anorexia nervosa. *International Journal of Eating Disorders* **39**: 677–684.
21. Lock J, Couturier J, Bryson S, et al. (2006). Predictors of dropout and remission in family therapy for adolescent anorexia nervosa in a randomized clinical trial. *International Journal of Eating Disorders* **39**(8): 639–647.
22. Lock J, Le Grange D, Agras WS, et al. (2010). Randomized clinical trial comparing family-based treatment with adolescent-focused individual therapy for adolescents with anorexia nervosa. *Archives of General Psychiatry* **67**(10): 1025–1032.
23. Treasure J and Russell G. (2011). The case for early intervention in anorexia nervosa: theoretical exploration of maintaining factors. *The British Journal of Psychiatry* **199**: 5–7.
24. Moniz-Cook E, Agar S, Gibson G, et al. (1998). A preliminary study of the effects of early intervention with people with dementia and their families in a memory clinic. *Aging and Mental Health* **2**(3): 199–211.
25. Banerjee S and Wittenberg R. (2009). Clinical and cost effectiveness of service for early diagnosis and intervention in dementia. *International Journal of Geriatric Psychiatry*, www.interscience.wiley.com (accessed 9 April 2014).
26. Brodaty H, Green A, Koshera A. (2003). Meta-analysis of psychosocial intervention for caregivers of people with dementia. *Journal of the American Geriatric Society* **51**: 657–664.
27. Mittleman M, Haley WE, Clay OJ, et al. (2006). Improving care-giver well-being delays nursing home placements of patients with Alzheimer disease. *Neurology* **67**: 1592–1599.
28. Moniz-Cook E, Manthorpe J, Carr I, et al. (2006). Facing the future: A qualitative study of older people referred to a memory clinic prior to assessment and diagnosis. *Dementia* **5**(3): 375–395.
29. Kouri KK, Ducharme FC and Giroux F. (2011). A psycho-educational intervention focused on communication for caregivers of a family member in the early stage of Alzheimer's disease: Results of an experimental study. *Dementia* **10**(3): 435–453.
30. McGorry P, Johanessen JO, Lewis S, et al. (2010). Early intervention in psychosis: keeping faith with evidence-based health care. *Psychological Medicine* **40**: 399–404.
31. Gleeson J, Jackson HJ, Staveley H, et al. (1999). Family intervention in early psychosis. In: P.D. McGorry, and H.J. Jackson (eds), *The Recognition and Management of Early Psychosis*, pp. 376–406. Cambridge: Cambridge University Press.
32. Fadden G, Birchwood M, Jackson C, et al. (2004). Psychological therapies: implementation in early intervention services. In: P. McGorry and J. Gleeson (eds), *Psychological Interventions*

in Early Psychosis: A Practical Treatment Handbook, pp. 261–279. Chichester: John Wiley & Sons Ltd.

33. Addington J, Collins A, McCleery A, et al. (2005). The role of family work in early psychosis. *Schizophrenia Research* **79**: 77–83.

34. Fisher H, Theodore K, Power P, et al. (2008). Routine evaluation in first episode psychosis services: feasibility and results from the MiData project. *Social Psychiatry and Psychiatric Epidemiology* **43**: 960–967.

35. Singh SP and Grange T. (2006). Measuring pathways to care in first-episode psychosis: A systematic review. *Schizophrenia Research* **81**: 75–82.

36. Boydell KM, Gladstone BM and Volpe T. (2006). Understanding help-seeking delay in the prodrome to first episode psychosis: A secondary analysis of the perspectives of young people. *Psychiatric Rehabilitation Journal* **30**(1): 54–60.

37. De Haan L, Peters B, Dingemans P, et al. (2002). Attitudes of patients toward the first psychotic episode and the start of treatment. *Schizophrenia Bulletin* **28**(3): 431–442.

38. De Haan L, Welborn K, Krikke M, et al. (2004). Opinions of mothers on the first psychotic episode and the start of treatment of their child. *European Psychiatry* **19**: 226–229.

39. McCann TV, Lubman DI and Clark E. (2011). First-time primary caregivers' experience accessing first-episode psychosis services. *Early Intervention in Psychiatry* **5**: 156–162.

40. Fadden G and Smith, J. (2009). Family work in early psychosis. In: F. Lobban and C. Barrowclough (eds), *A Casebook of Family Interventions for Psychosis*, pp. 23–45. Chichester: John Wiley & Sons, Ltd.

41. Lester H, Marshall M, Jones P, et al. (2011). Views of young people in early intervention services for first-episode psychosis in England. *Psychiatric Services* **62**(8): 882–887.

42. Killackey E. (2009). Psychosocial and psychological interventions in early psychosis: essential elements for recovery. *Early Intervention in Psychiatry* **3**: 517–521.

43. Bird V, Premkumar P, Kendall T, et al. (2010). Early intervention services, cognitive-behavioural therapy and family intervention in early psychosis: systematic review. *The British Journal of Psychiatry* **197**: 350–356.

44. Jones K. (2009). Addressing the needs of carers during early psychosis. *Early Intervention in Psychiatry* **3**: S22–S26.

45. Gerson R, Davidson L, Booty A, et al. (2009). Families' experience with seeking treatment for recent-onset psychosis. *Psychiatric Services* **60**: 812–816.

46. Wong C, Davidson L, Anglin D, et al. (2009). Stigma in families of individuals in early stages of psychotic illness: family stigma and early psychosis. *Early Intervention in Psychiatry* **3**(2): 108–115.

47. Lafond V. (2009). Coming to terms with mental illness in the family – working constructively through its grief. In: F. Lobban and C. Barrowclough (eds), *A Casebook of Family Interventions for Psychosis*, pp. 167–184. Chichester: John Wiley & Sons, Ltd.

48. Knock J, Kline E, Schiffman J, et al. (2011). Burdens and difficulties experienced by caregivers of children and adolescents with schizophrenia-spectrum disorders: a qualitative study. *Early Intervention in Psychiatry* **5**: 349–354.

49. Jones DW. (2004). Families and serious mental illness: working with loss and ambivalence. *British Journal of Social Work* **34**(7): 961–979.

50. Iyer SN, Loohuis H, Pawliuk N, et al. (2011). Concerns reported by family members of individuals with first-episode psychosis. *Early Intervention in Psychiatry* **5**: 163–167.

51. Newman S, Simonds LM and Billings J. (2011). A narrative analysis investigating the impact of first episode psychosis on siblings' identity. *Psychosis: Psychological, Social and Integrative Approaches* 1752–2447.

52. Sin J, Moone N, Harris P, et al. (2012). Understanding the experiences and service needs of siblings of individuals with first-episode psychosis: a phenomenological study. *Early intervention in Psychiatry* **6**: 53–59.

53. McCrone P, Knapp M and Dhanasir S. (2009). Economic impact of services for first-episode psychosis: a decision model approach. *Early Intervention in Psychiatry* **3**: 266–273.
54. Linszen D, Dingemans P, Van der Does J.W, et al. (1996). Treatment, expressed emotion and relapse in recent onset schizophrenic disorders. *Psychological Medicine* **26**: 333–242.
55. Leavey G, Gulamhussein S, Papadopoulos C, et al. (2004). A randomized controlled trial of a brief intervention for families of patients with a first episode psychosis. *Psychological Medicine* **34**: 423–431.
56. Riley G, Gregory N, Bellinger J, et al. (2011). Carers education groups for relatives with a first episode of psychosis: an evaluation of an 8 week education group. *Early Intervention in Psychiatry* **5**: 57–63.
57. Reed M, Peters S, Banks L, et al. (2010). Sharing Care with Families. In: P. French, J. Smith, D. Shiers, M. Reed and M. Rayne (eds), *Promoting Recovery in Early Psychosis: A Practice Manual*, pp. 226–234. Oxford: Wiley-Blackwell.
58. Zhang M, Wang M, Li J, et al. (1994). Randomised-control trial of family intervention for 78 first-episode male schizophrenic patients. An 18-month study in Suzhou, Jiangsu. *British Journal of Psychiatry* **165**(24): 96–102.
59. O'Brien MP, Zinberg JL, Bearden CE, et al. (2007). Psychoeducational multi-family group treatment with adolescents at high risk for developing psychosis. *Early Intervention in Psychiatry* **1**: 325–332.
60. Rossberg JI, Johannessen JO, Klungsoyr O, et al. (2010). Are multi family groups appropriate for patients with first episode psychosis? A 5-year naturalistic follow-up study. *Acta Psychiatrica Scandinavica* **122**: 384–394.
61. Onwumere J, Bebbington P and Kuipers E. (2011). Family interventions in early psychosis: specificity and effectiveness. *Epidemiology and Psychiatric Science* **20**(2): 113–119.
62. Askey R, Gamble C and Gray R. (2007). Family work in first-onset psychosis: a literature review. *Journal of Psychiatric and Mental Health Nursing* **14**: 356–365.
63. Alvarez-Jimenez M, Parker AG, Hetrick SE, et al. (2011). Preventing the second episode: a systematic review and meta-analysis of psychosocial and pharmacological trials in first-episode psychosis. *Schizophrenia Bulletin* **37**(3): 619–630.
64. Schlosser DA, Miklowitz DJ, O'Brien MP, et al. (2011). A randomized trial of family focused treatment for adolescents and young adults at risk for psychosis: study rationale, design and methods. *Early Intervention in Psychiatry* **6**(3): 283–291. doi: 10.1111/j.1751-7893.2011.00317.x
65. Addington J and Burnett P. (2004). Working with families in the early stages of psychosis. In: JFM Gleeson and PD McGorry (eds), *Psychological Interventions in Early Psychosis: A Treatment Handbook*, pp. 99–116. Chichester: John Wiley & Sons, Ltd.
66. Crisp K and Gleeson J. (2009). Working with families to prevent relapse in first-episode psychosis. In: F. Lobban and C. Barrowclough (eds), *A Casebook of Family Interventions for Psychosis*, pp. 67–90. Chichester: John Wiley & Sons, Ltd.
67. Onwumere J Smith B and Kuipers, E. (2009). Family intervention with ethnically and culturally diverse groups. In: F. Lobban and C. Barrowclough (eds), *A Casebook of Family Interventions for Psychosis*, pp. 211–231. Chichester: John Wiley & Sons, Ltd.
68. Burbach F Fadden G and Smith J. (2010). Family interventions for first-episode psychosis. In: P. French, M. Reed, J. Smith, M. Rayne and D. Shiers (eds), *Early Intervention in Psychosis: Promoting Recovery in Early Psychosis*, pp. 210–225. Oxford: Blackwell Publishing Ltd.
69. Smith J, Fadden G and O'Shea M. (2009). Interventions with siblings. In F. Lobban and C. Barrowclough (eds), *A Casebook of Family Interventions for Psychosis*, pp. 185–210. Chichester: John Wiley & Sons, Ltd.
70. Smith J, Fadden G and Taylor L. (2010). The needs of siblings in first-episode psychosis. In: P. French, M. Reed, J. Smith, M. Rayne and D. Shiers (eds), *Early Intervention in Psychosis: Promoting Recovery*, pp. 235–244. Oxford: Blackwell Publishing Ltd.

71. Miklowitz DJ, Chang KD, Taylor DO, et al. (2011). Early psychosocial intervention for youth at risk for bipolar I or II disorder: a one-year treatment development trial. *Bipolar Disorders* **13**: 67–75.

72. Macneil CA, Hasty MK, Berk M, et al. (2011). Psychological needs of adolescents in the early phase of bipolar disorder: implications for early intervention. *Early Intervention in Psychiatry* **5**: 100–107.

73. Lucksted A, McFarlane W, Downing D, et al. (2012). Recent developments in family psychoeducation as an evidence-based practice. *Journal of Marital and Family Therapy* **38**(1): 101–121.

74. Le Grange D and Loeb KL. (2007). Early identification and treatment of eating disorders: prodrome to syndrome. *Early Intervention in Psychiatry* **1**: 27–39.

75. Cardemil EV, Kim S, Pinedo TM, et al. (2005). Developing a culturally appropriate depression prevention program: the family coping skills program. *Cultural Diversity and Ethnic Minority Psychology* **11**: 99–112.

4
Do Early Intervention Services for Psychosis Represent Value for Money?

Paul McCrone[1] and Martin Knapp[1,2]

[1]*Centre for the Economics of Mental and Physical Health, Health Service and Population Research Department, Institute of Psychiatry, King's College London, UK*
[2]*Personal Social Services Research Unit, London School of Economics and Political Science, UK*

Introduction

Mental health problems typically affect individuals in many ways and the detrimental impact is reflected in the large economic cost of these conditions. Cost can be divided into the direct effects of mental health problems that lead to service responses from care providers and the indirect effects, for example a reduced ability to work, study or to engage in recreational activities. As such, a plethora of agencies are frequently involved in providing care. Recent estimates have suggested that the total health and social care costs associated with mental health problems in England are £20 billion, with a further £29 billion and £51 billion due to lost employment and human costs, respectively [1]. Previously, McCrone et al. [2] demonstrated that of £23 billion service costs (including social care and support from families), around 17% could be attributed to care and treatment responses to schizophrenia, bipolar disorder and other psychoses.

Recognising that mental health problems have major economic impacts should encourage us to consider the 'value for money' of alternative interventions, treatments and services. Economic evaluations are crucial because the resources required to provide inpatient beds, psychological therapies, medication and other interventions could be used to treat different patients with mental health problems and indeed patients with other conditions (e.g. cancer, asthma and diabetes). Health care resources are limited in their supply and yet the demand for these resources is almost unlimited. This has always been the case,

Early Intervention in Psychiatry: EI of nearly everything for better mental health, First Edition.
Edited by Peter Byrne and Alan Rosen.

but is particularly important when countries are going through periods of economic austerity. Ensuring that economic evaluations are conducted in a way such that decision makers are able to organise care using the best available evidence is imperative.

The onset of psychosis in adolescence or early adulthood is associated with disruption of education, low rates of post-school training, poor educational outcomes, impoverishment of social life, poor social functioning, lower-than-average employment and marriage rates, and higher-than-average rates of receipt of disability pensions [3–8]. Other things being equal, the longer the duration of untreated psychosis, (DUP) the higher the rates of occupational inactivity and suicide [9, 10].

One response across many countries has been the development of early intervention (EI) services. Policy makers in England have generally been very supportive of EI and recommended that EI teams should be set up in each local mental health system to provide intensive support for young people who are developing a first episode of psychosis. What policy makers need to know is whether these teams are effective and cost-effective.

Approaches to economic evaluation

It is important to adopt a comprehensive perspective when considering the costs associated with EI services. Clearly, it is crucial to measure the costs of the EI team itself, but an evaluation should also measure the cost of inpatient care, other mental health services, general health care, care provided by social services, inputs from education agencies and contacts with the criminal justice system. Furthermore, family members or friends will also often provide care and support. This will usually be unpaid but it clearly carries an economic cost given that unpaid carer time can usually be used for other purposes. These are all direct service costs. The indirect costs associated with time taken off work or school/college, or reduced productivity whilst at work, should also be measured for individuals served by EI teams. By measuring such direct and indirect costs, it is possible to see whether the extra costs associated with EI teams are offset by reduced costs elsewhere in the system, whether they are unchanged, or whether in fact they are increased as a result of EI teams improving access to other forms of care.

A variety of methods are available for combining cost data with information on outcomes and evaluating different interventions or policies. The different types of analyses are distinguished according to the way in which outcomes are measured, and the choice between them depends crucially on the purpose of the evaluation.

Cost-minimisation analysis

A misconception about economic evaluation is that it is only concerned with the cost of different interventions. Whilst this is generally wrong, there may be situations when one is prepared to measure costs and to favour an intervention that costs less than the alternative with which it is being compared. This would only be acceptable if it was already known that the two interventions – say EI and usual care – were equally effective. If that were the case then the least costly would be the most efficient, other things being equal. Whilst economists will tend to warn against conducting such cost-minimisation analyses, decision makers at local and national levels may be drawn toward them when resources are particularly tight.

Cost-benefit analysis

Like all forms of economic evaluation, cost-benefit analysis measures costs in monetary units, but it measures outcomes using monetary units also. In principle this makes cost-benefit analysis particularly powerful. If the monetised measure of outcome exceeds the costs then the intervention produces a 'surplus', and when comparing two or more interventions, the one with the greatest surplus should be favoured. Comparisons with interventions in other sectors can be made if their outcomes can also be measured using monetary units. However, the challenge with this method is that it is difficult to express mental health outcomes in monetary terms, and studies that have done so have tended to focus on the economic value of gains in employment rather than clinical outcomes, for example reduced symptoms or improved functioning. It might be possible to value these clinical outcomes in monetary units using methods such as 'willingness to pay' but these have seldom been applied in mental health research.

Cost-effectiveness analysis

This form of evaluation may be of especial relevance if the key question is how to provide appropriate care for a particular patient group, such as those with first-episode psychosis. Cost-effectiveness analysis requires that a single outcome measure be chosen and this will usually be condition-specific. For example, in an evaluation of EI it may be appropriate to use a measure of functioning or symptomatology, or the DUP. When comparing EI with an existing alternative like standard care, costs will be combined with the outcome measure so that the intervention that produces the greatest outcome improvement for every pound spent can be identified. Whilst cost-effectiveness is commonly used, it is not ideal for decision makers, including commissioners, who have to decide how to spend health care funds across many different areas.

Cost-consequences analysis

Mental health problems affect people in numerous ways and therefore, it may be inappropriate to focus entirely on one outcome measure as described earlier. Cost-consequences analysis does not attempt to formally combine cost data with information on outcomes, but presents cost and outcomes alongside each other to allow decision-makers to come to an overall conclusion regarding the different interventions being compared. Many evaluations will conduct a cost-consequences analysis to supplement a more rigorous cost-effectiveness analysis.

Cost-utility analysis

This last form of analysis uses a generic measure of outcome such that interventions across all areas of health care can, in principle, be compared. In the vast majority of cost-utility analyses the outcome measure is the quality-adjusted life year (QALY), where the time spent in a particular health state is adjusted according to the health-related quality of life (which is a proxy for utility) experienced during that time. Health-related quality of life is measured on a scale anchored by one (full health) and zero (death). Therefore, if someone spends two years in a health state and during that time their quality of life is rated as 0.7, they will have gained 1.4 QALYs (two times 0.7). Clearly, the challenge of this approach is to measure health-related quality of life in a meaningful way. One option is to use a simple rating scale, but more sophisticated methods are available such as defining health states according to the EQ-5D [11] or SF-36 [12] and then converting these into utility values.

What do we know?

There is an accumulation of evidence relating to the effectiveness of early detection (ED) and EI services. However, there have been fewer studies which have provided information on the relative cost-effectiveness of such services compared to the existing care. In the review that follows, we have included full economic evaluations (where costs are combined with outcomes), cost studies and studies which do not report costs but do provide relevant resource use information.

Early detection studies

ED services tend to be relatively small scale and are usually set up in the context of research studies rather than as routine care. Valmaggia et al. [13] have performed one of the few economic studies of an ED service. A decision model approach was used to map the care pathways for patients with prodromal symptoms who would receive either a specialist service or treatment as usual (assumed to be GP and counsellor contacts). Patients were assumed to either make a transition to psychosis or not, and if they did they would then have a probability of a long or short DUP and then a probability of inpatient or non-inpatient care. The model was run for 2 years. During the first year, the per-person costs were estimated to be £2596 for ED and £724 for usual care (at 2003/4 price levels). This 259% extra cost was due to the ED patients receiving input that would not be matched by alternative standard care. However, over the entire 2-year period the costs were estimated to be £4396 and £5357. This saving of 18% is due to reduced inpatient stays (because of reduced DUP) and increased time in work.

Early intervention studies

Substantially more evaluations have assessed the economic impact of EI services. This is likely to be the result of such services being introduced as part of clinical practice. For example, in England there have been official Department of Health guidelines regarding the setting up of EI teams across the country (http://www.dh.gov.uk/prod_consum_dh/groups/dh_digitalassets/@dh/@en/documents/digitalasset/dh_4058960.pdf.).

An economic evaluation of the EPPIC service in Melbourne compared 51 EPPIC patients treated in 1993 and 1994 with 51 matched controls who received the pre-EPPIC treatment model between 1989 and 1992 [14]. Costs included inpatient stays, outpatient appointments, medication, community mental health team contacts, general practitioner contacts and private therapy. Mean bed days were 42 for EPPIC and 80 for pre-EPPIC. The costs of the EPPIC intervention were $AUD 5147 and $AUD 2688 (at 1993/4 price levels) for pre-EPPIC community-based care. However, mean total costs were

$AUD 7110 less (30%) for the EPPIC patients compared to pre-EPPIC patients due to reductions in inpatient service use outweighing increases in community services.

More recently, the same group reported economic findings approximately 7.5 years later for these patients [15]. The mean annual costs were $AUD 3445 for EI and $AUD 9503 for standard care (difference of 64%; 2000/1 price levels). Inpatient costs were $AUD 1178 for EI and $AUD 3243 for standard care (difference of 64%). During the 2 years prior to follow-up assessment, 56% of EI and 33% of standard care patients had been in paid employment. EI patients also had significantly better clinical outcomes.

In another pre–post study (in Canada), Goldberg et al. [16] compared hospital use between 159 patients receiving an EI service and 146 receiving standard care in a period before the team was established. There were on average 2.3 admissions for EI patients and 2.9 admissions for standard care patients. Readmissions occurred for 41% of EI and 54% of standard care patients. The mean length of time in hospital was 43.7 days for EI patients and 60.2 days for standard care patients (difference of 27%). EI patients had significantly fewer involuntary admissions and emergency room visits. Total mean costs were $2371 for EI and $2125 (at 2002 price levels) for standard care patients. However, there were savings for acute beds and emergency room visits.

A similar study in England compared 75 patients receiving EI with 114 who received care before the EI team was established [17]. Mean admissions over 3 years were 0.9 for EI and 1.9 for standard care (a difference of 53%). Mean readmissions were 0.4 and 1.3, respectively (a difference of 69%) and mean bed days were 44.9 and 96.7 (a difference of 54%). This difference in bed days would equate to around £17,000 per patient (using costs from [18]). EI patients were also significantly more likely to remain engaged with the services after 1 year.

Larsen et al. [19] in a Norwegian/Danish study compared two areas which had an EI service with two areas without EI. The intervention consisted of a public awareness campaign and targeted campaigns at GPs, social workers and school health workers. The main aim was to reduce DUP. This paper reported follow-up at 1 year for around 280 patients. The mean length of the initial hospitalisation was 11.9 weeks for the EI group and 11.8 for the standard care group. EI patients spent on average 16.4 weeks in hospital during the year compared to 15.5 weeks for the standard care patients. Weeks of psychotherapy were similar (42.0 EI, 45.5 standard care) and medication duration was slightly less for EI (37.3 weeks) compared to standard care (41.7 weeks). Therefore, resource use was similar between the groups. However, total duration of psychosis was 22 weeks for EI and 44 weeks for standard care (EI 50% of standard care).

In the Danish OPUS study, Petersen et al. [20] showed that treatment was stopped during the first year despite a need for it for 1% of EI patients and 6% of those receiving standard care. The EI lasted for 2 years and consisted of assertive community treatment, family involvement and social skills training for 275 patients. A control group included 272 patients. The figures during the second year were 2% and 3%, respectively. Mean days in hospital were 62 for EI and 79 for standard care in year 1 and 27 EI and 35 standard care in year 2. There were on average 45 outpatient visits for EI patients and 18 for standard care patients in year 1 and 32 EI and 11 standard care in year 2.

A 5-year follow-up of the OPUS study was performed by Bertelsen et al. [21]. After 2 years of EI treatment patients would receive standard care (which may just be from their GP). At 2 years there were significant differences in favour of EI for psychotic symptoms and functioning. There were no significant differences at 5-year follow-up. There was no impact on suicidal behaviour at either follow-up. The proportion not hospitalised during the 2-year follow-up was 32% EI and 27% standard care. The figures were 57% and 54% during the 3–5-year period. Mean inpatient days during the first 2 years were 96 for EI and 123 for standard care (EI 22% less than standard care). The figures in the 3–5-year period were 58 EI and 71 standard care (18% less for EI), and in the entire 5-year follow-up they were 149 EI and 193 standard care (23% less for EI). During the 5-year period, 4% of EI patients and 10% of standard care patients lived in residential care. After 5 years, 61% of EI patients and 59% of standard care patients were not working.

Grawe et al. [22] compared EI and standard care for patients in Norway who had experienced their first symptoms not more than 2 years previously (but had not received treatment). EI did not attempt to reduce DUP. It consisted of pharmacotherapy, low caseload, family therapy, cognitive behavioural therapy (CBT), case management and crisis management. Follow-up was at 2 years and 50 completed the trial. Admissions to hospital occurred for 33% of EI and 50% of standard care patients (not significant). Suicide attempts were made by 13% of EI and 5% of standard care patients.

In Sweden, Cullberg et al. [23] compared patients with schizophrenia receiving EI with those receiving standard care (from a historical cohort) and another group receiving current social psychiatric care. The EI service focussed on crisis intervention, family support, continued engagement over a 5-year period, non-hospital-based residential care and low-dose medication. Clinical outcomes were better for the EI group than for the standard care group but similar compared to the social psychiatry patients. Compared to the latter, EI resulted in inpatient costs that were 94% lower in the first year of follow-up, 57% in year 2 and 55% in year 3. Outpatient costs were though 255%, 15% and 11% higher for these 3 years. Total costs for EI were lower by 29% in year 1, 55% year 2 and 61% in year 3.

The Lambeth Early Onset (LEO) study in south London found that EI, based on an assertive outreach model, resulted in a lower relapse rate than standard care [24]. Readmissions took place for 33% of EI patients compared to 51% of standard care patients, and the mean numbers of readmissions were 0.4 and 0.8, respectively. The EI group spent a mean 35.5 days in hospital during the 18-month follow-up compared to 54.9% in the standard care group (a difference of 35%). McCrone et al. [25] reported cost and cost-effectiveness findings from this trial. Total mean costs were £11685 in the EI group and £14062 in the standard care group (at 2003/4 price levels), with the difference (17%) not being significant. However, vocational outcomes and quality of life were both improved for the EI group and this combined with the (albeit non-statistically significant) costs savings resulted in a high likelihood of cost-effectiveness.

In a follow-up to the LEO study, Gafoor et al. [26] examined admissions in the period 3.5–5 years after entry to the study. They found that that 33% of EI patients and 39% of standard care patients had admissions. The mean number of bed days was 45.3 and 51.4 days respectively. After controlling for patent characteristics it was found that EI patients spent on average 2 more days in hospital than standard care patients. This study either suggests that EI does not have a long-term effect or that when patients are discharged back to standard care they have similar outcomes to others. Of course, what must be borne in mind is that the initial savings are not lost.

In another RCT of EI in London, Kuipers et al. [27] found that there were few differences between EI and standard care over a 9-month follow-up. Mean inpatient days were 9.3 for EI and 16.4 for standard care. This difference of 43% was not statistically significant. However, this was a small trial of just 59 patients.

Using a Markov modelling approach, McCrone et al. [28] compared EI to standard care over 1- and 3-year periods. In the 2-month cycles of the model, EI patients were assumed either to stay with the EI team, be referred to standard care teams, to be involuntarily admitted or to be voluntarily admitted. For standard care, the options were to stay with the standard care services or to receive either type of admission. Data for the model were obtained from trials, routine datasets and local service information. EI input was estimated to be more expensive than standard care input, but total costs were 35% less (£9422 vs. £14394 over 1 year and £26568 vs. £40816 over 3 years; 2003/4 price levels). The costs savings were due to lower initial admission and readmission rates.

Employing economic evidence

There are many reasons for wanting to see readily available and robust evidence on the costs and cost-effectiveness of EI services. As budgets tighten and the needs for treatment and support continue to grow, so health care and other decision makers are increasingly wanting to know how to squeeze more services and better outcomes from available (or shrinking) resources. Unsurprisingly, they are often seeking economic evidence to inform their actions. At the same time, lobbying groups are using cost and other economic data to press the case for treatment changes or system reforms.

The manufacturers or suppliers of health technologies (such as medications or medical devices) have long employed economic arguments to help sell their products, while the purchasers of those technologies and the commissioners of treatments and services are keen to secure value for money. Of course, 'technologies' such as EI are non-proprietory and do not have companies to champion them. Regulatory and other bodies are also using economic data to help monitor the consequences of policy and practice change.

In many countries, there are now formal over-arching mechanisms to examine the cost-effectiveness of new technologies in order to feed into national or regional reimbursement and coverage decisions [29]. In England and Wales, the National Institute for Health and Clinical Excellence (NICE) evaluates technologies (often *groups* of technologies and whole classes of medications such as second-generation antipsychotics) as a basis for drawing up clinical guidelines to support local commissioning and prescribing decisions. NICE has expert committees to look at evidence on both clinical effectiveness and cost-effectiveness. It has, for example, scrutinised the economic evidence on EI in its work on schizophrenia: www.nice.org.uk

A notable characteristic of many mental health problems, especially psychoses, is that they can have an impact across many facets of an individual's life, often resulting in a need for support from a range of different agencies and systems. These will have cost implications. From our summary of economic studies mentioned earlier, it was clear that the economic consequences of EI can include impacts on social care, education, housing, criminal justice and social security benefit systems. EI can also affect an individual's ability to get and retain paid employment, with economic consequences for individuals, families and communities, as well as for the national economy. Economic studies can provide evidence that spans these various systems, feeding into (usually much-needed) efforts to improve collaboration [30].

At an international level, bodies such as the European Commission (EC) make use of economic evidence to bolster the case for action. Along with the EU Member States, the EC endorsed a *Mental Health Pact* a few years ago to promote mental wellbeing and address mental health needs. In developing the case for the *Pact*, the Commission employed a range of arguments highlighting the economic impacts of poor mental health [31]. The World Health Organization's (WHO) *Choosing Interventions that are Cost Effective (CHOICE)* programme (http://www.who.int/choice/en/) collated information for each of the 17 WHO sub-regions on the costs, impact on population health and cost-effectiveness of different health interventions [32], including a range of mental health interventions [33, 34].

There are never enough resources to meet all needs or satisfy all wants, which is why decision-makers up and down health care and other systems find it helpful to examine evidence on costs and cost-effectiveness to inform their discussions and guide their decisions. The economics evidence base on EI services has been slow to develop but is now offering the kind of information that is so necessary at a time of economic austerity. This evidence suggests that EI services have the potential to be cost saving and cost-effective. However, they do require 'up-front' investment and so with the austerity being faced by many countries in the second decade of this century such services cannot be seen as necessarily secure. If EI services are protected it is likely that they will nonetheless change over time. Such change may well see key elements of EI become integral to standard care services, much in the same way as has happened with assertive community treatment. This in itself will represent a new pattern of working and this will require thorough evaluation including assessment of value for money.

References

1. Centre for Mental Health. (2010). The economic and social costs of mental health problems in 2009/10 http://www.centreformentalhealth.org.uk/pdfs/Economic_and_social_costs_2010.pdf (accessed 11 April 2014).
2. McCrone P, Dhanasiri S, Patel A, et al. (2008). *Paying the price: the cost of mental health care in England to 2026.* London: King's Fund.
3. Ang YG and Tan HY. (2004). Academic deterioration prior to first episode schizophrenia in young Singaporean males. *Psychiatry Research* **121**: 303–307.
4. Cannon M, Jones P, Huttunen MO, et al. (1999). School performance in Finnish children and later development of schizophrenia: a population-based longitudinal study. *Archives of General Psychiatry* **56**: 457–463.
5. Hollis C. (2000). Adult outcomes of child- and adolescent-onset schizophrenia: diagnostic stability and predictive validity. *American Journal of Psychiatry* **157**: 1652–1659.
6. Jarbin H, Ott Y and Von Knorring AL. (2003). Adult outcome of social function in adolescent-onset schizophrenia and affective psychosis. *Journal of the American Academy of Child and Adolescent Psychiatry* **42**: 176–183.
7. Lenior M, Dingemans PM, Linszen DH, et al. (2001). Social functioning and the course of early-onset schizophrenia: five-year follow-up of a psychosocial intervention. *British Journal of Psychiatry* **179**: 53–58.
8. Schothorst P, Emck C and van Engeland H. (2006). Characteristics of early psychosis. *Comprehensive Psychiatry* **47**: 438–442.
9. Clarke M, Whitty P, Browne S, et al. (2006). Suicidality in first episode psychosis. *Schizophrenia Research* **86**: 221–225.

10. Norman R, Mallal AK, Manchanda R, et al. (2007). Does treatment delays predict occupational functioning in the first episode psychosis? *Schizophrenia Research* **91**: 259–262.
11. Williams A. (1995). *The Role of the EuroQoL Instrument in QALY Calculations*. Centre for Health Economics, University of York.
12. Ware J, Snow KK, Kosinski M, et al. (1993). *SF-36 Health Survey, Manual and Interpretation Guide*. The Health Institute, New England Medical Centre, Boston, MA.
13. Valmaggia LR, McCrone P, Knapp M, et al. (2009). Economic impact of an early intervention service for people with an at risk mental state for psychosis. *Psychological Medicine* **39**: 1617–1626.
14. Mihalopoulos C, McGorry PD and Carter RC. (1999). Is phase-specific, community-oriented treatment of early psychosis an economically viable method for improving outcome? *Acta Psychiatrica Scandinavica* **100**: 47–55.
15. Mihalopoulos C, Harris M, Henry L, et al. (2009). Is early intervention in psychosis cost-effective over the long term? *Schizophrenia Bulletin* **35**: 909–918.
16. Goldberg K, Norman R, Hoch J, et al. (2006). Impact of a specialized early intervention service for psychotic disorders on patient characteristics, service use, and hospital costs in a defined catchment area. *Canadian Journal of Psychiatry* **51**: 895–903.
17. Dodgson G, Crebbin K, Pickering C, et al. (2008). Early intervention in psychosis service and psychiatric admissions. *Psychiatric Bulletin* **32**: 413–416.
18. Curtis L. (2012). Unit costs of health and social care. Canterbury, PSSRU.
19. Larsen TK, Melle I, Auestad B, et al. (2006). Early detection of first-episode psychosis: the effect on 1-year outcome. *Schizophrenia Bulletin* **32**: 758–764.
20. Petersen L, Jeppesen P, Thorup A, et al. (2005). A randomised multicentre trial of integrated versus standard treatment for patients with a first episode of psychotic illness. *British Medical Journal* **331**: 602–605.
21. Bertelsen M, Jeppesen P, Petersen L, et al. (2008). Five-year follow-up of a randomized multi-center trial of intensive early intervention vs standard treatment for patients with a first episode of psychotic illness: the OPUS trial. *Archives of General Psychiatry* **65**: 762–771.
22. Grawe RW, Falloon IRH, Widen JH, et al. (2006). Two years of continued early treatment for recent-onset schizophrenia: a randomised controlled trial. *Acta Psychiatrica Scandinavica* **114**: 328–336.
23. Cullberg J, Mattsson M, Levander S, et al. (2006). Treatment costs and clinical outcome for first episode schizophrenia patients: a 3-year follow-up of the swedish 'Parachute Project' and two comparison groups. *Acta Psychiatrica Scandinavica* **114**: 274–281.
24. Craig TKJ, Garety P, Power P, et al. (2004). The Lambeth Early Onset (LEO) Team: randomised controlled trial of the effectiveness of specialised care for early psychosis. *British Medical Journal* **329**: 1067.
25. McCrone P, Craig TKJ, Garety P, et al. (2010). Cost-effectiveness of an early intervention service for people with psychosis in south London: the LEO study. *British Journal of Psychiatry* **96**: 377–382.
26. Gafoor R, Nitsch D, McCrone P, et al. (2010). Effect of early intervention on 5-year outcome in non-affective psychosis. *British Journal of Psychiatry* **196**: 372–376.
27. Kuipers E, Holloway F, Rabe-Hesketh S, et al. (2004). An RCT of early intervention in psychosis: Croydon Outreach and Assertive Support Team (COAST). *Social Psychiatry and Psychiatric Epidemiology* **39**: 358–363.
28. McCrone P, Knapp M, Dhanasiri S. (2009). Economic impact of services for first episode psychosis: a decision model approach. *Early Intervention in Psychiatry* **3**: 266–273.
29. McDaid D, Cookson R, ASTEC Group. (2003). Evaluating health care interventions in the European Union. *Health Policy* **63**: 133–139.
30. McDaid D, Oliveira MD, Jurczak K, et al. (2007). Moving beyond the mental health care system: an exploration of the interfaces between the health and non-health sectors. *Journal of Mental Health* **16**: 181–194.

31. McDaid D. (2008). Mental health reform: Europe at the cross-roads. *Health Economics, Policy and Law* **3**: 219–228.
32. Hutubessy R, Chisholm D, Tan-Torres Edejer T, et al. (2003). Generalized cost-effectiveness analysis for national level priority setting in the health sector. *Cost Effectiveness and Resource Allocation* **1**: 8.
33. Chisholm D, Sanderson K, Ayuso-Mateos JL, et al. (2004). Reducing the global burden of depression: population-level analysis of intervention cost effectiveness in 14 world regions. *British Journal of Psychiatry* **184**: 393–403.
34. Chisholm D, van Ommeren M, Ayuso-Mateos JL, et al. (2005). Cost-effectiveness of clinical interventions for reducing the global burden of bipolar disorder. *British Journal of Psychiatry* **187**: 559–567.

II

Early Intervention Across the Lifespan

5
Perinatal Preventive Interventions in Psychiatry: A Clinical Perspective

Martin St-André[1], Hannah Schwartz[2] and Keiko Yoshida[3]
[1] *Sainte-Justine University Health Center, Université de Montréal, Montreal, Canada*
[2] *St. Mary's Hospital Center, McGill University, Montreal, Canada*
[3] *Department of Child Psychiatry, Kyushu University Hospital, Fukuoka City, Japan*

Introduction

The early years are a critical time of development during which multiple transformations take place for both infant and family. Infants experience enormous brain development ante- and postnatally, making them both highly receptive and highly vulnerable to environmental influence. For example a recent review suggested that 'the fetal period is ripe for renewed focus in child psychiatric conditions. The field of developmental origins has come into its own in much of medicine, with strong programs of research investigating fetal and placental effects related to subsequent heart disease, diabetes mellitus, and cancer' [1]. Families, and especially mothers, experience multiple changes that may have a lasting impact on their well-being and on the development of their child. This chapter will describe how a better understanding of the trajectory of individuals during the perinatal period provides rich entry point for trying to prevent perinatal psychiatric disorders, early relationship disorders and child psychiatric conditions.

The perinatal period: a critical transition

The transition to parenthood is a developmental crisis. The future mother experiences profound neurohormonal, intrapsychic and interpersonal challenges that redefine her sense of identity and her capacity for intimacy and nurturing. This intense period involves

Early Intervention in Psychiatry: EI of nearly everything for better mental health, First Edition.
Edited by Peter Byrne and Alan Rosen.

reworking attachment relationships, reconsidering one's identity to accommodate the parental role, experiencing various losses, transforming marital intimacy, establishing a parental alliance, defining the ideals and goals of becoming a new parent, and reconsidering one's family and cultural heritage. The parental alliance gets progressively established in the context of various types of behavioural and socioemotional interactions within the family.

During pregnancy and the first year of their child's life, parents normally encounter a broad range of affects: feelings of joy, awe and wonder, but also of strangeness, ambivalence and helplessness. Self-doubts about the capacity to nurture a child and feelings of ambivalence towards the infant or the marital partner are also part of the experience. Postnatally, as mutual affective regulation gets established in the family system, both parents and infant become better able to enjoy their interaction and to repair their communicative difficulties. This period brings about new strengths but also new vulnerabilities in parents, including the onset or exacerbation of psychiatric disorders. If psychopathology surfaces during this period, not only will the mother suffer from her condition but she will also be affected in her parental role through changes of affects, perceptions and behaviours.

Developmental trajectories get established early for children

Multiple longitudinal studies have shown that various childhood conditions, notably aggressive behaviour and even some child psychiatric conditions, can be prevented when intervention starts early and even antenatally [2]. Indeed, intervening early during pregnancy allows the establishment of a therapeutic alliance with vulnerable families and helps parents increase their sense of security during this period.

The attachment literature has demonstrated that attachment patterns are transmitted across generations but also that transmission gets established very early, even antenatally. For example in a seminal and replicated study, maternal attachment organisation was assessed during pregnancy and was shown to predict mother–infant attachment at 1 year of age [3].

At the family level, triadic interactions between mother, father and child have also been shown antenatally and significantly predict the postnatal triadic interactions [4]. This data points towards the possibility of intervening antenatally with the family, not only to improve parental well-being and to facilitate the parental alliance, but also to directly help the triadic relationship with the infant.

Prenatal characteristics of the infant, such as sex, the presence of multiple foetuses or various medical conditions also impact the early relationship. Parents develop internal representations of their infants antenatally and these representations influence how the parent behaves towards the infant. Studies with the Working Model of the Child Interview have shown that parental representations of the unborn infant – considering for example richness or distortions of representations – were linked to infant perception postnatally, hence influencing the various levels of parent–infant interactions postnatally [5].

The infant is very interactive after birth and the characteristics of the infant will be very influential on the early parental affective states and vice versa. This concept has been extensively studied through the transactional model of development. Hence infants born with various risk factors such as a difficult temperament, 'colic', medical problems or various neurosensory difficulties will create specific challenges to the 'goodness-of-fit' between parent and infant.

The antenatal environment: stress during pregnancy and the impact of untreated psychopathologies

In various cultures, traditional beliefs have emphasised the importance of protecting both mothers and foetuses against negative or stressful life events. This important intuition has been borne out by an increasing number of empirical studies clarifying the role of stress on maternal and infant neurodevelopmental outcomes.

Social stress is central to stressful environmental circumstances; it includes migration, racial discrimination, domestic violence, trauma, young or advanced maternal age. In addition, special clinical obstetrical circumstances will lead to a higher risk of psychiatric complications. These include pregnancy after perinatal loss or infertility, high-risk pregnancy (including multiple pregnancy), perinatal trauma, prematurity, foetal conditions or early temperamental difficulties in infants.

The perinatal stress literature has emphasised the role played by elevated transplacental cortisol. Cortisol is a hormone that is essential for the development of the foetal central nervous system. It crosses the placental barrier after being metabolised and 'buffered' by a placental dehydrogenase. An increasing number of prospective, well-controlled studies – but not all – have found that foetal exposure to elevated cortisol is associated with a higher risk of negative neurodevelopmental outcomes in infants. These effects range from emotional, cognitive, motor and language effects, in addition to a higher risk of childhood and adolescent conditions such as ADHD or conduct disorder [6]. In these studies, the link between antenatal stress and outcomes still holds after many confounding variables are controlled, such as life habits, SES and postnatal depression. More recently, studies have suggested that not all foetuses are affected equally and that the epigenetic impact of stress on the developing foetus could be related to genetic predispositions, notably the variants of the serotonin transporter gene. Moreover, developmental outcomes are strongly modulated by the quality of the attachment relationship [7].

The risk of elevated stress not only affects maternal and family well-being but also obstetrical follow-up and outcomes. Multiple studies suggest an increased risk of low birth weight, preterm delivery and pregnancy complications [8].

Although the effects of stress appear to be significant on infant neurodevelopment, the effects of stress are neither linear nor necessarily clinical. Indeed many clinical situations demonstrate apparently few observable effects on the infants, tending to confirm the fact that infants are neuroplastic and able to recover well. Hence, expectant mothers should not be made to feel guilty. However, this data highlights that stress should be considered a risk factor that justifies preventive maternal and familial interventions.

Psychopathology during the perinatal period
General considerations

Perinatal psychiatric conditions are common in mothers and fathers; these conditions are reciprocally influenced by pregnancy. The costs of an untreated psychiatric condition during this period are high. A psychiatric decompensation can lead to impulsivity and lack of judgment, substance use, increase the risk of suicide and infanticide and interfere with prenatal care and birth preparation. A relapse can also negatively impact the physiology of pregnancy, the social network and the marital relationship. Ultimately, the cumulative impact greatly increases the risk of mother–infant relationship disorders.

For at-risk populations, notably parents with a prior history of mental illness or a history of high psychosocial risk, screening is now regularly offered in various primary care and more specialised settings. The most common mental health screening tool in obstetrical populations is the Edinburgh Postnatal Depression Scale [9].Various factors will influence the accessibility to mental health care for these at-risk populations, including service availability and modes of interdisciplinary communication that will facilitate reference and coherence of approaches across settings.

After screening and referral, personalised recommendations for expectant or new families will depend on a proper assessment of the symptoms and severity of the parental illness. Important determinants will be patient's knowledge about the illness, duration of asymptomatic functioning, identified precipitants, number of prior episodes, frequency, type and duration of prior decompensations, time elapsed since the last episode, prior response to treatment, presence of various comorbidities such as substance use or, importantly, personality disorder [10]. The partner and extended family network will often be solicited as key partners for treatment planning. Importantly, the clinician who is asked questions about treatment should also be ready to explore and frankly discuss the patient's readiness for parenthood, especially among very vulnerable patients.

In higher-risk populations, such as parents with severe mental illness, the assessment of parental capacities is a consideration during the perinatal period. Generally, the assessment of risk factors should start during pregnancy and includes the mental status of the mother, her psychosocial environment, her support network. The assessment needs to address key risk factors such as the maternal perceptions, affects and behaviours with the infant as well as infant-specific factors such as twin pregnancies, medical status and temperamental characteristics. Although the first goal of prevention should always be family preservation, it is essential that the infant's basic and emotional needs be met. In some instances, this might necessitate an intensive psychosocial early intervention approach involving the family. In more severe cases, the consideration of a temporary child placement, concurrent family planning or adoption may be necessary.

Cultural aspects are sometimes overlooked but are extremely important and fundamental to the health care worker's understanding of the situation. Poverty, overcrowding, diminished social support, conflicting recommendations regarding pregnancy care and infant rearing, integration of traditional modes of accompaniment, cultural taboos and the incorporation of healing methods within a medical context pose unique challenges for migrant families. Often, using an interpreter/culture-broker is necessary for facilitating communication with migrant families and for clarifying their views and expectations regarding perinatal and infant care.

Depression and anxiety during pregnancy

Description   Pregnancy can be a time of happiness, personal reflection, maturation and interpersonal development. However, pregnancy does not protect against depression or anxiety. Across studies, perinatal depression prevalences are estimated to be between

10% and 30% Moreover, many women report the new onset or the exacerbation of a pre-existing anxiety disorder (such as panic disorder or obsessive–compulsive disorder). Fathers are now receiving more attention when it comes to perinatal mental health issues. A recent meta-analysis [11] demonstrated that perinatal depressive symptoms reach 10% in expectant fathers. This underlines the importance of addressing the father's need in preventive approaches during this critical transition.

'Baby blues' is common in the postpartum period and affects 30–80% of women. It is characterised by mild symptoms of depression that last up to 2 weeks, resolve spontaneously, do not affect maternal functioning and have not been shown to have long-term sequelae. Perinatal depression should be suspected when symptoms are more severe and enduring. In addition to the typical symptoms of depression, such as sadness, guilt, and disturbed sleep or appetite, lack of concentration, interest and psychomotor changes, it is imperative to discuss whether the mother has any suicidal or infanticidal thoughts in order to intervene immediately. Intrusive, distressing thoughts of accidental or intentional harm involving the newborn are common among women with postpartum-onset depression and can lead to avoidance of caring for the baby which can impair the development of the mother–child relationship. In contrast to delusional thoughts, obsessions associated with nonpsychotic depression or obsessive–compulsive disorder are not associated with an increased risk of aggression towards the child. Fear of 'becoming crazy' in the postpartum is usually a symptom of anxiety for women with no risk factors for bipolar or psychotic disorders and can be treated with reassurance.

For infants, prolonged exposure to maternal depressive and anxiety disorders has been associated with an increased risk of negative developmental outcomes in the cognitive, language and socioemotional domains. [12] Infants born to depressed mothers have higher cortisol levels, experience more negative and less positive parenting and require extra attention from health care professionals. Descriptions of parental interactions most commonly associated with parental depression are well captured by the clinical relationship disorders described in the DC:0-3R Classification [13].

Prevention and treatment planning for perinatal depression and anxiety Among future-mothers presenting with current or past history of depression during pregnancy, many will be at risk of presenting a postnatal episode. This highlights the privileged position that health care workers have in preventing postpartum episodes and improving the outcomes of children and families. In women who are at increased risk, prenatal counselling and planning is crucial to optimise preventive interventions. For the patient, the family and the clinical team, the challenge will be to maintain a high degree of vigilance for a recurrence of symptoms, while considering the possibility that many of the anxiety or depressive symptoms presented during pregnancy may reflect a challenging transition to parenthood and may not be a harbinger of psychopathology. Health professionals should make sure that conditions requiring treatment are screened for and assessed, without unnecessarily medicalising and pathologising the transition to parenthood. Nonetheless, pregnancy-related anxiety should not be dismissed as a simple transient state and interdisciplinary efforts should be made to increase maternal feelings of security and safety [8, 14].

The prevention of perinatal depression necessitates a variety of approaches. Raising public awareness is often the first step in the population and among obstetrical, paediatric and psychiatric teams. Increasing the level of emotional security among expectant mothers facilitates maternal well-being and diminishes risk factors. In more targeted groups, various psychotherapeutic approaches, usually involving the family as a whole, can be considered. Medical interventions are described in the treatment section.

Nonmedical intervention Psychotherapy and psychosocial interventions have an important place in the treatment and prevention of antenatal and postpartum depression. A recent review article summarised the psychological and psychosocial treatments for perinatal depression. [15] Psychotherapy as well as psychosocial interventions for postpartum depression is supported in research with good results. Psychosocial interventions (peer support, nondirective counselling) as well as psychological interventions (cognitive behavioural therapy and interpersonal therapy) are all effective in decreasing depressive symptoms [16]. Partner support has been identified by women who have recovered from postpartum depression as an important factor in their recovery and they should be included in treatment planning. All psychological interventions seem to have moderate effect sizes and there does not appear to be a difference between the different forms of interventions [17].

Anxiety disorders and their treatment during pregnancy have not been as extensively studied as depressive disorders and the empirical data on the efficacy of therapy for anxiety disorders in pregnancy are lacking. However, clinical experience and studies in the general population tend to confirm the effectiveness of psychotherapy in this population, using mainly cognitive behavioural therapy but also complementary approaches such a clinical mixture of bodily approaches, individual and systemic work, targeted nursing accompaniment and liaison work with obstetrical teams.

Mother and infant have the potential to improve the mother's interactions with her baby and increase the positive feedback from these exchanges. This can increase the pleasurable moments with the baby, improve the mother's self-esteem and indirectly her mood.

Preventive interventions, including family, mother, couple, parent and youth-group-based interventions, have been shown to decrease by 40% the risk of transmission of a mental disorder in children aged 3–18 years [18].

Medical intervention A description of the various psychopharmacotherapies for the perinatal psychiatric condition is beyond the scope of this chapter. However, several general comments can be made. First, the risks of psychopharmacologic treatments during pregnancy should always be weighed against the risk of not treating the maternal condition with reference to maternal well-being, pregnancy outcomes, parent–child relationship, infant neurodevelopmental impacts and marital outcomes. Hence drug therapies for perinatal conditions can be thought of not only as remedial but also as preventive. Second, the vast literature on psychopharmacological treatments during pregnancy does not always take into full consideration the impact of an untreated or partially treated maternal condition on infant outcomes. Third, the perception of psychopharmacological treatment is greatly influenced by the developmental issues during pregnancy: autonomy, transmission, filiation, heritages and identifications. Hence any discussion of psychopharmacological treatment with patients should necessarily go beyond the evidence base to include the subjective perception of receiving a psychotropic medication at a most vulnerable developmental period. Fourth, treatment recommendations will be determined after a careful analysis of the clinical trajectory of the mother-to-be and of the risks and benefits of receiving and not receiving the medication according to the stage of pregnancy. Since the psychopharmacological literature is particularly dynamic and evolving, the reader is referred to recent reviews on the subject [19, 20].

Antidepressants during pregnancy have been extensively studied and have generally been shown not to increase the 3% baseline risk of major malformations. There has, however, been some concern about a possible increased risk of septal defects with some molecules, thus requiring a careful assessment in each case. Various perinatal outcomes have also been studied and shown to demonstrate a slightly increased risk of persistent pulmonary hypertension of the neonate [21] and more commonly a syndrome of neonatal adaptation among exposed infants, which is not severe and is self-limited in a majority of cases [22]. Neurobehavioral outcome measures have been reassuring in the majority of studies.

Bipolar disorder, schizophrenia and postpartum psychosis

Description

Bipolar disorder   Bipolar disorder has a prevalence in the general population of 1–2%. Because this disorder is usually diagnosed in women in their late teens to early 20s, during prime reproductive years, it can have a significant impact on mothers and children, both antenatally and postnatally. In a population-based cohort study of almost 30 000 women, the period between days 10 to 19 postpartum was when women were at their peak risk of a psychiatric readmission and a diagnosis of bipolar disorder was the strongest risk factor for readmission. In a review article, the risk of a postpartum episode was even higher at 30–50% [23]. The postpartum period is a particularly vulnerable time for bipolar women, even among those who did not present mood changes during their pregnancy. Women may present with bipolar depression or with hypomanic or even full blown psychotic episodes. Symptoms in the postpartum period often develop rapidly. This information highlights that childbirth and the first year postpartum are significant risk factors for the recurrence of a bipolar episode. Women who opt to discontinue medication are at a higher risk than those who continue their medication during pregnancy and postpartum. This highlights the importance of identifying women with bipolar disorder, providing them with prenatal monitor and counselling – even during adolescence – and instituting close follow-up. Although the effects of a manic or mixed episode on the developing foetus is not as rigorously studied as depression, these undoubtedly are stressful events which may involve at-risk behaviour; substance use, unprotected sexual contacts, unhealthy diet and lack of obstetrical follow-up. A postpartum event may impact the parent–child relationship if there is a rupture in contact with the mother and a disorganised environment that results from a manic episode poses a difficulty for an infant to adapt to its new home and challenges the child's sense of security.

Schizophrenia   Although about 30% of mothers with schizophrenia report some improvement of their condition, close to 60% of mothers report deterioration. Cessation of medication during pregnancy has been associated with a relapse risk of 65% [24]. The risk of noncompliance to medical treatment is often elevated and may require the use of depot antipsychotic medication.

Independently of exposure to antipsychotics, schizophrenia has been recognised as a risk factor for congenital malformations in some studies. Especially when untreated, this illness may lead to inadequate prenatal care, the use of alcohol, tobacco and substance, spontaneous abortions, low birth weight and still birth [24].

Mothers with schizophrenia experience distinct challenges when confronted with parenting and some will lose custody of their children due to their illness. The positive symptoms of schizophrenia, such as command hallucinations and delusions, are more readily apparent and therefore quickly identified, but the negative symptoms may also be detrimental to the child's development and can diminish the capacity of the mother to stimulate and communicate with her infant sufficiently [25].

Postnatally, delusions or command hallucinations always constitute very serious symptoms that interfere greatly with infant care and may lead to severe neglect, infanticide or maternal suicide. The prevention of perinatal decompensation among affected mothers is thus critical and may necessitate calling forth the extended family network.

Postpartum psychosis   Postpartum Psychosis (PPP) is seen after 0.1–0.2% of all deliveries and has its onset during the first few days after birth. Women characteristically present with disorganization, agitation, delusional thoughts, hallucinations, irritability; in many cases, their severe confusion may mimic delirium. PPP is often the first manifestation of a bipolar disorder. Bipolar disorder being a recurrent condition, recurrence risk of PPP is 57% if the patient presented a prior episode of PPP and probably worse if the patient presented a prior episode of PPP and has a family history of the disease [26].

PPP is a psychiatric emergency. It is associated with a significant risk of maternal suicide and infanticide, especially when the infant is part of the mother's delusional thinking, which is often the case. The illness requires urgent hospitalization and antipsychotic medication. In contrast to ancient practices, the contact with the infant should be maintained under close supervision. Depending on the underlying psychiatric condition, the prognosis is often good, with full recuperation of maternal functioning.

For women who have suffered from a previous PPP, a new pregnancy is often experienced as potentially reparative but is often associated with increased anxiety and fragmented traumatic memories about the previous episode. Preventive interventions with this population not only involve medical prophylaxis but must also provide extra support to help the family cope with the difficult memories related to a prior psychotic episode.

Prevention and Treatment planning of patients with bipolar disease and schizophrenia   The high relapse rate of bipolar illness justifies in most cases a prophylactic psychopharmacological intervention, especially postnatally. Indeed, preventing PPP, which is often associated with a diagnosis of bipolar disorder, necessitates in the vast majority of cases reintroducing or continuing a mood stabiliser.

Mothers with schizophrenia should be accompanied carefully throughout the perinatal period for relapse prevention and for securing the parent–infant relationship – even when hospitalised. For many mothers with this condition, the coordination of work with teams that are specifically targeting the mother–infant relationship will be critical for preventing neglect and abuse among children.

Nonmedical intervention   There are currently no published studies on the efficacy of psychotherapy in treatment of bipolar disorder and its effectiveness at preventing a perinatal episode of depression or mania. However, psychoeducation, stress management, sleep preservation and facilitation of interpersonal support are clinical cornerstones of preventing decompensation.

For women with schizophrenia, short-term psychotherapy can be considered when the mother-to-be has specific worries about pregnancy or parenting, has a history of abuse, prior death of a child or loss of custody of a child, difficulties with asserting themselves and having their needs understood by their partners or those who have delusions that are amplified by stress [27].

Medical intervention   Mood stabilisers during pregnancy fall into three main categories: lithium, anticonvulsants and antipsychotics. Lithium is the most extensively utilised mood stabiliser during pregnancy and is used to treat relapse and to have significant preventive effect for PPP. Most anticonvulsants used during pregnancy are associated with an increased risk of neural tube defects, nonspecific anomalies or various cognitive changes, although studies do not always specify the role played by the medication [28].

Antipsychotics come in two main categories: conventional and novel. The conventional antipsychotics are unsurprisingly the most studied and are thought in the majority of cases to be compatible with pregnancy, including the injectable forms. The data regarding the novel antipsychotics are slowly accumulating and do not demonstrate thus far major risks or typical patterns of malformations. However, care must be exercised since the data are still fragmentary. In addition, neonatal adaptation syndromes have been described with the new antipsychotics [29].

Finally, a word should be said regarding electroconvulsive therapies. Electroconvulsive therapy has been shown to be safe during pregnancy and can have life-saving potential in the rare case of severe refractory depression, mania or psychosis [30].

Substance use during pregnancy

Substance use during pregnancy can have devastating effects on the child, mother and family system. In addition, social difficulties and risky behaviour associated with substance abuse can have detrimental effects on the foetus and infant. However, substance using mothers are often motivated to work on addiction during pregnancy. Screening women of childbearing age, educating and treating those who have substance use problems is the ultimate preventative measure. Preventive programs offer youth protection support even antenatally, frequently facilitating a therapeutic alliance and the integrated delivery of services. There are a multitude of negative effects on foetal outcomes when expectant mothers abuse substances including low birth weight, miscarriage, preterm labour and placental abruption. A recent review article highlighted that maternal alcohol use, smoking and cannabis use is related to neurobehavioural and cognitive outcomes such as ADHD, increased externalizing behaviour and decreased general cognitive functioning [31]. It has even been shown that marijuana use during pregnancy affects reading comprehension and is associated with underachievement at the age of 10 [32]. However – and this is also the case for other conditions – when considering transmission of disease it is often difficult to disentangle what was caused by other aspects of the maternal condition, by genetic factors and other environmental factors. The underlying message from these studies is that the environment is an important risk factor for infants and therefore must be addressed by substance use programs in order to change the child's outcome.

Heroin, cocaine, stimulants are all other common substances abused during pregnancy. A discussion of these substances is beyond the scope of this chapter [33]. Fetal Alcohol Spectrum Disorders encompass dysmorphic features, neurological and behavioural sequelae and learning difficulties. It is important to identify and quantify substances that have been used by expectant mothers in order to plan for complications during pregnancy and delivery. Newborns may need to have specialised treatment for withdrawal symptoms soon after birth.

Perinatal programs

Various preventive programs have been designed starting during pregnancy. The efforts range from health promotion programs for the general population, such as in Japan [34], to programs specifically targeting at-risk populations [35]. An example of a hallmark preventive perinatal program is the Nurse-Family partnership pioneered by David Olds [36] which essentially supports high-risk parents during their pregnancy through the early childhood of their infant. The program is built on complementary theoretical models, notably human ecology, self-efficacy and attachment theory. The goals of the program are to facilitate the optimal development of children, particularly preventing abuse and neglect. The targeted population is 'high risk' which includes first-time single mothers who are often very young and poor. The program provides 9 prenatal visits and 23 postnatal visits until the age of 2. The results show a decrease of abuse and neglect during childhood, fewer accidents and ingestions of poisons, improved maternal behaviour, longer interpregnancy intervals, more return to work and less dependency on state support. The 15 year follow-up of the population shows significant long-term effects: less alcohol and drug abuse, less problems with the law and of early sexual activity.

This program has influenced numerous programs in the world, such as the SIPPE program (integrated perinatal and early childhood programs), universally applied in Quebec as part of socialised medicine. In France, the Montpellier model has had a large influence by closely involving obstetrical teams and carefully linking their work with postnatal services [14].

Conclusion

The challenge of preventive intervention during the perinatal period involves not only the screening and identification of at-risk populations, the careful assessment of targeted patients, the delivery of treatments addressing the needs of parents and infants but most importantly the difficult work of coordinating interventions and training across various domains of services. Too often, the various levels of services for pregnant women and their family tend to be fragmented as antenatal, postnatal, community, frontline, child psychiatric and paediatric services which strive to establish lines of communication and to integrate their specific roles. Although much work remains to be done, various initiatives are attempting to better integrate services with the ultimate goal of providing complementary, seamless preventive interventions at a most sensitive developmental period for infants and families.

References

1. Nigg J. (2012). Environment, developmental origins, and attention-deficit/hyperactivity disorder. *Archives of Pediatrics and Adolescent Medicine,* doi:10.1001/archpediatrics.2011.905
2. Tremblay RE, Hartup WW and Archer J (eds) (2005). Developmental origins of aggression. *Guilford.*
3. Fonagy P, Steele H and Steele M. (1991). Maternal representations of attachment during pregnancy predict the organization of infant-mother attachment at one year of age. *Child Development* **62**: 891–905.
4. Fivaz-Depeursinge E and Corboz-Warnery A. (1999). The primary triangle: A developmental systems view of mothers, fathers and infants. *Basic books.*
5. Zeanah CH, Benoit D, Hirschberg L, et al. (1994). Representations of attachment in mothers and their one year-old infants are concordant with infant classifications. *Developmental issues in psychiatry and psychology* **1**: 9–18.
6. Talge NM, Neal C and Glover V. (2007). Antenatal maternal stress and long-term effects on child neurodevelopment: how and why?. *Journal of Child Psychology and Psychiatry and Allied Disciplines* **48**(3–4): 245–261.
7. Bergman K, Sarkar P, Glover V and O'Connor TG. (2010). Maternal prenatal cortisol and infant cognitive development: moderation by infant-mother attachment. *Biological Psychiatry* **67**(11): 1026–1032.
8. Dunkel Schetter C and Tanner L. (2012). Anxiety, depression and stress in pregnancy: implications for mothers, children, research and practice. *Current Opinion in Psychiatry* **25**(2): 141–148.
9. Cox JL, Holden JM and Sagovsky R. (1987). *Detection of postnatal depression. Development of the 10-item Edinburgh Postnatal Depression Scale. The British Journal of Psychiatry.* **150**: 782–786.
10. Apter-Danon G and Candilis-Huisman D. (2005). A challenge for perinatal psychiatry: therapeutic management of maternal borderline personality disorder and their very young infants. *Clinical Neuropsychiatry* **2**(5): 302–314.
11. Paulson JF and Bazemore SD. (2010). Prenatal and postpartum depression in fathers and its association with maternal depression: A meta-analysis. *JAMA: The Journal of the American Medical Association* **303**(19): 1961–1969.
12. Yonkers KA, Wisner KL, Stewart DE, et al. (2009). The management of depression during pregnancy: a report from the American Psychiatric Association and the American College of Obstetricians and Gynecologists. *General Hospital Psychiatry* **31**, 403–413.
13. Diagnostic Classification of Mental Health and Developmental Disorders of Infancy and Early Childhood: Revised Edition (DC:0-3R) (2005). Zero to three.
14. Molénat F. (2009). *Prévention Précoce: Petit Traité Pour Construire Des Liens Humains.* Paris: Érès.
15. Fitelson E, Kim S, Baker AS and Leight K. (2011). Treatment of postpartum depression: clinical, psychological and pharmacological options. *International Journal of Women's Health* **3**, 1–14.
16. Dennis CL and Hodnett ED. (2007). Psychosocial and psychological interventions for treating postpartum depression. *Cochrane Database of Systematic Reviews*, Issue 4. Art. No.: CD006116. doi:10.1002/14651858.CD006116.pub2
17. Cuijpers P, Brännmark J and van Straten A. (2008). Psychological treatment of postpartum depression: a meta-analysis. *Journal of Clinical Psychology* **64**(1): 103–118.
18. Siegenthaler E, Munder T and Egger M. (2012). Effect of preventive interventions in mentally ill parents on the mental health of the offspring: systematic review and meta-analysis. *Journal of the American Academy of Child and Adolescent Psychiatry* **51**(1): 8–17. e8.

19. St-André M and Martin BZ. (2010). Psychopharmacological treatments during pregnancy: risks and benefits for the mother and her infant. In: S. Tyano, M. Keren, H. Herrman and J. Cox (eds), *Parenting and Mental Health: a Bridge Between Adult and Infant Psychiatry*, pp. 129–146. London: Wiley-Blackwell.

20. Massachusetts General Hospital Center for Women's Mental Health. Women's Mental Health.org [Internet]. http://www.womensmental health.org/ (accessed 6 May 2014).

21. http://www.fda.gov/Safety/MedWatch/SafetyInformation/SafetyAlertsforHumanMedical Products/ucm283696.htm (accessed 13 February 2012).

22. Ferreira E, Martin B, Carceller AM, et al. (2007). Effects of SSRIs and Venlafaxine during pregnancy in term and preterm neonates. *Pediatrics* **119**: 52–59.

23. Chaudron LH and Pies RW. (2003). The relationship between postpartum psychosis and bipolar disorder: a review. *Journal of Clinical Psychiatry* **64**(11): 1284–1292.

24. Trixler M, Gati A, Fekete S, et al. (2005). Use of antipsychotics in the management of schizophrenia during pregnancy. *Drugs* **65**, 1193–11206.

25. Solari H, Dickson KE and Miller L. (2009). Understanding and treating women with schizophrenia during pregnancy and postpartum. *Canadian Journal of Clinical Pharmacology*, **16**(1): e23–e32.

26. Robertson E, Jones I, Haque S, et al. (2005). Risk of Puerperal and non-puerperal recurrence of illness following bipolar affective puerperal psychosis. *British Journal of Psychiatry* **186**: 258–259.

27. Doucet S, Jones I, Létourneau N, et al. (2011). Interventions for the prevention and treatment of post-partum psychosis: a systematic review. *Archives of Women's Mental Health* **14**: 89–98.

28. Palac S and Meador KJ. (2011). Antiepileptic drugs and neurodevelopment: An update. *Current Neurology and Neuroscience Reports* **11**: 423–427.

29. Gentile S. (2010). Antipsychotic therapy during early and late pregnancy. A systematic review. *Schizophrenia Bulletin* **36**(3): 518–544.

30. Forray A and Ostroff B. (2007). The use of electroconvulsive therapy in postpartum affective disorders. *The Journal of ECT* **23**(3): 188–193.

31. Huizin AC and Mulder E. (2006). Maternal smoking, drinking or cannabis use during pregnancy and neurobehavioural and cognitive functioning in human offspring. *Neuroscience & Biobehavioral Reviews* **30**(1): 24–42.

32. Goldschmidt L, Richardson GA, Cornelius MD and Day NL. (2004). Prenatal marijuana and alcohol exposure and academic achievement at age 10. *Neurotoxicology and Teratology* **26**: 521–532.

33. Boris NW. (2009). Parental substance use. In: CHZ Zeanah (ed.), *Handbook of Infant Mental Health*, 3rd edition, pp. 171–179. Guilford Press.

34. Kamibeppu K, Furuta M, Yamashita H, et al. (2009). Training health professionals to detect and support mothers at risk of postpartum depression or infant abuse in the community: a cross-sectional and a before and after study. *Bioscience Trends* **3**(1): 17–24.

35. Gauthier Y. (2009). *L'avenir de La Psychiatrie de L'enfant*. Paris: Érès.

36. Olds DL, Sadler L and Kitzman H. (2007). Programs for parents of infants and toddlers: recent evidence from randomized trials. *Journal of Child Psychology and Psychiatry and Allied Disciplines* **48**: 355–391.

6
Psychiatry and Intervention in Infancy and Early Childhood

Jane Barlow

Mental Health & Wellbeing, Warwick Medical School, University of Warwick, UK

Introduction

During the past two decades there has been an increase in evidence across a range of disciplines (e.g. genetics, neuroscience, developmental psychology, infant mental health, psychotherapy) to suggest that the early parent–child relationship has a significant role in the origins of childhood psychiatric disorder. This chapter will present research which suggests that the pathway linking the two is the child's attachment organisation, and the impact of this on the child's capacity for emotion regulation and on their rapidly developing nervous system. The chapter will focus specifically on the evidence in relation to disorganised and traumatic attachment relationships, which are now recognised to be significant precursors of a range of clinical phenomena including borderline personality disorder. Psychiatric disorder in adults is strongly associated with childhood psychiatric disorder, and this evidence therefore has significant implications in terms of the development of mental health problems across the lifespan.

The first part of the chapter examines the relationship between a range of child psychiatric problems and the emerging evidence in terms of the aetiological processes involved. The specific focus is on recent theories and evidence about the origins of such problems in terms of early maladaptive intersubjective experiences between the parent and infant. The second part of the chapter examines a number of innovative interventions that involve working 'dyadically' to address a range of childhood disorders whose origins, it will be argued, lay in such early relationship experiences. We focus in particular on evidence-based approaches that target both the parent and the child with a view to

Early Intervention in Psychiatry: EI of nearly everything for better mental health, First Edition.
Edited by Peter Byrne and Alan Rosen.
© 2014 John Wiley & Sons, Ltd. Published 2014 by John Wiley & Sons, Ltd.

changing parent–child interaction, and/or parental and child representational systems, in order to target child attachment security. It will be argued that the evidence strongly points to the need for a range of secondary/tertiary level services for children presenting with problems that have their origins in the early parent–child relationship.

The aetiology of child psychiatric disorder

Young children experience a range of problems during childhood and these begin early with functional (eating and sleeping) and behavioural disorders being the primary reason for referral of children under the age of 3 years to child mental health clinics [1]. Recent studies have found a prevalence rate of around 10% for behavioural disorders in preschool children [2] with some estimates being as high as 30% [3, 4]. Many of these problems show evidence of comorbidity, and one study found that 45% of referred children between the ages of 18–47 months had signs of both internalising and externalising problems [5]. The research also suggests considerable continuity between early problems and later psychiatric disorder. Emotional and behavioural problems in children aged 3 and 4 years are highly stable, approximately 50% of children still having problems in adolescence [6], and are also strongly associated with later psychopathology [7] including antisocial behaviour and conduct disorder [8].

Genetic and environmental risk factors have long been implicated in the development of childhood psychiatric disorder, but recent evidence has also suggested a role for epigenetic mechanisms, in relation, for example to conditions such as autism [9] and ADHD [10]. Knowledge about the genetic and the epigenetic contribution to disorder is important in terms of our understanding about resilience (i.e. why it is that some children exposed to high risk environments do not go on to develop problems later) and the environmental factors that can be targeted to prevent problems occurring in the case of epigenetic processes. The concerns of this paper, however, are with identifying recent research about the direct influence of early environmental factors and in particular the parent–infant/toddler relationship, which can be targeted as part of secondary and tertiary service/provision.

Although abusive parenting has long been recognized to be strongly associated with a wide range of mental-health problems in children (including anxiety, depression, post-traumatic stress, dissociation, oppositional behaviour, suicidal and self-injurious behaviour, substance misuse, anger and aggression, and sexual symptoms and age-inappropriate sexual behaviour) [11], over the past decade, increasing attention has been given to the influence of wider parenting practices on child development. Developmental research during the 1980s showed a strong association between parenting practices characterised by harsh and inconsistent discipline, little positive parental involvement with the child, poor monitoring and supervision, and behaviour and conduct problems in early childhood [12]. More recently, research in the fields of developmental psychology, infant mental health and neuropsychology has begun to highlight the importance of early parent–child interaction in terms of its impact on a child's capacity for emotion regulation, and it has been postulated that the key task of very early childhood and in particular, infancy, is the regulation of emotional states [13]. Research on attachment has developed significantly since Bowlby (1982) [14] first identified its role in promoting a sense of safety and security in the child. Perhaps most importantly attachment is now recognized to be a significant bio-behavioural feedback mechanism with a key role in the dyadic regulation of emotion. Research in the field of infant mental health suggests that this dyadic regulation takes place in repeated moments of 'affect synchrony' in which the parent and baby are emotionally attuned, and is facilitated by parents who are able to repair ruptures that occur following dyadic misattunement [15]. Neuroscientific research shows that these moments of synchrony impact on the limbic and cortical areas of the developing right cerebral brain [16]. Perhaps most importantly, by the end of the first year of life these early interactions have significantly shaped the right cortical–subcortical circuits via implicit-procedural memory [16], the main consequence being the development of unconscious strategies of affect regulation that have considerable stability over time [17].

Optimal parent–infant interaction thus enables the child 'to develop an internal system that can adaptively regulate arousal and an array of psychobiological states (and thereby affect, cognition and behavior)' [18]. Schore (2010) [16] writes the following regarding suboptimal parenting:

'In contexts of relational trauma this caregiver is emotionally inaccessible, given to inappropriate and/or rejecting responses to her infant's expressions of emotions and stress and provides minimal or unpredictable regulation of the infant's states of over-arousal. Instead she induces extreme levels of stimulation and arousal (i.e. the very high stimulation of abuse and/or the very low stimulation of neglect). And finally, because she provides no interactive repair, she leaves the infant to endure extremely stressful intense negative states for long periods of time' [16].

The discovery of a 'disorganised' category of attachment [18] gave rise to a body of research which showed that it was a significant risk factor for later psychopathology across childhood [19]. Disorganised attachment refers to behaviours that appear to be contradictory in terms of the child's approach to the attachment figure and examples include where the child approaches but with the head averted or with fearful expressions, oblique approaches or disoriented behaviours such as dazed or trance-like expressions or freezing of all movement [18].

Disorganized attachment is found in around 80% of children who experience abusive parenting [20]. However, it is also found in 15% of population samples [21] and as such occurs outside the context of abuse [22]. Although there appears to be a genetic basis (i.e. a polymorphism of the DRD4 gene) for disorganized attachment [23], disorganisation has also been found to be associated with parenting behaviours that have been characterized as frightened and frightening (Fr-behaviour) [24] or hostile and helpless [22], and recent research suggests that it is the maternal behavior that 'amplifies or offsets the risk conferred by the genotype' [25]. Such parenting behaviours include affective communication errors (e.g. mother positive while infant distressed); disorientation (frightened expression or sudden complete loss of affect); and negative-intrusive behaviours (mocking or pulling infants wrist) [23]. A recent meta-analysis of 12 studies confirmed the strength of the association between such atypical or 'anomalous' parenting at 12/18 months and disorganised attachment [26].

There is a high stability between disorganisation in infancy and wide-ranging problems in later childhood including compulsive coercive/caregiving behaviours [21], social and cognitive difficulties, and psychopathology [27]. A recent study of older children (aged 8–12 years) also found that a disorganised attachment was associated with symptoms that met clinical criteria [28].

Research examining developmental pathways suggests that disorganised attachment maybe a significant factor (often alongside metacognitive deficits such as mentalisation) linking early traumatic interpersonal experiences with dissociative problems [29, 30], personality disorder [31, 32] and schizophrenia [33].

Methods of working with childhood psychiatric disorder

The above research suggests the importance of understanding the early parenting experiences of children presenting with psychopathology, and points to the need for a comprehensive assessment of the extent to which a child's capacity for affect regulation and the defensive relational structures associated with insecure or disorganised attachment, are impinging on their broader functioning. This body of research also suggests that for interventions to be optimally effective, they need to address these issues, alongside the needs and parenting abilities of the primary caregiver.

The next section examines a number of innovative approaches to treatment that are aimed directly or indirectly at improving the infant's attachment security. We examine briefly what each approach comprises alongside the evidence base to support their use.

Dyadic treatment approaches

Parent–child psychotherapy Parent–infant/child psychotherapy involves parent–infant/child psychotherapists working with both mother and baby/child using psychotherapeutic principles by focusing on the relationship between the parent and infant/child, parental representations and parenting practices (see Box 6.1 for further details).

Box 6.1   *Parent–child psychotherapy*

The approach is supportive, nondirective and nondidactic, and includes developmental guidance based on the mother's concerns. During the session, the mother and therapist jointly observe the infant, and the therapist aims to 'allow distorted emotional reactions and perceptions of the infant as they are enacted during mother–infant interaction to be associated with memories and affects from the mother's prior childhood experiences. Through respect, empathic concern and unfailing positive regard, the therapeutic relationship provides the mother with a corrective emotional experience, through which the mother is able to differentiate current from past relationships, form positive internal representations of herself and of herself in relationship to others, particularly her infant. As a result of this process, mothers are able to expand their responsiveness, sensitivity and attunement to the infant, fostering security in the mother–child relationship and promoting emerging autonomy in the child' [33].

Although parent–infant/child psychotherapy has its origins in 'representational' approaches, which focus primarily on understanding and changing the mothers mental representations about the infant/child and their relationship to the parents own experiences of being parents, more recent approaches have introduced the use of concomitant 'behavioural' strategies. Watch, Wait and Wonder (WWW) is 'a child led psychotherapeutic approach that specifically and directly uses the infant's spontaneous activity in a free play format to enhance maternal sensitivity and responsiveness, the child's sense of self and self-efficacy, emotion regulation, and the child-parent attachment relationship. The approach provides space for the infant/child and parent to work through developmental and relational struggles through play. Also central to the process is engaging the parent to be reflective about the child's inner world of feelings, thoughts and desires, through which the parent recognizes the separate self of the infant and gains an understanding of her own emotional responses to her child' [34].

Box 6.2 Watch, wait and wonder

The WWW approach involves a therapy room with standard toys (e.g. doll, tea set, wild and domestic animal farm set, doctor's kit, soft toys). Each session begins with the parent being asked to 'get down on the floor' and observe and follow their child's lead in activities. During the first half of the therapy session, the therapist sits in the room but does not interact with the dyad. The second half of the session involves a discussion between the parent and therapist about the activities initiated by the child and the parental understanding of their child's behaviour and play [34].

A rigorous (RCT) evaluation compared infant-led psychotherapy (WWW) with a standard representational mother–infant psychotherapy (PPT) with 67 clinically referred mothers and infants aged 10–30 months [35]. The study found that both WWW and PPT were successful in reducing infant presenting problems, decreasing parenting stress, and reducing maternal intrusiveness and mother–infant conflict, but that the WWW group showed a greater shift toward a more organised or secure attachment relationship, and a greater improvement in cognitive development and emotion regulation than infants in the PPT group. Mothers in the WWW group reported a larger increase in parenting satisfaction and competence, and decrease in depression compared to mothers receiving PPT. However, these differences had disappeared by the 6-month follow-up, by which time the PPT group had achieved the same outcomes as the WWW group [36].

There is increasing evidence from rigorous studies highlighting the benefits of parent–child psychotherapy particularly in terms of children exposed to severely compromised or traumatising environments [37, 38] and with parents who are emotionally abusive [39] or who have major depressive disorder [40]. Preliminary clinical studies have also examined the value of this approach with parents with borderline personality disorder [41].

Video-interaction guidance

Video-interaction guidance (VIG) is a behavioural approach that focuses on the relationship between the parent and infant, and involves the use of videotaped interactions being used by the therapist to help the mother to recognise her own positive responses and interactions with her infant, and to elaborate appropriate responsiveness. Mutual enjoyment and pleasurable interactions are identified and encouraged with a view to building maternal confidence [42].

Box 6.3   Video-interaction guidance

One of the leading proponents and trainers of VIG in the United Kingdom writes regarding this approach that:

'... the guider is using micromoments of the film to activate the parent to explore their and their infant's thoughts, feelings and intentions in a supportive atmosphere. The guider pays attention to the rhythm of the interaction leaving "spaces" for the parent to think. This enables them to develop new thoughts, feelings and intentions that can trigger new narratives about themselves as parents and their view of their own parenting. VIG believes that long lasting change takes place when parents develop their own new narratives and are motivated to change their behaviours in line with their new belief in themselves' [43].

A meta-analysis evaluating the impact of video-interaction guidance with wide-ranging problems (i.e. hyperactivity, faltering growth, disabilities, parents with eating disorders, etc) identified 29 studies of which 21 involved a controlled comparison, and 9 were randomised controlled trials [44]. The children in the families had an average age of 2.3 years, ranging from 0 to 8 years old. This review found significant positive effects on both the parenting behaviour and attitude of parents and the development of the child. It should be noted, however, that this review did not present the findings separately for RCTs.

Video Feedback Intervention to promote Positive Parenting (VIPP) [45] is another variation of this intervention (see Box 6.4).

Box 6.4   Video feedback intervention to promote positive parenting (VIPP)

'VIPP is delivered in the home over four sessions. Each session starts with making the videotape that will be used in the next session. Activities are standardised and involve playing together, the mother bathing the infant and cuddling. In each intervention session video-feedback is implemented around a specific given theme. VIPP highlights "chains" of interaction with at least three turns: signal from the baby, mother's sensitive response and baby's positive reaction to this response' [46].

One study found positive short-term effects of VIPP on maternal sensitivity and insecure–disorganized infant attachment in adoptive families [47] although this was not a randomised controlled trial. There is, however, some uncertainty with regard to the mechanism by which this intervention works. For example although a recent study found an impact on preschool externalising but not internalising problems this did not appear to be mediated by maternal sensitivity or infant attachment [48].

Attachment-based parent-training programmes Parent–child interaction therapy (PCIT) is a short-term, parent-training programme, based on both attachment and social learning theory. It is directed at families with 2- to 6-year-old children experiencing behavioural, emotional or family problems – see Box 6.5 [49].

Box 6.5 Parent–child interaction therapy

'PARENT-CHILD INTERACTION THERAPY (PCIT) is a manualized parent training program has two discrete phases, Child-Directed Interaction (CDI) and Parent-Directed Interaction (PDI). CDI concentrates on strengthening parent-child attachment as a foundation for PDI, which emphasizes a structured and consistent approach to discipline. Throughout treatment, emphasis is placed on the interaction between the parents and their child due to the specific theoretical assumptions about the development and maintenance of externalizing behavior 1 in children. The protocol is assessment driven and is not time limited; progress in the parent–child interactions is coded at each session, and treatment is completed when parents have mastered the skills of CDI and PDI and the child's behavior is within normal limits' [49].

There is rigorous research evidence about its effectiveness with depressed [50] and abusive [51–53] parents, alongside victims of interparental violence [54], and children with behavioural problems [55, 56].

The Circle of Security is a 20-week group-based parent education and psychotherapy programme based on attachment theory and 'designed to help caregivers re-evaluate their internal representations of the child and the self to match the emotional needs of their children' [57]. It involves the delivery of an individualized treatment plan which consists of (a) identification of caregiver–child interaction patterns, including child attachment classification; (b) identification of caregiver developmental history and internal working models of self and child; and (c) identification of a key ("linchpin") issue that forms the focus of the therapeutic work [46].

Box 6.6 Circle of security

Five key goals of the protocol are to (a) establish the therapist and the group as a secure base from which the caregiver can explore his or her relationship with the child; (b) increase caregiver sensitivity and appropriate responsiveness by providing caregivers a map of children's basic attachment needs; (c) increase caregivers' capacity to recognize and understand both the obvious and more subtle verbal and nonverbal cues that children use to signal their internal states and needs when using the caregiver as a secure base for exploration and as a haven of safety; (d) increase caregiver empathy by supporting reflection about both the caregiver's and the child's behaviours, thoughts, and feelings regarding attachment-oriented interactions and (e) increase caregiver reflection about how his or her own developmental history affects current caregiving behaviour (Hoffman et al. 2006, p. 1018) [56].

Although there is, as yet, no RCT evidence available, early evaluation of the programme suggests its effectiveness in improving children's attachment classifications [57].

Conclusions

The past two decades had witnessed the development of an extensive body of research from a range of disciplines, which has greatly enhanced our understanding about the importance of early parent–child interactions in the aetiology of childhood psychiatric disorder. This research has built on what was already known about the relationship between abuse and later psychiatric disturbance, highlighting the importance of the first 3 years of life, in terms of the association between a wide range of 'atypical' or 'anomalous' parenting practices and the child's later capacity for affect regulation.

Improved knowledge about the importance of early relationship experiences in the aetiology of childhood psychiatric disorders has given rise to a number of new approaches to treatment that are underpinned by a recognition of the importance of working 'dyadically' during the first 5 years of a child's life, and are aimed at changing parental behaviours and/or parental representations, in order to promote a secure attachment relationship. It has also given rise to a number of innovative ways of working with children based on recognition of the role that their experiences of early parenting have had in terms of their later development. Such approaches target the child's attachment organisation, with a view to enhancing their capacity for affect regulation, and reducing the defensive structures associated with insecure and disorganised attachment patterns.

The new 'dyadic' approaches that are emerging in response to increased awareness both about disorganised attachment and trauma-based pathology, involve innovations to existing and widely used evidence-based approaches. Perhaps most importantly, they include both parent and child in the treatment programme. Practitioners across a range of disciplines will need to develop new skills to enable them to deliver these methods of treatment.

References

1. Keren M, Feldman R and Tyano S. (2001). Diagnoses and interactive patterns of infants referred to a community based infant mental health clinic. *Journal of the American Academy of child and Adolescent Psychiatry* **40**(1): 27–35.
2. Furniss T, Beyer T and Guggenmos J. (2006). Prevalence of behavioural and emotional problems among six year old preschool children: baseline results of a prospective longitudinal study. *Social Psychiatry and Psychiatric Epidemiology* **41**(5): 394–399.
3. Lavigne JV, Binns HJ, Christoffel KK, et al. (1993). Behavioral and emotional problems among preschool children in paediatric primary care: prevalence and paediatricians' recognition. *Pediatrics* **91**(3): 649–655.
4. Charlton T, Abraham M and Jones K. (1995). Prevalence rates of emotional and behavioural disorder among nursery class children in St Helen, South Atlantic: an epidemiological study. *Journal of Social Behavior and Personality* **10**: 273–280.
5. Thomas JM and Guskin KA. (2001). Disruptive behavior in young children: What does it mean? *Journal of the American Academy of Child and Adolescent Psychiatry* **40**: 44–51.
6. Campbell SB. (1995). Behaviour problems in preschool children: a review of recent research. *Journal of Child Psychology and Psychiatry* **36**(1): 113–149.

7. Caspi A, Moffitt TE, Newman DL and Silva PA. (1996). Behavioural observations at age 3 years predict adult psychiatric disorders. *Archives of General Psychiatry* **53**: 1033–1039.

8. Robins LN. (1991). Conduct disorder. *Journal of Child Psychology and Psychiatry* **32**(1): 193–162.

9. Nguyen A, Rauch TA, Pfeifer GP and Hu VW. (2010). Global methylation profiling of lymphoblastoid cell lines reveals epigenetic contributions to autism spectrum disorders and a novel autism candidate gene, RORA, whose protein product is reduced in autistic brain. *Federation of American Societies for Experimental Biology Journal* **24**: 3036–3051.

10. Elia J, Laracy S, Allen J, et al. (2011). Epigenetics: genetics versus life experiences. *Current Topics in Behavioral Neuroscience* **9**: 314–340.

11. Gilbert R, Widom CS, Browne K, et al. (2009). Burden and consequences of child maltreatment in high-income countries. *Lancet* **373**: 68–81.

12. Patterson GR, DeBaryshe D and Ramsey E. (1989). A developmental perspective on antisocial behavior. *The American Psychologist* **44**(2): 329–335.

13. Schore AN. (1994). Affect regulation and the origin of the self: the neurobiology of emotional development. In: Lawrence Erlbaum Associates (ed.), *Relational Trauma in Infancy*, pp. 19–47. Hillsdale, NJ: Routledge Press.

14. Bowlby J. (1982). *Attachment*, 2nd edition. Vol. 1: *Attachment and Loss*. New York: Basic Books.

15. Beebe B and Lachmann FM. (2002). *Infant Research and Adult Treatment: Coconstructing Interactions*. Hillsdale, NJ: Analytic Press.

16. Schore A. (2010). Neurobiology of attachment. In: Tessa Baradon (ed.). *Relational Trauma in Infancy*, p. 22. London: Routledge.

17. Waters E, Merrick S, Treboux D, et al. (2000). Attachment security in infancy and early adulthood: A twenty-year longitudinal study. *Child Development* **71**: 684–689.

18. Main M and Solomon J. (1986). Discovery of an insecure disorganized/disoriented attachment pattern: procedures, findings and implications for classification of behaviour. In: MW Yogman and T.B. Brazelton, *Affective Development in Infancy*, pp. 95–124. Norwood, NJ: Ablex.

19. Lyons-Ruth K and Jacobvitz. (2008). Attachment disorganization: Unresolved loss, relational violence and lapses in behavioral and attentional strategies. In: J Cassidy and PR Shaver (eds.), *Handbook of Attachment*, 2nd Edition, pp. 520–554. New York: Guilford.

20. Carlson V, Cicchetti D, Barnett D and Braunwald K. (1989). Disorganized/disoriented attachment relationships in maltreated infants. *Development and Psychopathology* **25**: 525–531.

21. van IJzendoorn MH, Schuengel C and Bakermans-Kranenburg M. (1999). Disorganized attachment in early childhood: Meta-analysis of precursors, concomitants, and sequelae. *Development and Psychopathology* **11**: 225–250.

22. Lyons-Ruth K, Yellin C, Melnick S and Atwood G. (2005). Expanding the concept of unresolved mental states: hostile/helpless states of mind on the Adult Attachment Interview are associated with disrupted mother–infant communication and infant disorganization. *Development and Psychopathology* **17**: 1–23.

23. Lakatos K, Nemoda Z, Toth I, et al. (2002). Further evidence for the role of the dopamine D4 receptor gene (DRD4) in attachment disorganization: interaction of the III exon 48 bp repeat and the 521 C/T promoter polymorphisms. *Molecular Psychiatry* **7**: 27–31.

24. Jacobvitz D, Hazen NL and Riggs S. (1997). Disorganized mental processes in mothers, frightened/frightening behavior in caregivers, and disoriented, disorganized behavior in infancy. Paper presented at the biennial meeting of the Society for Research in Child Development, Washington, DC.

25. Barry RA, Kochanska G and Philibert RA. (2008). G x E interactions in the organization of attachment: Mothers' responsiveness as a moderator of children's genotypes. *Journal of Child Psychology and Psychiatry* **49**: 1313–1320.

26. Madigan M, Bakermans-Kranenburg M, van Ijzendoorn G, et al. (2006). Unresolved states of mind, anomalous parental behaviour and disorganized attachment: A review and meta-analysis of a transmission gap. *Attachment and Human Behavior* **8**: 89–111.

27. Green J and Goldwyn R. (2002). Annotation: attachment disorganisation and psychopathology: new findings in attachment research and their potential implications for developmental psychopathology in childhood. *Journal of Child Psychology and Psychiatry* **43**: 835–846.

28. Borelli JL, David DH, Crowley MJ and Mayes LC. (2010). Links between disorganised attachment classification and clinical symptoms in school-aged children. *Journal of Child and Family studies* **19**(3): 243–256.

29. Dutra L, Bureau JF, Holmes B, et al. (2009). Quality of early care and childhood trauma: A prospective study of developmental pathways to dissociation. *Journal of Nervous and Mental Disease* **197**(6): 383–390.

30. Liotti G (1999). Disorganization of attachment as a model for understanding dissociative psychopathology. In: J Solomon and C George. (eds). *Attachment Disorganization*, pp. 291–317. New York: Guilford Press.

31. Agrawal HR, Gunderson J, Holmes BM and Lyons-Ruth K. (2004). Attachment studies with borderline patients: a review. *Harvard Review of Psychiatry* **12**(2): 94–104.

32. Bateman AW and Fonagy P. (2007). Mentalising and borderline personality disorder. *Journal of Mental Health* **16**(1): 83–101.

33. Liott G and Gumley A. (2008). Annotation: attachment disorganisation and psychopathology: new findings in attachment research and their potential implications for developmental psychopathology in childhood. *Journal of Child Psychology and Psychiatry* **43**: 853–846.

34. www.watchwaitandwonder.com (accessed 12 September 2011).

35. Cohen N, Muir E, Lojkasek M, et al. (1999). Watch, wait and wonder: testing the effectiveness of a new approach to mother-infant psychotherapy. *Infant Mental Health Journal* **20**: 429–451.

36. Cohen NJ, Loikasek M, Muir E, et al. (2002). Six-month follow-up of two mother-infant psychotherapies: convergence of therapeutic outcomes. *Infant Mental Health Journal* **23**: 4361–4380.

37. Lieberman AF and Van Horn P. (2008). *Psychotherapy With Infants and Young Children: Repairing the Effects of Stress and Trauma on Early Attachment*. New York, NY: Guilford Press.

38. Lieberman AF, Van Horn P and Ippen CG. (2005). Toward evidence-based treatment: child-parent psychotherapy with preschoolers exposed to marital violence. *Journal Of The American Academy Of Child and Adolescent Psychiatry* **44**(12): 1241–1248.

39. Cicchetti D, Rogosch FA and Toth SL. (2006). Fostering secure attachment in infants in maltreating families through preventive interventions. *Development and Psychopathology* **18**: 623–649.

40. Toth SL, Rogosch FA, Cicchetti D and Manly JT. (2006). The efficacy of toddler–parent psychotherapy to reorganise attachment in the young offspring of mothers with major depressive disorder: a randomised preventive trial. *Journal of Consulting and Clinical Psychology* **74**(6).

41. Newman L and Stevenson C. (2008). Disorder parent psychotherapy for mothers with borderline personality issues in infant clinical child psychology and psychiatry copyright ©. *SAGE Publications* **13**(4): 505–514.

42. McDonough SC. (2000). Interaction guidance: understanding and treating early relationship. In: CH Zeanah (ed.), *Handbook of Infant Mental Health*. New York: Guilford Press.

43. Kennedy H, Landor M and Todd L. (2010). Video interaction guidance as a method to promote secure attachment. *Educational and Child Psychology* **27**(3): 59–72.

44. Fukkink RG. (2008). Video feed back in the widescreen: a meta-analysis of family programmes. *Clinical Psychology Review* **28**(6): 904–916.

45. Juffer F, Bakermans-Kranenburg MJ and van Ijzendoorn MH. (2005). The importance of parenting in the development of disorganised attachment: evidence from a preventive intervention study in adoptive families. *Journal of Child Psychology and Psychiatry* **46**(3): 263–274.

46. HoffmanKT, Marvin RS, Cooper G and Powell B. (2006). Changing toddlers' and preschoolers' attachment classifications: the Circle of Security Intervention. *Journal of Consulting and Clinical Psychology* **74**(6): 1017–1026.

47. Juffer F, van IJzendoorn MH and Bakermans-Kranenburg MJ. (2008). Supporting adoptive families with video-feedback intervention'. In: F. Juffer, M.J. Bakermans-Kranenburg and M.H. van IJzendoorn (eds), *Promoting Positive Parenting: An Attachment-based Intervention (Monographs in Parenting)*, New York: Psychology Press.
48. Velderman MK, Bakersmans-Kranenburg FJ., van IJzendoorn MH, et al. (2006). Preventing pre-school externalising problems through video-feedback intervention in infancy. *Infantile Mental Health* **27**(5): 466–493.
49. Herschell AD, Calzada EJ, Eyberg SM and McNeil CB. (2002). Parent child interaction therapy: new directions in research. *Cognitive and Behavioral Practices* **9**(1): 9–15.
50. Timmer SG, Ho LK, Urquiza AJ, et al. (2011). The effectiveness of parent–child interaction therapy with depressive mothers: the changing relationship as the agent of individual change. *Child Psychiatry and Human Development* **42**(4): 406–423.
51. Chaffin M, Silovsky JF, Funderburk B, et al. (2004). Parent-child interaction therapy with physically abusive parents: efficacy for reducing future abuse reports. *Journal of Consulting and Clinical Psychology* **72**(3): 500–510.
52. Hakman M, Chaffin M, Funderburk B and Silovsky JF. (2009). Change trajectories for parent-child interaction sequences during parent-child interaction therapy for child physical abuse. *Child Abuse & Neglect* **33**(7): 461–470.
53. Thomas R and Zimmer-Gembeck MJ, (2011). Accumulating evidence for parent–child interaction therapy in the prevention of child maltreatment. *Child Development* **82**(1): 177–192.
54. Timmer SG, Ware LM, Urquiza AJ and Zebell NM. (2010). The effectiveness of parent–child interaction therapy for victims of interparental violence. *Violence and Victims* **25**(4): 486–503.
55. Berkovits MD, O'Brien KA, Carter CG and Eyberg SM. (2010). Early identification and intervention for behavior problems in primary care: A comparison of two abbreviated versions of parent-child interaction therapy. *Behavior Therapy* **41**(3): 375–387.
56. Zisser A and Eyberg SM. (2010). Treating oppositional behavior in children using parent-child interaction therapy. In: AE Kazdin, and JR Weisz (eds), *Evidence-based Psychotherapies for Children and Adolescents*, 2nd edition. pp. 179–193. New York: Guilford.
57. Powell B, Cooper G, Hoffman K and Marvin R. (2007). The *Circle of Security* Project: A case study–"It hurts to give that which you did not receive". In: D Oppenheim, DF Goldsmith (eds). *Attachment theory in clinical work with children bridging the gap between research and practice.* pp. 172–202. New York: Guilford Press.

7
Early Intervention for Young People with Mental Illness

Tom Callaly

Barwon Health, Geelong, Victoria, Australia; School of Medicine, Deakin University, Geelong, Victoria, Australia

Introduction

In this chapter I will explore current ideas on the value of early intervention for young people between the ages of 12 and 24 years, arguments for and against establishing a youth mental health service stream and describe the elements of such a service. The chapter finishes with short descriptions of some youth health and mental health services in Australia. While there may be reference to specific illnesses, early intervention approaches for specific illnesses are addressed in other sections of this book and this chapter addresses service delivery across diagnoses. This chapter focuses on the 12–24 years age-band rather than on the usual adolescent age-band (12–18 years). There is increasing support for the argument that the health and developmental needs of all 0–12 year olds differ sufficiently from adolescents and young people to justify separate services. Those aged between 12 and 24 years are emerging adults who are sexually mature, are in the final stages of their educational career or the first stages of their employment career, are embarking on socially accepted adult activities such as using alcohol and tobacco and commencing intimate relationships [1]. As society changes and the adolescent stage effectively lengthens with a longer period of dependence on family and longer periods preparing for a workforce, the traditional Child and Adolescent Mental Health Services (CAMHS) cut-off point of 18 years of age is less suited to older adolescents and young adults. As will be argued below, young people require treatment models that differ substantially from those suitable for children and older adults.

Early Intervention in Psychiatry: EI of nearly everything for better mental health, First Edition.
Edited by Peter Byrne and Alan Rosen.
© 2014 John Wiley & Sons, Ltd. Published 2014 by John Wiley & Sons, Ltd.

The need

Mental ill-health is the largest contributor to the health burden of young people. The arguments in favour of increased attention to earlier intervention for young people with mental illness are therefore now well established. In a recent Access Economic report in Australia, it is estimated that 24.3% of all Australians between 12 and 24 years of age suffered from a mental disorder in 2009 [2]. There is also evidence that the prevalence of mental illness in young people in Western societies is increasing and that the age of onset of mental illnesses is decreasing. There are many hypotheses put forward to explain this. Increasing use of drugs and alcohol at earlier ages, sociological changes in relation to the protective role of families and independence at a younger age, decreasing levels of exercise, smoking and dietary factors may all contribute [3–5]. The peak onset for severe mental illnesses is in youth: a recent American study reported that half of all life-long mental disorders start by 14 years of age, and three-quarters by 24 years of age [6].

As might be expected, the cost to society is enormous. The Access Economics report referred to above estimated that the financial cost for each young person affected by mental illness in Australia equates to AU$10,544 per annum, with the majority of this cost due to lost productivity because of higher unemployment, absenteeism and premature death [2]. Of great concern is the National Survey of Mental Health and Well-being Study Data, which shows that only 25% of young people and only 15% of males, aged 16–24 years who have a mental illness receive any treatment compared with 35% of the total population with mental illness [7]. Barriers to access and reluctance to access treatment in youth, a period of important growth and developmental milestones including educational attainment, career and family building, are particularly detrimental. Young adults with mental illness are at greater risk of suicide, self-harm and substance addiction. In addition, illness interrupts the attainment of critical age related developmental milestones [8]. Thus, at the time of greatest vulnerability and risk, when perhaps most could be done to prevent the development of more serious illness, young people frequently fail to access other primary care or specialist services for mental health care.

Early intervention in youth mental health – what does it mean?

The meaning of early intervention may seem self-evident; however, it needs to be carefully considered before conclusions can be reached about the effectiveness, including cost-effectiveness, of early intervention, the dangers associated with early treatment and approaches to the most effective design of services for the early stages of illness. The rationale behind early intervention is that, particularly for serious disorders such as schizophrenia, bipolar disorder and eating disorders, the longer a person goes untreated the greater the risk of psychosocial consequences due to disruption of education, family stress or breakdown, loss of friendships, use of drugs and alcohol to self-medicate, stigma and disruption of personality development. It is also increasingly understood that there is an active process of neuroprogression in major psychiatric disorders with structural brain changes and neurocognitive consequences [9]. With psychosis, the period between first experiencing symptoms and receiving treatment is referred to as the duration of untreated psychosis (DUP) and its reduction is a major aim of early intervention and specialised services are provided focusing on recovery as early as possible [10]. In addition, it makes sense that families and other carers are provided with an explanation (re-presented and repeated as necessary) and support from specialist health providers as early as possible rather than being left confused, distraught and uninformed which is too often the case.

Early intervention refers to the use of interventions in those displaying the early signs and symptoms of a mental health problem or disorder and contrasts with interventions around the early signs of recurring mental disorder, best referred to as relapse prevention or reduction [11, 12]. Early intervention is described as the 'fuzzy interface', between indicated prevention and case identification, and occurs at the point on the pathway to a mental disorder where there are signs and symptoms suggesting an at-risk mental state or indicating a first episode of mental illness. Early intervention must start with early identification, which may in turn mean seeing many people with symptoms that prove to be transitory and not indicative of the development of more serious disorder. Of course this is made much more difficult by the fact that in clinical practice, particularly with young people, symptom complexes are often transient and even when the individual is destined to develop a serious disorder, it is often extremely difficult or impossible to identify the trajectory or the length of time involved during the prodromal phase. Early identification is also complicated by the more diffuse and nonspecific nature of early forms of many disorders. Supporters of early intervention for psychosis argue that all young people with symptomatology should be offered help (whether in schools or workplace, primary care or specialist care) and the models of care which allow for this will, in turn, facilitate early identification and treatment of the minority of people who are on a trajectory to severe illness.

The major sources of disagreement between those who favour early intervention in psychosis and those who do not are whether or not prodromal illness can be identified and ought to be treated (if indeed that is possible) and whether a focus on early intervention for young people has led to resources being drained away from other mental health services where the evidence base is argued to be stronger. Critics of early intervention in the prodromal phase argue that services designed to offer help to all who present with symptoms may lead to 'pathologising' adolescents, increasing the risk of using medications with serious side effects when there is no illness, and wasting money that could be more usefully spent boosting services for those who have identified illness. In addition, they argue that there is no evidence that early intervention leads to better symptom outcomes in the long run [13].

Supporters of early intervention for psychosis argue that specialised services for first episode psychosis patients are needed to deliver the intensive biopsychosocial care that is required. The first and very well known of these in Melbourne was named the Early Psychosis Prevention and Intervention Centre (EPPIC). Such services have been shown to be superior to generic services at 12 months, 2 years and up to 5 years after entry to the service [14]. There is debate as to whether or not these improvements are maintained after the person leaves the service. However if specialist treatment can be maintained, even at a lower level of intensity, there is evidence that these good outcomes can not only be maintained but can continue to improve over 5 years [15]. Critics of specialist early psychosis services argue that specialist service treatment plans are no different from those that would be considered best practice by generic multidisciplinary psychiatry teams. This is good where it is true. But many generic teams in public mental health services are not adequately resourced for this sort of care and the crisis-driven nature of these services means that clinicians are required to keep people in case management for shorter periods than would be required to ensure the sort of intensive biopsychosocial care they need.

Those who favour early intervention point out that much of the deterioration seen in patients with schizophrenia and other psychotic disorders is not due to some inevitable biological process but due to psychosocial factors that operate in the years following first onset of illness. These psychosocial factors include disruption of education and preparation for a job or career, family stress caused by the illness, breakdown of friendships, the effects of stigma, the effects of substance use often used to relieve symptoms and the constant fear of relapse [16, 17]. These factors may well be preventable or at least ameliorated with early attention and support. Also, as mentioned above, families are usually in great distress during this early period and they desperately need education about illness and support in managing crisis which is often a major issue. When these factors are considered, whether or not the outcome in terms of symptoms a year or two later is no different for those who receive intensive care than for those who do not is somewhat academic. The longer a person remains severely ill in the community without treatment, the greater the likelihood that he or she will damage whatever supportive relationships they have and drop out of school or work. There is evidence that a lengthy DUP is at least associated with poorer outcome in terms of symptoms and functioning up to 10 years after the young person has received early intensive care [18].

These are all complex arguments to evaluate and further research will undoubtedly clarify matters over the coming years. What is clear to many of us who have worked in traditionally designed services is that the shorter the duration of established illness before treatment, the better. Indeed in our service, we often talk about 'earlier intervention'. While figures will vary from service to service, a mean DUP of 24 months has been described even in a modern and well-resourced Melbourne service [19]. It is difficult to imagine the community accepting that we should wait until the existence of breast cancer or cardiac disease is definitively established before any interventions are attempted.

Barriers to accessing services

It makes sense that an understanding of the reasons why young people do not seek help for psychological problems or do not or cannot access treatment would be helpful in making decisions about the design of services for young people. A number of studies show that young people are reluctant to seek professional mental health care. The Australian national survey mentioned above found that only 29% of children and adolescents with a mental health problem had been in contact with professional services of any type in a 12-month period [20]. In another Australian study, of 3092 young people aged between 15 and 24 years, 39% of the males and 22% of the females reported that they would not seek help from formal services for personal, emotional or psychological problems [21]. In this study 30% of young men, compared with only 6% of young women, reported they would not seek help from anyone. This gender difference in health seeking is of special concern given the substantially higher rates of completed suicide in young men.

Health seeking is not a simple process of experiencing psychological difficulties and then seeking help [22]. When a young person first becomes aware (or other family or friends become aware) of psychological difficulties, the next step is to conclude that it is a problem which the person should seek help for. Despite appraising the situation as a problem, the person or family and friends may be unwilling to seek help. And even if willing to seek help, they may simply not know where to go. Determinants of help-seeking behaviour may relate to the individual experiencing the psychological difficulties such as mental health literacy, attitudes and perceived stigma, and to the individual's environment such as family, school, community support systems, health system structures and payment systems.

Young people are more likely to seek help when they recognise that they have a mental health problem. Mental health literacy comprises the ability to recognise mental health problems, and knowledge of how to seek mental health information and services. Mental health literacy is poor among young Australians, particularly young men [23]. A certain amount of emotional competency is required to seek mental health help and this competence appears less developed in young men.

There have been many initiatives in Australia, the United States, the United Kingdom and Norway to increase mental health literacy in the community [23]. Research in the area emphasises how difficult this work is and how important it is to use the media which young people will be exposed to. In the Compass project in Australia, for example young people were consulted about the format of information material and where it should be made available. Youth-friendly material was made available in selected cinemas, registrations and places where young people would congregate [24]. In Australia, a major initiative has been the development of partnerships between schools and general practices and material has been produced to support practices with this [25].

Younger adolescents will share their concerns with parents and family, but parents must be able to recognize mental health problems, be willing to seek help and know how to access it. For young people aged up to 16 years, school is central and is the ideal setting in which to reach out to them. Hence having friendly and confidential access to psychological support, such as counsellors or well-informed supportive teachers at school is of critical importance. General practice is the initial point of contact with professional services. However there is concern that GPs do not always recognise mental health problems in young people and older youth who visit the GP on their own are often reluctant to mention their personal emotional problems because of concerns about confidentiality or being viewed as weak or abnormal [22].

Some of the barriers to help seeking are purely physical. The location of services may make them difficult to access (young people rely on public transport to a greater extent than adults). Facility opening times will be a barrier if restricted to school hours. Young people often find the design and decor of traditional health services youth-unfriendly and sterile.

Stigma associated with mental health problems is a major concern for young people and there is evidence that young people tend to have more discriminatory attitudes to mental health problems than adults [26]. This can lead to an unwillingness to admit problems or ask for help from friends, parents or professionals. Young people have less experience attending GPs because their physical health is usually good. Those of us with experience in parenting will be well aware that young people expect and need to feel respected and listened to by health professionals in contrast to the acceptance we parents had for the more paternalistic approach typical of health professionals in the past. Certainly, young people today usually will not come along to an appointment just because their parents or doctor thinks it is a good idea. Unhelpful past experiences of seeking help where the young person felt that they were not listened to, their problems were not taken seriously or worse, where confidentiality was breached, also contribute to negative attitudes towards mental health services including school counsellors and general practitioners [27, 28].

The model of service provision is very important. Barriers to seeking help early on from specialist mental health services including drug and alcohol services can be particularly strong. The traditional model of offering appointments at certain times within the health facility will not suit many young people who want flexibility about attendance. The traditional approach to history taking is too rigid for many and an approach to the young person which supports engagement with the clinician is essential. It is also essential that they not have to continually repeat their stories (as they are usually expected to when referred from one traditional service to another e.g. drug treatment services to mental health services). Overall, engaging the young person is very important and requires a particular style and therapeutic skill, which is often lacking in traditional services [8].

The weaknesses of traditional service age-bands

Debate continues as to how specialist services for young people should be organised and delivered.

On the one hand it is argued that it makes more sense developmentally, legally and socially to group adolescents with children as in traditional CAMHS services and that the creation of a separate youth service will create two transition points: child to youth service and youth service to adult service) instead of the traditional one (from child and adolescent services to adult services) which further increases difficulties with continuity of care [29]. Thus, it is argued by proponents of this view, what is required is for CAMHS and adult services to receive more support and funding. Others argue that the traditional CAMHS model does not serve adolescents well, and that equally the traditional adult model fails to serve young adults well. What is needed, this group argues, is youth services which integrate mental health, drug and alcohol and physical care [30]. Discontinuity of care provision for 'graduates' of CAMHS who are not accepted by adult services is common and well recognised and is a further argument for separate youth services [31].

What would an ideal framework for identifying illness as early as possible and delivering effective youth-friendly services to young people look like?

Figure 7.1 illustrates the continuum of service provision which must be created if we are to provide a comprehensive framework and identify those who are destined to develop more serious illnesses at the earliest possible time. An effective framework must include elements ranging from measures directed at the whole youth population to the provision of specialised youth mental health services. Figure 7.1 illustrates the need for close connection and collaboration between the different elements of the continuum so that young people can move from one element to another with ease.

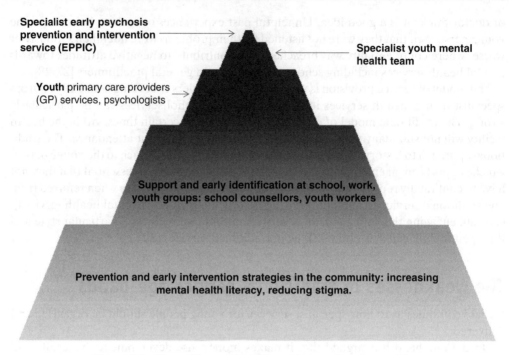

Figure 7.1 The youth mental health continuum of service provision

For specialist mental health services, one of the most challenging considerations in this field is whether or not to establish specialist services for young people separate from current CAMHS and adult services. If a decision is made to establish separate services, another consideration is whether the separation should be based on age-band (e.g. a service for 12–24 year olds, 16–30 year olds etc) or disorder (e.g. psychotic disorders, personality disorders). Inevitably there are inherent tensions around disorder or age-specific services as against broader and more generic services which must be recognised. Benefits for a separate service based on age-band include clinicians gaining experience and expertise in working with young people and the elimination of troublesome service transition point at 18 years of age. These benefits must be weighed against acceptance of what are inevitable arbitrary age cut-offs, narrowness of focus, artificial parsing of comorbidities and resource implications associated with minimum team size. Issues to be considered if setting up a separate service include the national and state context, the political will of the local level to make such changes, the maturity of local service collaboration and the size of the service (it may be too inefficient for a small rural service to establish a separate youth mental health service and too inefficient for a medium-sized service to establish an EPPIC). For all the reasons put forward above, we in the Barwon Mental Health, Drug and Alcohol Services concluded that the ideal vehicle for the provision of mental health and drug and alcohol services is an integrated health service geared towards young people from early teens to mid-20s. We originally concluded that our service did not serve a large enough population to merit establishing an EPPIC but have recently commenced work to establish an EPPIC in collaboration with a neighbouring Area Mental Health Service which serves an additional population of 150,000.

Clockwork young people's health service

Clockwork, a good example of an integrated GP youth health service, was set up in 1994 by general practitioners with an interest in adolescent health who recognised that the traditional general practice is not usually youth friendly or easily accessed by young people. They recognised a need for a youth service that linked health care needs with social difficulties to overcome the barriers often encountered when young people try to access the traditional health system; a system all too often lacking either the capacity or sensitivity to handle the complex problems of youth. Instead they established a service in central Geelong, Victoria, Australia operated from a youth art and culture venue where interested GPs could spend most of, or part of their practice seeing young people.

Important features of Clockwork include: the target age range is 12–25 years, the service is free, young people were consulted in the design of the premises and the operation of the service and confidentiality is guaranteed [32]. Clockwork has since become the core partner in *headspace* Barwon in 2006 as described in the next section.

Headspace

Headspace is Australia's National Youth Mental Health Foundation. It was established in response to the recognised weaknesses of the system as described above. Its aim is to provide a national, coordinated focus on youth mental health and related drug and alcohol problems in Australia, to improve access for young people aged 12–25 years to services and to ensure better coordination between services. *headspace* is funded by the Commonwealth Government of Australia [33]. Effectively, *headspace* has been providing funding to regions that have made a successful application to *headspace*, to establish a platform for integrating existing primary care services as well as establishing new services (including GPs, psychologists, youth workers) for young people. Since 2006, *headspace* has funded the establishment of 30 integrated youth-friendly *headspace* sites across the country and there are more promised in the 2010 Federal Budget. The 2011–2012 budget measure provides funding for 90 fully sustainable *headspace* sites across Australia by 2014–2015.When all 90 sites are fully established, *headspace* is expected to help up to 72,000 young people each year.

To be successful in gaining *headspace* funding and approval to use the *headspace* brand, each local area must form a partnership with local health providers such as GPs, youth services, drug and alcohol services and public specialist mental health services and commit to providing access for young people aged 12–25 years to primary mental health care, alcohol and drug counselling, and vocational and social support. In Geelong in 2006, the GP Association of Geelong, which operates Clockwork Youth Health Service, became the lead agency for the consortium of services which was successful in gaining *headspace* funding.

Headspace also fosters community awareness and improves mental health literacy on young peoples' mental health issues across Australia through designing and funding national multimedia campaigns. It also works to increase the knowledge, understanding and skills of GPs and other service providers through the development and dissemination of evidence-based education, training and resources.

Jigsaw: specialist mental health services for young people in the Barwon region, Australia

Barwon public Mental Health and Drug and Alcohol Services (MHDAS) provide mental health and drug and alcohol services for a large regional section of south-west Victoria, Australia which has a total population of approximately 300,000 people. As stated above, the executive of the Barwon MHDAS concluded that the ideal vehicle for the provision of mental health and drug and alcohol services is an integrated health service geared towards young people from 16 to 24 years of age collaboratively with other health and social agencies. We did not believe the child and adolescent services were effectively serving the specialist needs of adolescents including forming linkages with schools and paediatricians and simultaneously collaborating intensively with young peoples' health services. Nor did we believe that the adult services, which were once focused on 18–65 year olds, could easily tend to their older clientele and simultaneously focus on the needs of their younger adults.

In mid-2002, the Barwon MHDAS embarked on a 2 year process of planning and negotiation to bring together the Barwon health services for young people, including some sections of its CAMHS, adult mental health teams, drug treatment services and community counselling services to form one service for all 16–24 year olds in the region which was named Jigsaw. When this service re-engineering was complete, CAMHS provided services for children and adolescents up to 15 years of age and adult team responsibility was reduced to providing services for 25 to 65 year olds [34]. Jigsaw then formed partnerships with other young persons' health service providers in the region. A formal agreement was established with local Psychiatric Disability Rehabilitation and Support Services (PDRSS), a nongovernment organisation, and Clockwork, the already established GP young persons' health service described above. A memorandum of understanding committed services to work together towards providing integrated services. This new service shared premises on the first floor of the major shopping centre within the North Geelong region. Young people were consulted in the design and decor of the reception area. The new integrated youth service utilised a single, shared electronic record and shared responsibility for funding different elements of the service including information technology developments and reception staff. Jigsaw, the public mental health service in Geelong, was then well positioned to become an active partner in *headspace* Geelong when it was formed in 2006.

One of the major areas of challenge that the consortium in Geelong has faced has been that of establishing and maintaining service integration [35]. The interagency and interclinician conflicts and challenges, which working closely together and relying on one another's commitment to a shared vision inevitably gives rise to, are often unanticipated and poorly prepared for. A shared interest in developing better services is not always sufficient to carry the collaboration through difficult times.

Conclusion

Improving the mental health care of our young people is a significant and growing challenge. For a plethora of reasons, including sociological and cultural changes outside of the control of health services, doing 'more of the same' will not address this challenge.

Increasing funding to CAMHS and traditional adult mental health services may improve things but do not address the fundamental difficulties of increasing morbidity combined with poor access to our services. Only bold and creative service redesign which involves close collaboration with other services for young people is urgently needed. There is no doubt that the sorts of innovations discussed in this chapter will need careful comparison and evaluation to establish the extent of their effectiveness as we move forward.

References

1. Arnett JJ. (2004). *Emerging Adulthood: The Winding Road From the Late Teens Through the Twenties*. New York: Oxford University Press.
2. Access Economics. (2009). *The Economic Impact of Youth Mental Illness and the Cost Effectiveness of Early Intervention*. Canberra: Access Economics.
3. Jacka FN, Pasco JA, Mykletun A, et al. (2010). Association between western and traditional diets and depression and anxiety in women. *American Journal of Psychiatry* **167**(3): 305–311.
4. Pasco JA, Williams LJ, Jacka FN, et al. (2008). Tobacco smoking as a risk factor for major depressive disorder: population-based study. *British Journal of Psychiatry* **193**(4): 322–326.
5. Pasco JA, Jacka FN, Williams LJ, et al. (2011). Don't worry, be active: positive affect and habitual physical activity. *Australian and New Zealand Journal of Psychiatry* **45**(12): 1047–1052.
6. Kessler RC, Berglund P, Demler O, et al. (2005). Lifetime prevalence and age-of-onset distributions of DSM-IV disorders in the National Comorbidity Survey Replication. *Archives of General Psychiatry* **62**: 593–602.
7. Australian Bureau of Statistics. (2008). *National Survey of Mental Health and Well-Being. Summary of Results*. Canberra: Australian Bureau of Statistics.
8. Macneil CA, Hasty MK, Berk M, et al. (2011). Psychological needs of adolescents in the early phase of bipolar disorder: implications for early intervention. *Early Intervention in Psychiatry* **5**(2): 100–107.
9. Berk M, Kapczinski F, Andreazza AC, et al. (2011). Pathways underlying neuroprogression in bipolar disorder: focus on inflammation, oxidative stress and neurotrophic factors. *Neuroscience and Biobehavioral Reviews* **35**(3): 804–817.
10. Yung AR. (2012). Earlier intervention in psychosis: evidence gaps, criticism and confusion. *Australian and New Zealand Journal of Psychiatry* **46**(1): 7–9.
11. Berk M, Conus P, Lucas N, et al. (2007). Setting the stage: from prodrome to treatment resistance in bipolar disorder. *Bipolar Disorders* **9**(7): 671–678.
12. Berk L, Hallam KT, Colom F, et al. (2010). Enhancing medication adherence in patients with bipolar disorder. *Human Psychopharmacology* **25**(1): 1–16.
13. Bertelsen M, Jeppesen P, Petersen L, et al. (2008). Five-year follow-up of a randomized multicenter trial of intensive early intervention versus standard treatment for patients with a first episode of psychotic illness: the OPUS trial. *Archives of General Psychiatry* **65**(7): 762–771.
14. Bertlesen M, Jeppesen P, Peterson L, et al. (2008). Five-year follow-up of a randomized multicenter trial of intensive early intervention vs standard treatment for patients with a first episode of psychotic illness. *Archives of General Psychiatry* **65**: 762–771.
15. Norman RMG, Manchanda R, Malla AK, et al. (2011). Symptom and functional outcomes for a five-year early intervention program for psychosis. *Schizophrenia Research* **129**: 111–115.
16. Francey SM, Nelson B, Thompson A, et al. (2010). Who needs antipsychotic medication in the earliest stages of psychosis? A reconsideration of benefits, risks, neurobiology and ethics in the era of early intervention. *Schizophrenia Research* **119**(1–3): 1–10.
17. Kapczinski F, Dias VV, Kauer-Sant'Anna M, et al. (2009). Clinical implications of a staging model for bipolar disorders. *Expert Review of Neurotherapeutics* **9**(7): 957–966.

18. Marshall M, Lewis S, Lockwood A, et al. (2011). *Cochrane Database Systematic Reviews* (6): CD00 4718.
19. Petrakis M, Penno S, Oxley J, et al. (2012). Early psychosis treatment in an integrated model within an adult mental health service. *European Psychiatry* **27**(7): 483–488. doi:10.1016/j.eurpsy.2011.03.004
20. Andrews G, Hall W, Teesson M and Henderson S. (1999). *The mental health of Australians*. Canberra: Mental Health Branch, Commonwealth Department of Health and Aged Care.
21. Zachrisson HD, Rodje K and Mykletun A. (2006). Utilization of health services in relation to mental health problems in adolescents: a population-based survey. *BMC Public Health* **6**: 34–40.
22. Rickwood DJ, Deane FP and Wilson CJ. (2007). When and how do young people seek professional help for mental health problems? *Medical Journal of Australia* **187**(7 Suppl): S35–S39.
23. Kelly CM, Jorm AF and Wright A. (2007). Improving mental health literacy as a strategy to facilitate early intervention for mental disorders. *The Medical Journal of Australia* **187**: S26–S30.
24. Wright A, McGorry PD, Harris MG, et al. (2006). Development and evaluation of a youth mental health community awareness campaign. *BMC Public Health* **6**: 215. doi:10.1186/1471-2458-6-21.
25. MindMatters Plus. http://mmplus.agca.com.au/ (accessed 9 April 2014).
26. BMA. (2006). Child and adolescent. A guide for healthcare professional. *BMA Board of Science*, http://www.familieslink.co.uk/download/jan07/ChildAdolescentMentalHealth%202006. pdf (accessed 9 April 2014).
27. Coulson C, Ng F, Geertsema M, et al. (2009). Client-reported reasons for non-engagement in drug and alcohol treatment. *Drug and Alcohol Review* **28**(4): 372–378.
28. Berk M, Hallam K, Malhi GS, et al. (2010). Evidence and implications for early intervention in bipolar disorder. *Journal of Mental Health Administration* **19**(2):113–126.
29. Birlison P. (2009). Should youth mental health become a specialty in its own right? No. *BMJ: British Medical Association* **339**: b3371, doi:10.1136/bmj.b3371
30. McGorry P. (2009). Should youth mental health become a speciality in its own right? Yes. *BMJ : British Medical Association*, **339**: b3373, doi:10.1136/bmj.b3373.
31. Singh S P. (2009). Transition of care from child to adult mental health services: the great divide. *Current Opinion in Psychiatry* **22**: 386–390.
32. Gore C. (2005). Clockwork young people's health service. *Australian Family Physician* **34**(1/2), http://www.racgp.org.au/afp/200501/200501gore.pdf (accessed 30 January 2012).
33. McGorry PD, Tanti C, Stokes R, et al. (2007). headspace: Australia's National Youth Mental Health Foundation – where young minds come first. *Medical Journal of Australia* **187**: S68–S70.
34. Callaly T, Dodd S, Ackerly C, et al. (2009). Description and qualitative evaluation of Jigsaw, an integrated young persons' mental health program. *Australasian Psychiatry* **17**(6): 480–483.
35. Callaly T, von Treuer K, van Hamond T and Windle K. (2011). Forming and sustaining partnerships to provide integrated services for young people : an overview based on the headspace Geelong experience. *Early Intervention in Psychiatry* **5**(1): 28–33.

8

Transiting Out of Child and Adolescent Mental Health Services – Influences on Continuities and Discontinuities in Mental Health Care

Linda Dowdney[1] and Helen Bruce[1,2,3]

[1] University College London, Institute of Child Health, London, UK
[2] East London NHS Foundation Trust, London, UK
[3] Barts and the London School of Medicine and Dentistry, London, UK

Introduction

In the only major UK study of whether and how users of child and adolescent mental health services (CAMHS) transfer successfully to adult mental health services (AMHS), Singh and colleagues elucidate influences impinging upon this transition [1–3]. This study joins others in the National Institute for Health Research Service Delivery and Organization (NCCSDO) programme of research focusing on understanding continuities and discontinuities in care in a variety of UK health care systems, including severe mental health difficulties in adults, learning disabilities and paediatric health services [4, 5]. Singh and colleagues note that while there is much talk about transition between CAMHS and AMHS, there is little substantive research. Hence, while focusing on the latter transitions, we draw from this wider body of literature as relevant issues arise.

The challenges of providing children and families with continuity of care as they move vertically over time through various health and social care services, and horizontally between different service sectors have preoccupied policy makers, researchers and practitioners for some considerable time. In the United Kingdom, such concerns have led to a proliferation of policies and guidance from successive governments focusing on how best to achieve successful transitions between child and adult health, mental health and social care services (see, e.g. [6–10]). CAMHS–AMHS professional guidelines are also available – see e.g. [11].

It has been argued that clarity in the definition of continuity of care will improve communication across services, facilitate solutions to transition problems and encourage valid and reliable transition outcome research [12]. A variety of conceptual models incorporating organizational, structural, process, professional, service user and outcome variables are available in the NCCSDO studies [4, 13]. For the moment, we follow Singh and colleagues in focusing specifically on the *'health care transition defined as a formal transfer of care from CAMHS to adult services'* [3, p. 10]. We later consider how a wider and more dynamic definition could help identify aspects of service development and provision that would enhance this transition process.

Child and adolescent mental health disorders
Epidemiology

Nine per cent of British children will meet DSM-IV criteria for childhood disorder of a severity that impairs functioning and warrants treatment [14]. Rates of disorder increase with age and those first evident in childhood, such as anxiety, depression and conduct disorder, peak in adolescence – with increases in the rate of depression being most common in girls and of conduct disorder in boys. Other disorders show their peak *onset* in adolescence including psychosis, bipolar, eating and emerging personality disorders. While estimates of comorbidity vary across studies, depending in part upon diagnostic criteria, conservative estimates suggest that at least a quarter of children will experience comorbid disorders, these being particularly evident between anxiety and depression, between attention deficit and hyperactivity disorder (ADHD) and behaviour disorders and between depression and some behaviour disorders [14, 15].

Service provision – CAMHS

Specialist mental health care for children, young people and their families in the United Kingdom is provided within CAMHS, a public health service free at the point of delivery. Within England and Wales, the service is divided into four increasingly specialized tiers, with Tiers 3 and 4 (the focus of this chapter), providing multi-disciplinary team services for children and young people with the most serious problems. In practice, children and their families may be involved in different services across the tiers, concurrently or historically, as well as with other social and health agencies that come under the umbrella of children's services [7]. Consequently, multi-agency working, within and across health, education and social care sectors tends to be the rule rather than the exception. While the organization of CAMHS services may differ in Scotland and Northern Ireland, both countries offer multi-disciplinary CAMHS for children with the most serious mental health needs, and the transition from CAMHS to AMHS raises concerns similar to those elsewhere in the United Kingdom [16, 17].

The types of therapy provided in specialist services reflect their multi-disciplinary composition, and can include psychological, psychotherapeutic and systemic therapies as well as pharmacotherapy. The model of service delivery is developmental – reflecting children's biological, psychological, and social needs as well as the onset and course of differing disorders over childhood and adolescence. Families and careers are an integral part of therapeutic interventions, though the extent of their involvement and the role they play change as the child matures. With younger children, parents may act as 'co-therapists', while by the time their child reaches the legal age to give consent to treatment (16 years), parents will often be seen separately as a supportive adjunct to individualized treatment of their child. Across the age range, whatever the form of treatment employed, viewing the child within the context of the family and utilizing family resources to aid in the recovery process are integral to service provision.

Developmental needs for continuity of care

Both research and clinical experience support the need for a smooth transition between child and appropriate AMHS based on developmental trajectories evidencing continuities in psychopathology between childhood, adolescence and young adulthood.

Continuities in psychopathology and adult outcomes

Longitudinal epidemiological studies show that serious child and adolescent emotional and behavioural problems, and child mental health service use, predict adult psychiatric disorder [18, 19]. For example child and adolescent conduct/opposition problems predict anxiety and depression, antisocial personality and psychotic disorders in young adults [18, 20]. Retrospective analyses of adults with psychiatric disorder, drawn from a birth cohort study, indicate that about 73% had received a psychiatric diagnosis before 18 years of age, and 50% before 15 years of age. Up to 60% had a history of conduct and/or oppositional defiant disorder [21]. ADHD is now thought to persist in about 50–60% of adolescents, and recent evidence suggests a continuation into young adulthood, with prevalence rates in those previously diagnosed in childhood varying according to whether they met full diagnostic criteria (15%) or were in partial remission (65%) [22]. Vulnerability of those with emotional disorders continues into young adulthood [19]. World Health Organization figures reveal that suicide, uncommon in childhood and early adolescence, increases markedly from mid-adolescence to early adulthood. In the United Kingdom in 2003, suicide rates for those aged 15–24 years were 8 per 100,000 for males and 2.3 for girls [23]. Clearly, child and adolescent mental health problems represent a key risk factor for psychiatric problems in adulthood.

Broader-based outcome studies are also relevant. For instance, a recent longitudinal study of three successive cohorts of youth with serious emotional disturbance found a decline in rates of employment, and increases in employment instability and involvement in crime. Of those aged 21–25 in 2009, 60.5% had been arrested and 44.2% had been on probation or parole [24]. Similarly, adult outcomes for those with ADHD include educational and occupational failure, disturbed interpersonal relationships, delinquency and criminality [22].

The evidence for continuities in psychopathology and psychiatric disorder argues for the provision of, and smooth transition to, appropriate service support as adolescents transition into adulthood. Yet, both nationally and internationally, problems at the interface of child and adult mental health services are more likely to lead to discontinuities rather than continuities in care [25, 26].

Service transitions – difficulties at the interface
Service characteristics

CAMHS and AMHS differ markedly in a variety of ways, stemming from differences in their history, culture, models of care and service configurations. These differences can result in difficulties at the interface between services, such that Singh and colleagues found only 58% of those leaving CAMHS transferred into AMHS and less than 5% of them experienced an optimal transition [2]. Additional factors impacting on the transition process include client characteristics such as diagnostic profiles and variation in developmental and clinical needs.

Eligibility for services   Young people receiving care from CAMHS evidence a wide range of emotional and behavioural problems – problems often complicated in adolescence by the emergence of risk-taking behaviours, accommodation needs and early parenthood. Complex mental health, social and developmental needs are evident as they move into young adulthood. The main criteria for eligibility into CAMHS is essentially that the child or young person is experiencing a mental health difficulty that is impairing their own, and/or their family's functioning in daily life. In contrast, AMHS services, with their greater emphasis on biological disorders, are likely to have eligibility criteria resting upon the presence of 'a severe and enduring mental illness'. Singh and colleagues [2] found that those most likely to make the transition to AMHS were those who met this criterion and/or who had a history of admission to inpatient units. Many young people attending CAMHS, though in need of continuing mental health care, are unlikely to meet this diagnostic threshold. A situation further complicated in young people by the diagnostic uncertainty stemming from an overlap between normal adolescent turmoil and the nonspecific prodrome of serious mental illness.

Service entry and exit from mental health services is also determined by age criteria. Where these are inflexible, barriers between services arise. With the exception of specialized services such as early intervention services (EIS) for those experiencing the early onset of serious mental health disorders (see Chapter 15), AMHS are largely available from the age of 18 years – the age which government policy suggests as the upper limit for CAMHS [7]. Nonetheless, geographic variations results in some CAMHS services not being offered beyond the age of 16 years, unless the young person remains in full-time education [3].

Doubtless, these rigid boundaries reflect clinicians' attempts to operate within service and resource constraints. Yet the impact upon those needing services is a marked gap in service provision. The resource implications of providing a comprehensive CAMHS service to 16 and 17 year olds are significant [11]. Yet the alternatives can include some young people being rejected – even for AMHS waiting lists until age criteria are met; or not being considered suitable for AMHS until a mental health crisis is reached, with entry into adult services then being potentially traumatic and emotionally costly to the young person and their family.

Service ethos, therapeutic models and transition protocols   Treatments available to young people and their families in CAMHS, such as systemic family therapy and individual psychotherapy alongside supportive family work, are unlikely to be available in many AMHS. Those seeking a continuation of such therapies can therefore experience an abrupt end to their care. Also, the person-centred focus of AMHS with its greater emphasis on autonomy and self-determination can effectively exclude families/carers, even though they remain highly involved in the young person's care [27].

This change in ethos can interact unhelpfully with the developmental needs of young people. In eating disorders (ED), for example CAMHS treatment models are likely to involve parents and young people combining to 'fight the ED' [28]. Young CAMHS leavers entering Adult Eating Disorder Services seem particularly likely to have maturational issues [29]. A sudden, poorly co-ordinated move to AMHS that emphasise individual autonomy, the acceptance of personal responsibility for tackling disorder and the exclusion of families can be *bewildering and dangerous for patients and their families* [30, p. 399].

Achieving the right balance between respecting client confidentiality and utilizing family support is a difficult task. Within CAMHS negotiations as to what information can and cannot be shared with others both prior to and during therapy are common. While regular contact with carers during transition forms part of the care model of EIS services, in other AMHS services, confidentiality can be used as a 'smokescreen' functioning to exclude families and carers [31].

It is not surprising, therefore, that Singh and colleagues [3] conclude that differing service and therapeutic models, communication difficulties, differences in protocols relating to how care needs are assessed, and misperceptions and poor communication between child and adult services hamper smooth transition between the two. These difficulties are enhanced in services lacking clear transition policies and protocols to guide and set standards for the process. Singh and colleagues' survey [1] indicates that only a minority of CAMHS services had developed policies and protocols governing these service transitions. In others, the protocols either did not exist or were not followed – representing a failure to implement government policy guidelines.

Client characteristics

While some service characteristics impact negatively upon the transition process for those who are eligible for entry into AMHS, other difficulties derive from the absence of services, or of appropriate services, for young people whose psychiatric diagnostic profile does not qualify them for AMHS. We give one major illustrative example, focusing specifically on young people with the neurodevelopmental disorders ASD and ADHD. These groups are eligible for CAMHS services prior to diagnosis on the basis of impaired functioning either at home and/or in education. CAMHS services will undertake diagnosis, offer appropriate interventions and provide the cross-agency liaison essential for effective functioning in educational and other settings. The focus will be on acceptance and management of the condition so as to minimize emotional and behavioural sequelae as far as possible. Young people with neurodevelopmental disorders are particularly likely to experience transition difficulties [3]. These stem in part from their emotional and behavioural profiles, and in part from current service structures.

With respect to young people with ASD, two particular characteristics are pertinent to the current discussion. First, even daily life transitions in routines and contexts can provoke emotional and behavioural distress for them. Major transitions, such as between services, are therefore likely to be particularly problematic. Careful preparation of the young person, based on parental and clinical expertise around how contextual and relational transitions have previously been managed successfully, is essential should a service transition need to be negotiated.

Secondly, in adolescence, those with high-functioning ASD develop a more acute awareness of their social and relationship difficulties. The need in adolescence for understanding more nuanced social interchanges and the implicit perspectives of others, combined with the more sophisticated demands of adolescent friendships, can be particularly stressful for them. Marked emotional distress is one sequelae and it is not surprising that a recent study of high-functioning children and adolescents with ASD found that around 70% met the criteria for an additional psychiatric disorder [32].

Taken together, therefore, these particular characteristics suggest both a potential need for these young people to receive mental health services and for their transition into those services to be managed in a careful way. However, those with high-functioning ASD will find themselves ineligible for entry into either adult learning disabilities services or AMHS. They do not meet the intellectual impairment criteria for the former, or the 'severe and enduring' mental health disorder criteria of the latter. Furthermore, most UK AHMS lack staff with specific training and experience in working with individuals with ASD [32]. The gap in service provision and support occurs for these young people just as they reach the major developmental transition of leaving the structure imposed by secondary education and moving into the relatively unstructured adult life of independence, employment, college or further training opportunities and adult relationships. They are left unsupported, therefore, at a crucial point in their development, in a fashion likely to cause them and their families' great distress, with the possibility of an exacerbation of any pre-existing mental health difficulties.

A similar picture emerges with respect to ADHD, though here the picture is complicated by the developmental aspects of the disorder such that some key symptoms lessen markedly as adolescents progress into adulthood, with a diagnostic issue for ADHD in adults, namely that the '*age-appropriate expression of clinical symptoms has yet to be firmly established*' [22, p. 12]. Given this combination of diagnostic uncertainty and the impact of maturational processes, adult psychiatrists may well find it difficult both to recognize ADHD as a valid diagnosis and to understand the need of young people for AMHS [33]. A decline in pharmacological prescriptions for ADHD is apparent in adolescence, reflecting developmental transitions, independent adolescent decision making and a dropping out of services due to a lack of transition services [34]. In addition, once those with ADHD graduate out of child health services, pharmacological treatment is not straightforwardly available to them.

Clinical experience suggests that young people transiting from CAMHS, as opposed to paediatric health services, will involve a higher proportion of those with more complex presentations, including comorbid diagnoses and the social and behavioural concomitants of the disorder outlined previously. Their continued impulsivity, attention difficulties and chaotic lifestyles indicate a need for particularly clear referral procedures and easy to understand, coherent, interservice and interagency transition protocols. Careful discussion and negotiation with the young person and their families needs to pave the way for potential entry into adult services.

While particular aspects of their respective conditions may influence exactly how the transition process would best be managed, for those with neurodevelopment disorders, the overriding problem is that those with the greatest mental health needs may well face a lack of AMHS service provision, failing as they do to meet AMHS eligibility criteria.

Managing the interface – ways forward
Perspectives on continuity

Young people, families and professionals – moving on together We began this chapter with a definition of continuity focusing on the point of transfer between child and adult mental health services, a definition that led to analyses of service limitations at the transition interface. Parker and colleagues suggest that service user and family/carer experiences represent a defining aspect of continuity, such that *'service users, carers and professionals construct continuity dynamically between themselves'* [13, p. 576.]. If we accept this perspective, then user and carer views will need to influence future transition processes, whether at the interface of existing services or in new service developments.

Yet, there is limited primary research in this area at the CAMHS and AMHS interface [3]. Drawing on the wider paediatric health, and adult mental health literature, relevant points emerge or are confirmed, though it is worth noting that even where user/carer views are sought, professional views of continuity dominate the conceptual and research framework employed [13, 35].

Youth and young adults consistently value high-quality relationships with key professionals, and particularly with professionals who recognize and work with their developing maturity, personal agency and potential contribution to their own care. They value timely information, advance planning and good communication and coordination between users and involved services. Both young people and their carers value the young person being regarded in the round, rather than within a narrow diagnostic framework – i.e. as individuals simultaneously negotiating developmental, educational, employment, housing and other social transitions in addition to service transitions [36–39].

While mental health professionals also value interservice communication and coordinated care [3, 38], there is rather more emphasis on organizational and structural concerns such as empowering and effective leadership, workforce stability and geographic proximity [40]. Concerns have also been expressed about who bears clinical responsibility during the transition process [38]. All are valid concerns, particularly at a time of ongoing major structural changes and financial limitations in the NHS. What will be important in future service development is that services do indeed *'listen more'* to the views of users and carers [36, p. 638].

Yet, is such a potential co-construction of continuity sufficient for guiding future service development and delivery? Within child health, there is a recognized need for service models incorporating developmental continuity, i.e. going beyond meeting medical need to recognizing the accompanying psychosocial, educational and vocational needs of young people [41, 42]. This perspective recognizes continuity as, at least in part, *'managing the complex dynamics at work during the period of transition from child to adult care'* [5, p. 13]. This developmental focus has informed a variety of diagnostic specific child health transition services (see [43] for a review), and is influencing the development of some CAMHS–AMHS transition services.

Transition services

Guidelines for good practice   There is a plethora of complex legislation and policy documents that together form the basis of good practice guidelines. Useful summary guides for mental health professionals, public commissioners of CAMHS and AMHS services and service users/families are now available [44, 45]. Interestingly, these CAMHS guidelines concur with those suggested nationally and internationally for *all* children with chronic health needs (see [46] for a review).

Some of the guidelines are simply the obverse of impediments to optimal transitions already outlined, namely a need for forward planning and preparation of young people and their families for the service transfer; appropriate timing of transfer based on clinical or developmental need rather than age criteria; flexibility at service boundaries and individualized, person-centred transition pathways. As suggested earlier, 'standard' transition processes can be modified to meet the needs of particular groups, such as those with neurodevelopmental disorders – requiring the application of clinical understanding at the service interface.

Beyond this, particularly within the child health literature, recommendations incorporate an awareness of adolescent developmental trajectories, the lifestyle and psychosocial aspects of adolescence and the extent of adolescent maturity with respect to self-care.

Careful preparation for the differing service ethos and delivery of care models in adult services is desirable, as is the involvement of young people and their families in the design and delivery of transition services. Protocols, developed jointly between CAMHS and AMHS, outlining the process and standards for optimal transition are essential aspects of good practice – though, as research has already identified, these need to be implemented in practice.

Research demonstrating the deficiencies of the transition to AMHS for CAMHS users has thus been effective in generating guidelines for change and audit tools with which services can address transition difficulties. How has this impacted upon service delivery and development?

Some service models   The paucity of published literature makes it difficult to answer the above question. Occasional reports do appear, for instance Verity and Coates [47] describe a transition service for CAMHS leavers with ADHD. A 12-month follow-up comprises a diagnostic assessment, pharmacological treatment and medical assessment, with the frequency of appointments based on the young person's responses to the implementation or adjustment of medication. Perhaps reflecting the lack of multi-disciplinary resources available, none of the referrals into this service had comorbid diagnoses, as is so common in the CAMHS ADHD population, and the forward transition into AMHS is not described.

In a recent research/transition literature scoping exercise, McConachie and colleagues [32] found a complete absence of published service transition models for those with ASD. One brief service innovation report of a time-limited neurodevelopmental clinic for those with ADHD or ASD is described [48]. The authors note that the greatest limitation of this new service is the lack of adult service provision. Without such forward care pathways, there is a danger that these limited services may become 'holding' services until a crisis situation develops, or hoped for pathways into AMHS evolve at some stage.

An understanding of service developments, therefore, has to be derived from local knowledge or from 'good practice' examples presented by public or research bodies (see, e.g. [49]). Within the NHS, it is our experience that these can take a number of forms including, for example the appointment of 'key' personnel, such as 'transition workers' who have a responsibility for liaising with relevant adult services to ensure a smooth transition process; transition protocols developed jointly between CAMHS–AMHS, and transition 'handover' clinics involving staff from both CAMHS and AMHS. Here, young people and their families can meet AMHS professionals, and learn more about the service ethos and models of care they will encounter post transfer. These service practice components aimed at smoothing the transition process are not, of course, mutually exclusive.

NHS transition initiatives tend to focus on specific diagnostic groups, particularly those thought not to be benefitting from current AMHS, such as those with neurodevelopmental disorders. Other examples include forming a young people's service, for those aged 14–18 years, within an existing adult early intervention psychosis service to avoid early adolescent drop-out, or failure to utilize, mental health services [49]. Another nominated 'good practice' example can be found in Hackney, a disadvantaged area of inner London where an innovative service extends CAMHS type provision to 18–25 year olds referred into the new service by generic CAMHS [49]. An assertive outreach model includes features designed to engage those most likely to drop out of services, such as appointments in non-health settings, active follow-up by phone or text when appointments are missed, and flexible provision based on recognising that young people may prefer to dip in and out of services in a self-determined way. Interventions include direct work in a variety of therapeutic models; liaison and training with other agencies and CAMHS and AMHS.

In short, there are a variety of local initiatives that may be based on the creative use of current staff, new part-time joint adult–child service posts, or pilot services based on short-term funding. An awareness of a need to demonstrate cost-effectiveness, and continued funding concerns, seem commonplace.

Currently, service developments appear guided by a combination of national findings and audits of local need. National findings can highlight the groups, such as those with neurodevelopmental disorders, in need of AMHS, as well as good practice transition procedures that meet national policy directives. Local needs' analyses can highlight particular service gaps in the light of local service configurations and the resources needed to fill these. A potential disadvantage is that transition service provision may remain highly localized and variable both within and between NHS trusts, locally and nationally.

Whether and how such provision could become coherent at the national level is unclear, particularly given that the 'good practice' examples given above remain *the exception rather than the rule* [7, p. 84]. Much remains to be achieved, therefore, and at a time of funding constraints and major organizational change within the NHS.

Prevention and transition

A preventive focus seems to guide service development in this area – this may range from seeking to prevent service drop-out by disengaged youth to a hoped for prevention of adverse mental health outcomes stemming from lack of appropriate care. Even more broadly, some services for adolescents or young adults may also aim for psychosocial outcomes such as educational or training achievements, reduction in stigma, or functioning social networks. Yet, there is limited research on service transition outcomes. This is partly due to the early stage of practice developments and service models, and also perhaps that many local service initiatives are unlikely to meet research evaluation criteria such as the use of representative samples and control groups. Some care has to be taken, therefore, in advocating the 'best' ways forward.

There is, of course, the issue of exactly what outcome criteria should be – and whether we adopt definitions of continuity that both facilitate valid and reliable outcome measures and allow measurement of the outcomes we are interested in. If we take a narrow definition of continuity, then we could concentrate on the effectiveness of procedures and protocols at the point of transition. If we aim to provide continuity of care co-constructed by users and professionals, then their evaluations and inclusion are integral. If we want to evaluate whether conceptual models (e.g. of developmental trajectories on a variety of dimensions) are effectively transformed into coherent transition service models, then we are into a different set of outcome measures [46]. And beyond the point of transition between child–adult services are questions as to which services are best suited to young people whose complex profiles and adverse long-term psychosocial outcomes characterize many who will leave CAMHS without an appropriate AMHS service to transition into. Detailed answers to these questions are, of course, the focus of other chapters.

References

1. Singh SP, Paul M, Ford, T, et al. (2008). Transitions of care from child and adolescent mental health services to adult mental health services (TRACK study): a study of protocols in greater London. *BMC Health Services Research* **8**: 135.
2. Singh SP, Paul M, Ford T, et al. (2010). Process, outcome and experience of transition from child to adult mental healthcare: a multiperspective study. *The British Journal of Psychiatry* **197**: 305–312.
3. Singh SP, Paul, M, Islam, Z, et al. (2010). Transitions from CAMHS Adult Mental Health Services (TRACK): A Study of Service Organization, Policies, Process and User and Carer Perspectives Report for the National Institute for Health Research Service Delivery and Organization Programme January 2010.
4. Parker G, Corden A and Heaton J. (2009). Synthesis and conceptual analysis of the SDO Programme's research on continuity of care. Report for the National Institute for Health Research Service Delivery and Organisation programme HMSO 2009.

5. Forbes A, While, A and Ullman R. (2002). A multi-method review to identify components of practice which may promote continuity in the transition from child to adult care for young people with chronic illness or disability. Report for the National Co-ordinating Centre for NHS Service Delivery and Organization R & D (NCCSDO).

6. Department of Health (2004). National service framework for children, young people and maternity services.

7. Department of Health & Department for children schools and families (2008). Children and young people in mind: the final report of the National CAMHS Review.

8. Department of Health & Department for children schools and families (2007). A transition guide for all services.

9. Department for Children Schools and Families and Department of Health. (2008). Transition: Moving on Well. A Good Practice Guide for Health Professionals and their Partners on Transition Planning for Young People with Complex Health Needs or a Disability.

10. Department of Health (2010). 'Fulfilling and rewarding lives'. The strategy for adults with autism in England.

11. Lamb C, Hill D, Kelvin R and Van Beinum M. (2008). Working at the CAMHS/Adult Interface: Good Practice Guidance for the Provision of Psychiatric Services to Adolescents/Young Adults. A Joint Paper from the Interfaculty Working Group of the Child and Adolescent Faculty and the General and Community Faculty of the Royal College of Psychiatrists, May 2008. Royal College of Psychiatrists.

12. Haggerty JL, Reid RJ, Freeman GK, et al. (2003). Continuity of care: a multidisciplinary review. *British Medical Journal* **327**: 1219–1221.

13. Parker G, Corden A and Heaton J. (2011). Experiences of and influences on continuity of care for service users and carers: synthesis of evidence from a research programme. *Health and Social Care in the Community* **19**: 576–601.

14. Ford T, Goodman R and Meltze H. (2003). The British child and adolescent mental health survey 1999: the prevalence of DSM-IV disorders. *Journal American Academy Child Adolescent Psychiatry* **42**: 1203–1211.

15. Costello EJ, Angold A, Burns BJ, et al. (1996). The Great Smoky Mountains study of youth. Goals, design, methods, and the prevalence of DSM-III-R disorders. *Archives of General Psychiatry* **53**: 1129–1136.

16. The Mental Health of Children and Young People: A Framework for Promotion, Prevention and Care. (2005). The Scottish Executive, Edinburgh.

17. Department for Health Social Services and Public Safety, Northern Ireland (DHSSPSNI]. (2011). Service Framework for Mental Health and Wellbeing.

18. Sourander A, Multima, P, Nikolakaros G, et al. (2005). Childhood predictors of psychiatric disorders among boys: a prospective community-based follow-up study from age 8 years to early adulthood. *Journal of the American Academy of Child and Adolescent Psychiatry* **44**: 756–767.

19. Johnson JG, Cohen P and Kasen S. (2009). Minor depression during adolescence and mental health outcomes during adulthood. *The British Journal of Psychiatry* **195**: 264–265.

20. Copeland WE, Shanahan L, Costello J and Angold A. (2009). Childhood and adolescent psychiatric disorders as predictors of young adult disorders. *Archives of General Psychiatry* **66**: 764–772.

21. Kim-Cohen J, Caspi A, Moffitt TE, et al. (2003). Prior juvenile diagnoses in adults with mental disorder: developmental follow-back of a prospective-longitudinal cohort. *Archives of General Psychiatry* **60**: 709–717.

22. Nutt DJ, Fone K, Asherson P, et al. (2007). Evidence-based guidelines for management of attention-deficit/hyperactivity disorder in adolescents in transition to adult services and in adults: recommendations from the British Association for Psychopharmacology. *Journal of Psychopharmacology* **21**: 10–41.

23. Gledhill J and Hodes M. (2011). Depression and suicidal behaviour in children and adolescents. In: D Skuse, H Bruce, L Dowdney and D Mrazek (eds), *Child Psychology and Psychiatry Frameworks for Practice*, 2nd edition, Wiley-Blackwell.
24. Wagner M and Newman L. (2012). Longitudinal transition outcomes of youth with emotional disturbances. *Psychiatric Rehabilitation Journal* **35**: 199–208.
25. Pottick KJ, Bilder S, Vander Steop A, et al. (2008). US Patterns of mental health service utilization for transition-age youth and young adults. *The Journal of Behavioral Health Services & Research* **35**: 373–389.
26. Davis M and Sondheimer DL. (2005). State child mental health efforts to support youth in transition to adulthood. *The Journal of Behavioral Health Services & Research* **32**(1): 27–42.
27. Repper J, Nolan M, Grant G, et al. (2008). Family Carers on the Margins: Experiences of Assessment in Mental Health Care. Report to the National Coordinating Centre for NHS Service Delivery and Organization R & D (NCCSDO) NCCSDO 2008.
28. Winston A, Paul M and Juanola-Borrat Y. (2012). The same but different? Treatment of anorexia nervosa in adolescents and adults. *European Eating Disorders Review* **20**: 89–93.
29. Arcelus J, Bouman WP and Morgan JF. (2008). Treating young people with eating disorders: transition from child mental health to specialist adult eating disorders services. *European Eating Disorders Review* **16**: 30–36.
30. Treasure J, Schmidt U and Hugo P. (2005). Mind the gap: service transition and interface problems for patients with eating disorders. *The British Journal of Psychiatry* **187**: 398–400.
31. Gray B, Robinson C, Seddon D and Roberts A. (2008). 'Confidentiality smokescreens' and carers for people with mental health problems: the perspectives of professionals. *Health and Social Care in the Community* **16**: 378–387.
32. McConachie H, Hoole S and Le Couteur AS. (2011). Improving mental health transitions for young people with autism spectrum disorder. *Child: Care, Health and Development*, **37**: 764–766.
33. Moncrieff J and Timimi S. (2010). Is ADHD a valid diagnosis in adults? No. *British Medical Journal* **340**: c547.
34. McCarthy S, Asherson P, Coghill D, et al. (2009). Attention-deficit hyperactivity disorder: treatment discontinuation in adolescents and young adults. *The British Journal of Psychiatry* **194**: 273–277.
35. Munoz-Solamando A, Townley M and Williams R. (2010). Improving transitions for young people who move from child and adolescent mental health services to mental health services for adults: lessons from research and young people's and practitioners' experiences. *Current Opinion in Psychiatry* **23**: 311–317.
36. Rees Jones I, Ahmed N, Catty J, et al. (2009). Illness careers and continuity of care in mental health services: a qualitative study of service users and carers. *Social Science Medicine* **69**: 632–639.
37. Doug M, Adi Y, Williams J, et al. (2011). Transition to adult services for children and young people with palliative care needs: a systematic review. *Archives of Disease in Childhood* **96**: 78–84.
38. Hovish K, Weaver, T, Islam Z, et al. (2012). Transition experiences of mental health service users, parents, and professionals in the United Kingdom: a qualitative study. *Psychiatric Rehabilitation Journal* **3**: 251–257.
39. Lester H, Khan N, Jones P, et al. (2012). Services users' views of moving on from early intervention services for psychosis: a longitudinal qualitative study in primary care. *British Journal of General Practice* **62**: e183–e190.
40. Belling R, Whittock, M, McLaren S, et al. (2011). Achieving continuity of care: facilitators and barriers in community mental health teams. *Implementation Science* **6**: 23.
41. While A, Forbes A, Ullman R, et al. (2005). Good practices that address continuity during transition from child to adult care: synthesis of the evidence. *Child: Care, Health and Development*, **30**: 439–452.

42. Viner RM. (2008). Transition of care from paediatric to adult services: one part of improved services for adolescents. *Archives of Disease in Childhood* **93**: 160–163.
43. Crowley R, Wolfe I, Lock K, et al. (2011). Improving the transition between paediatric and adult healthcare: a systematic review. *Archives of Disease in Childhood* **96**: 548–553.
44. Child and Maternal Health Observatory (ChiMat) – CAMHS Transitions, http://www.chimat .org.uk/camhs/transitions (accessed 26 May 2014).
45. Young Minds CAMHS Transition Guides. (2011), http://www.youngminds.org.uk/about/our_ campaigns/transitions
46. Watson R, Parr JR, Joyce C, et al. (2011). Models of transitional care for young people with complex health needs: a scoping review. *Child: Care, Health and Development* **37**: 780–791.
47. Verity R and Coates J. (2007). Service innovation: transitional attention-deficit hyperactivity disorder clinic. *Psychiatric Bulletin* **31**: 99–100.
48. Fung NK. (2007). Transitional services for neuro-developmental disorders. *Psychiatric Bulletin* **31**: 272.
49. Sainsbury M and Goldman R. (2011). Mental health service transitions for young people. Social Care Institute for Excellence, http://www.scie.org.uk/publications/guides/guide44/files/ guide44.pdf

9
Adults of Working Age

Karl Marlowe

East London NHS Foundation Trust, London, England, UK

Why bother with adult preventative medicine?

The majority of those with enduring mental health disorders present for the first time to both primary care and secondary care services as adults. Therefore early intervention in mental health does not mean intervention at an early age, but intervention early in a patient's care pathway, even before a diagnosis is clear. However, the current secondary mental health systems do not facilitate this with high thresholds jealously guarding a limited capacity. This may make every day practical sense, but the paradigm shift of this book argues that specialist mental health consideration is needed at an earlier developmental stage of a diagnosis. This would lead to both improvement in health outcomes and a benefit to the wider health economy. This chapter will focus on early intervention (EI) at the earliest stages and also on mental health promotion, which can be seen at a general population level to promote mental well-being and happiness.

This chapter will also explore the basis of this new paradigm and how EI services fit within the wider provision of adult mental health services. The current threshold for accessing secondary care adult mental services often requires a diagnosis *and* significant disability. We need to contrast this to mental health services for adolescents, where a presentation of symptom and distress is usually sufficient to receive specialist input. This thinking incorporates secondary prevention with the focus of treatment and intervention at the early developmental stage of a mental disorder. Secondary prevention detects those with a discernible disorder, decreases the duration of symptomatic distress and thereby reduces functional decline due to ongoing active pathology.

The development of preventative medicine for mental health has been recognised by governments across Scandinavia, Australasia and in the United Kingdom. In the United Kingdom, the Department of Health published a mental health strategy policy in 2011

Early Intervention in Psychiatry: EI of nearly everything for better mental health, First Edition.
Edited by Peter Byrne and Alan Rosen.
© 2014 John Wiley & Sons, Ltd. Published 2014 by John Wiley & Sons, Ltd.

'*No Health Without Mental Health: a cross-government mental health outcomes strategy for people of all ages*' [1]. It notes:

- most mental disorders develop in childhood

- three-quarters of mental health problems first present by the mid-20s

- there is a need to improve the support for early detection and intervention for offenders

- there should be a parity with physical health care in the way mental health patients are treated ('parity of esteem')

- Improving Access to Psychological Therapies (IAPT) needs to be available nationally

- there is a need to promote mental health and well-being and prevent mental illness (this aim is further defined by an emphasis on public health developments, and the development of a mental well-being measure for the nation).

So as government policy drives change, those working in mental health services need to change practice at the front line.

Why mental illness prevention, now?

'*The Anatomy of Melancholy*' published by Robert Burton 1621, which was based on earlier medical teaching from Persia and Greece, made reference to mental illness prevention [2]. Burton pointed out that melancholia (black bile) in excess leads to a specific course of illness through one's life, while noting that it could also be a force of creativity. There was however a suggested way to prevent the associated disease in this case, with the advice of '*be not solitary, be not idle*'. This can be seen as a very important contemporary feature of primary prevention for mental illness and continues to be advice for mental well-being of behavioural activation and reducing social isolation. It is also interesting to note that, historically, disease of mind and body has had an interrelation within preventative medicine, and this is still fully incorporated in traditional Chinese medicine.

In recent decades, the drivers for preventative medicine in mental health for adults have come from a focus in the early identification of those with a schizophrenia illness. The last decade has seen a proliferation of EI services for psychosis right across the globe, and in the United Kingdom these services have been incorporated into the National Institute for Health and Care Excellence's (NICE) recommendations for psychotic illnesses including bipolar affective disorder (psychosis). The supportive evidence ranges from an economic benefit, service user satisfaction and carer satisfaction, to hard evidence of a decrease in the morbidity on quality of life and the impact of each relapse. The plethora of research papers on EI services in psychosis has led to many centres incorporating strategies for the early detection of mental illness rather than being specific to the diagnosis of schizophrenia. Services have started focusing on young adults and those at a wider risk of psychosis diagnoses. There is the recognition that the life transition from adolescence to adulthood has inherent stress-vulnerability and services can help navigate the young person through this life stage. It is noted that the individualisation of breaking from one's family, the financial and emotional independence, the first relationships' break up, all need to be felt and internalised to lead to future mental health resilience.

In addition, wealth creation and gross domestic product (GDP) do not lead to improved mental and physical health across a population. This is reflected in the rising prevalence in obesity, diabetes and depression in the developed and the developing world. The argument is for the development of national prevention programmes, rather than just fund end-stage disease treatment when the patient is economically unproductive. In the United Kingdom there are several government initiatives to improve the mental health capital of the adult population. This economic imperative has directly led to improved primary care access for psychological therapies (IAPT), with an increase in thousands of cognitive behavioural therapists nationally. Having easy access to CBT in primary care is argued to have an economic benefit to society, as well as to the individual's quality of life, with less people on financial benefits and more people in work. This programme is expected to pay for itself over a lifetime via a decrease in unemployment benefits and increased productivity of the working population.

What is happiness and well-being anyway?

Over the last two decades of individualism, with success measured in wealth, there has been a social movement towards well-being, which is different from the scientific epidemiological models of disease. Well-being is a rather catch-all phrase which includes someone's satisfaction in their work–life balance, or self-definitions of success. This can be seen as a personal shift in modern priorities away from the previous generations' definitions of success, e.g. marriage, children, a car, a secure job. How many of us satisfy that description? A life well lived, having a social network, having physical health, reaching one's potential. These are some of the British philosopher's Alain de Botton's agents of happiness as opposed to competition with one's neighbours. He was also the founder of 'The School of Life' in London and has shown that there is a demand from many young adults who are seeking an understanding of their happiness and have a desire to build a preventative strategy from future mental illness. It is noted that the stigma associated with seeking well-being at facilities such as *The School of Life*, which are not overtly a mental health clinic, is less than the stigma that is generally associated with adult mental health services and being seen by a psychiatrist.

A more scientific stance is taken by Seligman in the book, '*Flourish – A Visionary New Understanding of Happiness and Wellbeing*' (2011) [3]. His seminal works have included the theories of *learned helplessness* in the 1960s and that of positive psychology in the 1990s. In '*Flourish*', there are very practical ways to achieve happiness with the headlines being: engagement, positive emotions, positive relationships, meaning and accomplishment. There is a need for social connection to other people's experiences as well as appraisal of what failure is and the internal settings of mental discontent. This book has been on international best sellers' lists and show that there is a rare, unexpected demand from the public for mental health promotion and the understanding of mental well-being.

The first country to measure gross national happiness (GNH) as well as gross domestic product (GDP) is the Himalayan Kingdom of Bhutan. They will not be unique as the UK government has now developed a national happiness and well-being measure. We can see that any work on prevention of mental illness needs to start with an understanding of happiness and well-being, as this fits within the primary prevention strategy for mental health. By reporting and measuring happiness and well-being there is an opportunity to affect future mental health outcomes. This is also an area for adult mental health services to consider even in the absence of diagnosable mental disorder.

What is EI in adult mental health services?

The implementation of prevention for mental illness has been impaired by the difficulty in the definitions of '*Mental Health*' and '*Prevention*'. These terms are defined by the absence of illness, but for mental illness prevention this is too simplistic. The above discussion of happiness and well-being did not lend itself neatly to the practical day-to-day work for those working in adult mental health services. In these services, mental illness is seen as disorders with a specific diagnosis, but in reality are across a continuum of mental health symptoms. The concept of prevention of mental illnesses does not easily fit with much of the illnesses seen in the mental health clinics or in the hospital wards. For example the concept of prevention may fit for a patient presenting with Korsakoff's dementia (related to Vitamin B deficiency and chronic alcohol dependency), but for most patients with diagnoses, such as schizophrenia, there is no clear link to aetiology. The worst outcome, suicide, is not specifically linked to a diagnosis or a single aetiology, but despite the sociological and environmental context, it still comes under the general heading of mental illness. Conceptually using the diagnosis to focus on the aetiology does not lead to an easy prevention strategy in most mental illnesses presenting in adulthood.

In the previous chapters, there was a full description of the transition from adolescence to adult services and it can be seen why diagnosis is an issue. The barrier to receiving care from adult services, after the input from adolescent mental health services, often lies at the difference between symptom presentation and diagnosis. Adult mental health services offer ongoing input based on a diagnostic or aetiological basis whilst child and adolescent mental health services (CAMHS) are based on symptoms as part of a developmental life course. Three-quarters of adults with a mental illness first present to services for help before the age of 24. Therefore a preventative mental health service needs to consider that the early symptoms at early detection do not attract a clear diagnostic label. It is at this point of first presentation at help seeking point and with nonspecific symptoms, when the services need to intervene. This would require the prevention services to have a rapid, flexible and low threshold access to referral, assessment and intervention. There have been services developed in Australia, for such a wide symptom presentation. These are called *youth platforms* with an aim for early detection and intervention of mental illness across a large population, age range and geography, and overcome the transition and diagnosis barrier.

The NHS in England and Wales aims to transform health services into health promotion services that can be succinctly summed up with the policy '*No Health Without Mental Health*'. There is a need for parity in mental health commissioning, service esteem and understanding akin to that with physical health services for adults. Physical health presentation can have a mental illness unrecognised and untreated, while those with mental illness often have their physical illness untreated. For example a person with schizophrenia illness dies with a physical health condition 25 years earlier than the general population [1]. Physical health professionals need to gain good mental health literacy, while the mental health services need to see physical health outcomes as part of their remit. For this to be achieved, EI and prevention of adult mental illness has to be everyone's business in the health and social sectors. As well as the statuary health services, physical and mental well-being strategies need to include local government, employers, educational establishments, and the third sector nonstatutory organisations.

Further to diagnosis and physical symptom presentation, a perception which blocks service initiatives in mental illness prevention is that these services are seen to be far too expensive. It does not take a harsh economic climate for this cost-benefit argument to require careful consideration. The Department of Health in the United Kingdom analysed the economic modes for several EI services in the paper, '*Mental Health Promotion & Mental Illness Prevention-the Economic Case*' (2011) [4]. This paper describes a range of services and provides evidence for commissioners. The services are discussed in more detail with the full cost-benefit analysis in the earlier sections of this book. In summary, the evidence for many services provided across the age groups, for example from dementia to early detection for psychosis, is of clear cost effectiveness. On the other hand some services were not cost effective, for example universal health visiting to detect and intervene in postnatal depression (despite an improvement in quality of life for the mothers in the first year). For a £1 investment, the total return for early detection for psychosis was £10, for alcohol screening by primary care it was £11, for EI for psychosis it was £17, for training GPs to better detect suicide it was a £43, and for putting up suicide barriers on bridges it was £54. The school programmes to intervene before conduct disorder develops by the age of 5, there was a future saving in adulthood of up to £83 for each £1 invested, with large saving in both the criminal justice system and for the national health service (NHS). Looking critically at the methodology, and despite there being several flawed assumptions, there is nevertheless face validity in the economic argument for mental illness prevention. There are adult mental illness prevention services in other countries (Canada, Ireland, Australia) where the economic argument is not made to justify them.

Principles of EI services for adults

Age and gender are important in mental health promotion and for EI services. For example the suicide rate in England has wide variations based on age group and gender. It is greatest for younger men and middle-aged women. In addition to this, men are known to see their doctors less frequently than women. So for an EI suicide strategy for men there would need to be a differential care pathway for assessment as one of the EI service principles. The public health preventative strategies are influenced by the age and gender needs of the population. The principles of EI services include the influence of social media, primary care professional's awareness of illness, and public education, in relation to age and gender of the targeted population.

The third focus for any EI service would be to incorporate easily accessible care pathways, for example telephone help lines for suicide prevention. The principle of easy access and multiple referral sources has been adopted in the operation of the improved access to psychological therapy services and in mental health court diversion/probation services. See Table 9.1 for a list of the EI service principles. The ease of access to services also requires consideration of the referral process, geographic settings and the service's opening times.

Table 9.1 Principles of EI services

Principle 1	Specific gender consideration for the intervention and outcomes
Principle 2	Specific age group consideration for communication and needs
Principle 3	Easy referral and access for professional assessment
Principle 4	Comorbidity does not impede access to care e.g. substances use
Principle 5	Staging/phasing of the disorder relevant to intervention offered

Comorbidity is common in adults presenting to adult mental health services and it is extremely important when considering EI and prevention at the first contact. Exclusion from adult EI services should not occur due to substance misuse. For example increased cannabis and alcohol use are both aetiological factors for mental illness, while an early age of first use of cannabis increases the risk of a later development of a schizophrenic illness. For depression, life events are a significant vulnerability and are associated with substance misuse. For women presenting to maternity services with comorbid substance misuse, early access to psychiatric perinatal services is recommended. Also, pregnancy is commonly associated with the development of mental health problems and mental illness. For these women contact with both antenatal and postnatal health professionals could ease access to mental health professionals at a very early stage. This is especially relevant in the United Kingdom, where suicide is the leading cause of maternal deaths in the first year after birth. An EI principle is that comorbidity should not be a barrier to the referral and access to mental health services.

The EI principles of *staging* allow different interventions to be offered dependent on the stages of an illness. Identifying phases or stages of a mental illness can reduce the iatrogenic toxic effects of an intervention. By having an analogous schizophrenia phase to cancer staging can decrease the pessimism and stigma, while also indicating how radical the intervention should be (see Table 9.2). The ethical consideration of false positives can be discussed within the context that not all those at ultrahigh risk will develop a disorder, and that nonspecific symptoms are a good enough reason to have a check-up with mental health professionals. EI services for schizophrenia have had an impact of interest in mental health diagnostic services, especially at an early detection level and there is renewed interest in a prodrome diagnosis. The recent development in EI services has been in primary prevention (e.g. indicative prevention for those at ultrahigh risk of developing schizophrenia illness). There are now reliable tools in primary prevention of schizophrenia, for example the Structured Interview For prodromal syndromes (SIPS/SOPS) criteria [5]. This has led to a primary prevention intervention for those at risk by recommending fish oils, decreasing cannabis use, receiving of cognitive behavioural therapy or general

Table 9.2 Cancer staging analogous to schizophrenia phases after McGorry (2006)

Cancer Staging	Schizophrenia Phases
Pre-cancer	Prodrome and ultrahigh risk
Stage 1	Acute with a short duration of untreated psychosis
Stage 2	Residual symptoms with partial recovery
Stage 3	Chronic symptoms with functional impairment

psycho-supportive intervention. The staging principle of schizophrenia phases has also demonstrated a cost-benefit, with more engaged patients during the intervention and early help-seekers at the onset stage of the disorder.

How to do EI for adults

Adult preventative mental health services need to focus on neglected populations such as homeless people, offenders, those with multiple comorbidities, medically unexplained symptoms and those who are help seeking without a diagnosable mental disorder. There is a need for services to be provided for those seeking reassurance. This includes people with a genetic risk associated with a family member having mental illness, despite the individual being asymptomatic. Table 9.3 demonstrates the large numbers of adults affected by mental illness and at risk of developing an illness. This requires public health measures and social marketing to target those hard to reach as well as mental health professionals who might be the first port of call early in the development of an illness. The 'how to do' can be taken from some of the specific services described in Section 4 of this book, but it is hoped that the following descriptions whet the appetite of how services can be developed across different populations and disease profiles.

The earlier description of preventive strategies narrows from a population level to an at-risk population, but an adult preventative service has to also have a theoretical conceptualisation. This is based on aetiology (e.g. risk groups), environmental risks (e.g. cannabis use and psychosis), theoretical prodrome with a critical period of intervention and is not the same as relying on a confirmed diagnosis. Examples can be found in Table 9.4, where schizophrenia and bipolar affective disorder are compared on a theoretical basis relevant to the development of the disorder. In this example the EI service for bipolar disorder would be provide over at least ten years, while for schizophrenia it may be half of this. Consideration of public health prevention strategies in Table 9.1 and the theoretical differences in Table 9.4 are required in making the EI service operational. The EI services would need the theoretical concept to not only detect those at risk (primary prevention), but also for intervention at a secondary and tertiary prevention level. Mental health disorders have a significant comorbidity with mood dysregulation, substance misuse, family dynamics, generalised low mood and occur within a social context. Even when specific mental disorders are the theoretical focus of the EI service, the barrier of no clear diagnosis should not impede early detection and mental health promotion. Nonspecific problems need to be recognised at first presentation for those seeking help, with a heightened index of suspicion from others at educational establishments, workplaces and at home by family members.

Table 9.3 Population prevalence of mental illness

1:3	Prisoners with mental health diagnosis
1:4	Population with mental health problems
1:20	Population with an anxiety disorder
1:20	Population with a depressive disorder
1:100	Population with a bipolar disorder
1:100	Population with a schizophrenia disorder

Table 9.4 Theoretic considerations for two specific disorders

	Schizophrenia	Bipolar Affective Disorder
Epidemiology	• 1% prevalence • First presentation <26 years old • NHS cost £960M/year	• Prevalence 0.5% BPAD I, 1% BPAD II • Onset age 15–20 years • NHS cost £199M/year
Aetiology	• Urbanicity associated • Stress-vulnerability model is inclusive of genetic vulnerability • Early cognitive-neurological markers	• Manic psychosis not urbanicity associated • BPAD I aggregate in families (6%) vs. general population (0.5%)
Prodrome	• Screening instrument to predict those at high risk for schizophrenia • A significant functional decline with attenuated psychotic symptoms	• Aged 10–17 years • Difficulty in thinking, compulsions, decreased concentration, tiredness, labile mood, physical agitation • First episode usually depression

What do EI Service for adults look like?

The aetiological concepts in the development of mental illness need to be considered by EI services in the early identification of mental disorders. The EI services seeing help-seekers also need to have a parallel service arm directed at the risk populations. It is in this area that an EI service to prevent mental illness needs to be familiar with concepts such as population segmentation and behavioural modification. Social marketing is a broad banner, which is used in public health planning to identify and communicate with those at highest risk. Social marketing is defined as the use of marketing techniques to produce public benefit and good. The techniques include communicating to the right segment of the population, the use of a mix of media to get a message across and for this to be recognised by the targeted population or individual, with a resulting action. The marketing research for the EI service needs to analyse behaviour change with the EI service principles. The most appropriate language, stigma or obstacles to accessing the service, the population awareness of risk and different explanations of illness, all need to be tackled as part of the social marketing process.

Social marketing has particular importance to ethnic minorities who are marginalised: they may have increased risk of illness, might not seek help until very late in the progression of illness, and might not be able to communicate in the host countries' language. New immigrants to developed countries have increased rates of psychosis and may be suspicious of the mainstream health services. There may be negative attitudes towards help seeking and mental illness, reinforced by social exclusion. Any communication or mental health literacy campaigns need to target this group using social marketing techniques. So before any EI service starts seeing patients it need to communicate in a shared language of at-risk, help-seeking, normalisation and general health promotion. Such multifocal campaigns to increase mental health literacy would be more effective than campaigns solely targeting GPs.

An ideal adult EI service encompasses the 16–25 year old high-risk age group, who are at the first stage of an illness. The adult EI services need to bridge and aid the navigation during this period of transition to adulthood. This can also be considered via a social marketing perspective, with information and media campaigns at college or university level, and noting that this population is part of a social network with a large peer group influence. The EI services need to use emails for self-referrals, website for general communication and tele-assessments for initial flexible screening. In considering this age group, the CAMHS and professional regulatory bodies accept that the adult mental health services have the skill to alleviate distress, promote well-being and to promote resilience. The adult and child services need to move away from the categorical services offered and develop shared expertise with adult EI services.

An open and flexible EI service care pathway for help-seekers is of contrast to routine adult mental health services, which mostly require primary care to gatekeep. The gatekeeper at a primary care level is based on cost and capacity considerations, but on a negative side leads to barriers for help-seeking with delays in referrals and delays in initial contact with mental health professionals. The cursory 15 minutes assessment with the General Practitioner does not allow for a full assessment of the early development of a mental illness. Therefore, adult EI services should offer joint assessment and shared care with primary care. It is expected that adult EI service would ultimately divert patients from future secondary care and from ongoing primary care input and be cost efficient in the medium to long term.

Example of a preventative adult EI service

An example of an adult EI service, which incorporated all the principles above, is the Tower Hamlets Early Detection Service (THEDS) in London for early detection of psychosis, www.theds.org.uk. This service was developed via stakeholder consultation with third sector providers, commissioners, service users and carers as well as statutory mental health services. THEDS has a social marketing process with a mixed media campaign and ongoing research to correctly identify and communicate with the at-risk populations. The service offers a full assessment over a 3-month period to all those referred, and 2 year of case management for those identified as being at ultrahigh risk for schizophrenia. The marketing campaign has included advertisements in local fast food shops, phone boxes, in benefits' offices and in local newspapers with articles written by THEDS' service users. See Figure 9.1 for an example of a local bus stop poster from the social marketing campaign and also used in local newspaper adverts. The help-seekers were also able to self-refer to THEDS via the website. The key to self referral was the messages focus on well-being and mental health promotion.

Future developments for adult EI services

Some of the most significant developments in the prevention of illness have been articulated via social marketing and behavioural economics. Thaler and Sunstein (2008) discusses the evidence for this in '*Nudge: Improving Decisions About Health, Wealth and Happiness*' [6]. There is the big issue that many people could be at risk of an illness and a relatively small change in their behaviour could be preventative. **There does not have to be the identification of illness for preventative behaviour to have benefit in that illness' domain.** Nudges do not necessitate a government, health care system or indeed a well

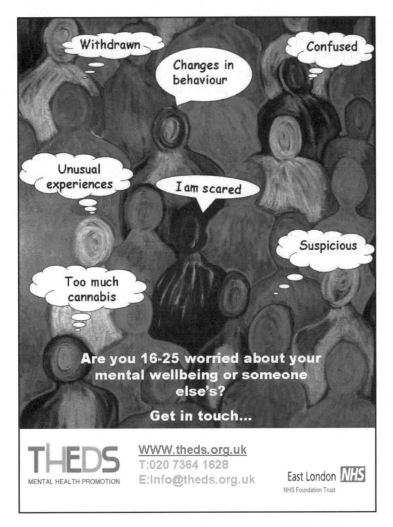

Figure 9.1 THEDS bus stop poster and newspaper advert. From an original painting courtesy of Janine Hodges & Karl Marlowe

meaning mental health professional being paternalistic telling a person not to do a high risk behaviour. We can enable social capital (which is social networks and shared values) to provide information to direct the behavioural changes for health benefit. For example in road safety, while crossing a road, there is a sign stating '*look right*', but individuals do not necessarily have to look at that sign, it is not coercive and allows choice. The result of the sign is that there is both public and individual benefit. Adult EI services need to continually develop messages and signs to influence behaviour for the prevention of mental illness.

The United Kingdom's NICE had as its focus the most effective treatments of illness. But is now issuing guidelines for menus, food labelling and lifestyle choices which directly affect physical and mental health. This preventative role for public health is expected to broaden as more evidence for the benefit of prevention becomes available. The advice to do exercise, which is well known to have a range of health benefit, is not coercive and is within paternal liberalism principles. However, there are areas relevant to EI for legislation to be part of public health strategy. In the case of smoking bans in all public places, this was introduced despite being unpopular and is now adopted in many countries with a significant population health improvement outcome. Health policy acknowledges that health risks are the government's responsibility, but there is a move towards greater individual personal responsibility.

Connecting the principles of public health medicine to the EI service principles (Table 9.1), and incorporating behavioural economics, will make EI practical for the wider population's better mental health.

References

1. Department of Health. (2011). No Health Without Mental Health: a cross-government mental health outcomes strategy for people of all ages'. COI, Crown, UK.
2. Burton R. The Anatomy of Melancholy, Introduction Gass W. (2001). The New York Review of Books, NY 10019.
3. Seligman M. (2011). *Flourish – A Visionary New Understanding of Happiness and Wellbeing.* Free Press: NY 10020.
4. Department of Health. (2011). *'Mental Health Promotion & Mental Illness Prevention-the Economic Case'.* M Knapp, D McDaid, M Parsonage (eds). UK: Crown.
5. McGlashan T, Walsh B and Woods S. (2010). Structured Interview For Prodromal Syndrome (Version 5). Prime Research Clinic, Yale School of Medicine New Haven, Connecticut, USA.
6. Thaler RH and Sunstein CR. (2008). *Nudge: Improving Decisions About Health, Wealth and Happiness.* New Haven and London: Yale University Press.

10

Early Intervention in Older Adults – A Focus on Alzheimer's Dementia

Brian Lawlor[1] and Celia O'Hare[2]

[1] Mercer's Institute for Research on Ageing; Trinity College Dublin; St Patrick's and St James's Hospitals, Dublin, Ireland
[2] The Irish Longitudinal Study on Ageing (TILDA), Department of Medical Gerontology, Trinity College Dublin, Ireland

Early intervention in the elderly, for those unfamiliar with the speciality of old age psychiatry, may appear to be a contradiction in terms. The parallels with the early intervention movement in psychosis are many. It is notable, for example that the Kraepelinian term 'dementia praecox' has been proposed as typifying the therapeutic nihilism endemic in the once accepted clinical approach to psychosis. Similarly, the raison d'être for an early intervention movement in geriatric psychiatry could be reaction to the current pervading view that brain failure is an inevitable consequence of the ageing process. It thus appears that the same seismic shifts in youth mental health as heralded by Pat McGorry and his contemporaries are coming to old age psychiatry [1].

It is, of course, the seismic shifts in population trends that have given a new urgency to the search for better ways to diagnose and treat the common mental health problems of later life. If the population of those over the age of 65 continues to increase in line with current demographic trends, so too will the prevalence of all age-related mental health problems [2]. It is, however, in no small part what some see as the impending 'dementia emergency' that has crystallised research efforts and siphoned public funding.

At the time of writing, the best estimates indicate that there are over 5 million people living with dementia in the USA [3]. In 30 years time it is predicted that this figure will have trebled. Governments around the world are finally taking note of such seemingly

Early Intervention in Psychiatry: EI of nearly everything for better mental health, First Edition.
Edited by Peter Byrne and Alan Rosen.
© 2014 John Wiley & Sons, Ltd. Published 2014 by John Wiley & Sons, Ltd.

apocalyptic predictions and top heavy demographic charts, where the proportion of younger generations is so graphically dwindling; the bottom pillars seem to shrink beneath the weight of this potential future burden. In the UK the 'Dementia Strategy' has highlighted the key targets of early diagnosis along with changes to both public and professional attitudes to dementia and its treatment [4].

The economic arguments

The current economic cost of dementia is estimated to be 1% of global GDP [5]. In 2010, the World Alzheimer's Association estimated that if dementia were a country it would be the world's eighteenth largest economy. In no other fatal illness would a diagnosis rate of 30% be tolerated yet this is the current standard in the UK [6]. Unfortunately however, even when a diagnosis does come, it is often when the illness is already advanced; too late to prevent harm and crises [4].

There are persuasive economic arguments in favour of early diagnosis and intervention. It is reported that despite significant upfront investments to establish early intervention services, these will quickly prove cost effective [7]. Early intervention in older adults makes sound fiscal policy, in particular given its potential to delay institutionalisation – perhaps the most prescient outcome in older adults.

Moving towards a staging model
'Symptomatic' Alzheimer's disease (AD)

As we have seen, in our current system even those with frank dementia may struggle to achieve a diagnosis. Whereas in specialist centres the accurate diagnosis of dementia is reported as above 90% [8], the patient presenting to their GP may still fail to be referred for further specialist assessment, let alone receive an accurate diagnosis. Such is the discrepancy between the pace of research and the standard of care most of our patients can expect, even the symptomatic treatments which are available remain out of reach for most patients. As is widely noted, until the advent of a disease-modifying treatment many nonspecialists may be reluctant to diagnose a terminal neurodegenerative disorder [9]. It is critical therefore to translate recent leaps in knowledge not only into a source of empowerment and optimism for patients and carers, but also into concrete changes to the care received by some of our most vulnerable patients.

Making a better, earlier diagnosis

In 2011, diagnostic guidelines which had remained fit for purpose since 1984 were finally revised to reflect new understandings gleaned from the intervening decades of research [10]. Now the diagnostic criteria for mild cognitive impairment (MCI) and AD incorporate 'biological markers', or biomarkers, although these remain outside of current standard clinical practice and remain a source of debate. Some, for example consider that the temporal ordering of biomarkers needs to be more convincingly determined [11].

The amyloid hypothesis remains the most accepted understanding of the neuropathological changes leading to AD. The theory posits that once the toxic amyloid-beta (Aβ)

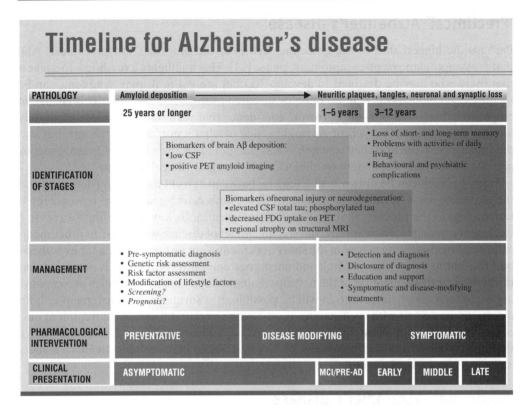

Figure 10.1 Timeline for Alzheimer's disease

peptide begins to aggregate, a cascade of events is triggered that produces the classical phenotype of AD [12]. Biomarkers now in use, and most of those in development, are each considered to reflect different points in the underlying pathophysiology.

As demonstrated in Figure 10.1, five AD biomarkers are currently considered sufficiently robust to be included in the new guidelines. These can be separated into two distinct categories; the major biomarkers of brain Aβ deposition (low cerebrospinal fluid (*CSF*) Aβ42 and positive *positron emission tomography* [PET] amyloid imaging) and the biomarkers of neuronal injury or neurodegeneration (elevated CSF total tau and phosphorylated tau, decreased *fluorodeoxyglucose* [FDG] uptake on PET in the temporoparietal cortex and regional atrophy on structural MRI).

To definitively determine if these biomarkers accurately reflect the temporal progression of the disease, longitudinal studies spanning 30–40 years would in theory be required [13]. In the absence of such data it can only be assumed that the biomarkers drawn from individuals at different clinical stages represent the changes along the continuum of the disease. Based on such models, change in CSF Aβ is proposed as the earliest available marker – correlating best with the asymptomatic phase. The markers of neuronal injury occur later and tally better with changes in cognitive function.

The clinical implications of the availability of such data are immense – we may soon be in a position to estimate time to clinical onset of symptoms and thus perhaps identify those in whom therapeutic interventions should be targeted.

'Preclinical' Alzheimer's disease

Perhaps the biggest shift in the guidelines comes in the proposals for 'preclinical' AD, that is asymptomatic or presymptomatic phase [14]. This highlights a readiness to suggest that those who may be destined to develop AD but are yet to display symptoms can be identified via biomarkers – albeit only for research purposes at this time. This change in emphasis is based not only on a growing confidence that such biomarkers can accurately identify those who have levels of amyloid outside of what is normal for their age, but also the imperative to ensure that research is less hampered by the effects of heterogeneous cohorts often overly dependent on subjective reports and clinical acumen.

Many parallels can be drawn, and often are, between current thinking on dementia and the pervading view of cancer 40 years ago. These days carcinoma '*in situ*' is an accepted terminology – the preclinical stage at which intervention is key and definitive curative treatment is possible. Increasingly, the staging model of disease so familiar to other medical specialities is gaining favour in the study of dementia not just as a schema for hypothesis building but to invigorate research and encourage early intervention. It is proposed that through accurate delineation of the neuropathological and cognitive features accompanying each stage, timely intervention will be possible. It is surmised that movement in both directions may occur with such staging also helping to accurately evaluate treatment outcome. The beckoning biomarkers will make AD diagnosis easier and faster, and ensure that disease-modifying treatments can be targeted where they are most likely to make a difference – prior to the symptomatic phase.

'Prodromal' Alzheimer's disease

At present, those with amnestic MCI (considered by many to be the symptomatic 'prodromal' phase of AD intervening between asymptomatic and overt dementia) are the target intervention group of choice. Studies consistently show a substantial yearly rate of transition from MCI to AD [15]. The ethical considerations of trialling novel treatments in this group (who in a research paradigm are also likely to demonstrate more than one positive putative biomarker) may seem simple. There are however many remaining questions: why for example do some people transition back to normal functioning and still others never convert [16]? Thus the ethics of treating those with an, as yet, ill-defined clinical trajectory should not be underestimated. As discussed in more detail below, flaws in the trial design and diagnostic variation across centres are again thought to account for at least some of these discrepancies. The foremost current clinical indication for biomarkers however, may indeed be in the MCI phase, and despite such apparent anomalies, research indicates that those with the clinical syndrome of MCI together with a positive Aβ biomarker and a positive biomarker of neuronal injury are the most likely to have underlying AD neurodegeneration with only a relatively short time before progression to dementia occurs.

Intervening in Alzheimer's disease – *a life course perspective*

Genetic risk

Each of us is born with a specific genetically determined risk profile for many diseases including genes that will help to determine our personal cognitive trajectory. AD genetic risk can be broadly divided into autosomal dominant mutations (encoding for 'familial' AD which classically presents before the age of 65) and genes which increase risk for the sporadic form of the disorder. The best defined of the latter is apolipoprotein E (APOE); two copies of the ε4 allele will increase risk while having the ε2 allele decreases risk for future AD [17]. As with most psychiatric disorders many other genes are implicated to a lesser extent and it is surmised that despite an inherent genetic risk profile it is ultimately gene–environment interactions which determine expression of the AD phenotype [18]; an underlying heterogeneity of genetic risk combined with an ever varying array of lifestyle exposures and idiosyncratic responses.

Those with familial forms of AD have a predictable age at which clinical symptoms will become apparent. Researchers evaluating biomarkers in probands of varying ages were able to distinguish a pattern of gradual accumulation of the hallmark features of AD. Studies following those with the autosomal dominant forms of AD, suggest that the characteristic pathological brain changes in this group begin much earlier than previously thought – most likely decades prior to a formal diagnosis with AD [19].

Cognitive testing has also proven sensitive in small cohorts in discriminating those with hereditary forms of AD from sporadic and normal ageing cohorts. Impairment in 'shape colour binding' has been posited as a possible specific early cognitive marker of AD [20].

Targeting the genes that code for the abnormal proteins may be the earliest intervention point feasible. Stem cell therapy and therapies targeting epigenetic mechanisms may make this possible in the future, although none have as yet progressed to clinical stage trials [21].

Although studying those with the genetically determined form of AD undoubtedly adds to our overall knowledge and understanding of AD, to extrapolate these findings to the sporadic cases of AD (which make up over 95% of cases) may be unsound.

Indeed not all genetic mutations necessarily confer an increased risk of AD; recent exciting research from Iceland has identified a rare mutation in amyloid-β precursor protein (APP) which is in fact protective against AD [22]. It is present in approximately 0.5% of the Icelandic population and has a similar prevalence in the other Scandinavian countries. It appears that this mutation reduces build up of amyloid in the brain (demonstrating a 40% reduction in the formation of amyloidogenic peptides in *in vitro* models) leading to improved cognitive outcomes – not just a reduced incidence of AD but also improved resilience to the cognitive decline associated with normal ageing.

Normal ageing

Studies charting the course of normal age-related cognitive change suggest that the initial changes may begin as early as the third or fourth decade – with a peak in cognitive performance around 20 years followed thereafter by a slow but inevitable decline [23]. Indeed it is suggested that up to 50% of the age-related decline in cognitive ability that occurs before 90 years is already established by the age of 60.

Epidemiological observational studies which point to universal age-related decrements have sparked headlines with their findings, as the decline once seen as the reserve of the decrepit moves perilously close to the rest of us [24]. Sensitive cognitive testing as administered in the Whitehall cohort studies following thousands of British civil servants, detected significant decline between the beginning of testing when a person was in their thirties and follow-up 10 years later. What triggers such decline and how it starts remains unknown. Thus discerning normal ageing from the subtle early pathological processes of AD is difficult (never more so than with the MMSE – which is the extent of the cognitive testing with which most clinicians are familiar). What we do know however is that undoubtedly the biggest risk factor for pathological decline in cognition is increasing age [25].

No cognitive health without physical health and social integration?

The fallacy of the mind–body dichotomy is laid bare in the latter decades as the brain and mind are revealed as one as we age. Early intervention in older adult mental health spans not just conventional psychiatric expertise but necessitates cross disciplinary input, for example in cardiovascular and cerebrovascular health, while equally requiring a knowledge and understanding of the social implications of ageing.

Following individuals who manage to resist functional decline despite the aggregates of normal ageing and ever increasing risk of AD pathology may provide an insight into ways to maintain cognitive health in the ageing population. Although at present interventions at population level cannot yet be recommended, research points to a number of key lifestyle factors that may interact with genetic predisposition to increase individual risk – as we often highlight to our own service users in the Mercers Institute (see Box 10.1: Seven Secrets). Specifically, increased levels of physical activity [26] and better social integration [27] are associated with a lower incidence of dementia. Furthermore research indicates that working to maintain the emotional and social network of people as they age is likely to reap rewards beyond better mental well-being towards helping to maintain cognitive health and independence [28].

Primary prevention

As psychiatrists we are well versed in risk. Stroke risk and ischemic heart disease risk are arguably more readily assessed, and indeed managed, than any other type of risk in a psychiatric population. Here, perhaps the role of the psychiatrist is as physician first is to acknowledge and manage these prime targets for possible primary prevention. Be that alone or with the support of the patient's primary care physician or geriatrician. The path to a healthy heart may also lead to a healthy brain. Research points to mid-life hypertension, obesity, smoking and diabetes as potentially sowing the seeds for AD in later life [29]. There is substantial overlap between AD and cerebrovascualar disease. Cerebral hypoperfusion resulting from ischaemia and cerebrovascular disease may accelerate accumulation of amyloid thus potentially playing a pivotal role in the pathogenesis of AD [30], indeed elevated levels of microinfarction are a consistent finding at autopsy in individuals with AD [31].

Secondary prevention

Secondary prevention may be promoted by an increased awareness of physical 'frailty' – no longer simply an imprecise clinical impression in geriatric medicine but an increasingly well-defined phenotype [32]. Indeed the proposed underlying mechanisms leading to physical frailty have much in common with those mentioned in this chapter in relation to

AD – from oxidative stress to cardiovascular risk. Autopsy studies have also revealed significantly elevated levels of AD neuropathology in those with the highest levels of frailty close to death – leading some to further argue a common underlying pathophysiology [33]. Again it is unclear which precedes which but intervening in either the physical or cognitive domain may have knock-on benefits in overall function.

Tertiary prevention

Keeping physical function in mind once symptomatic AD is established is also particularly important. Optimisation of physical health is likely to help maintain function, quality of life and delay institutionalisation, as well as lessen carer burden [34].

Cognitive reserve – a lifetime in the learning?

Just as with cancer, the ever elusive cure may simply reflect individual complexity [35]. Thus the parallels with oncology continue as the definitive AD treatment is unlikely to be a 'one solution fits all'. Multifactorial origins will likely mean complex multifaceted treatments are required just as the course of a malignancy and the response to treatment is rarely readily predictable. Explanations for such variation range from associated environmental risks to a person's personality and positivity. Such diverse explanations are also mooted for the variations observed in the clinical presentation of AD. Two people – one of whom in life lived with dementia, the other who remained independent and self-reliant, may display equivalent levels of plaque and neurofibrillary tangles at post mortem [36]. This may be a sobering thought for those for whom biomarkers are the panacea in the judicious targeting of treatment.

Cognitive reserve has been highlighted as one explanation for such variation [37]. Those whom in life remained well despite potentially pathological levels of neurodegenerative changes have been found to have higher levels of education, to have been more socially engaged and quite simply to have had larger brains. It is suggested that such factors enable the brain to cope with greater levels of AD pathology for a longer period of time, meaning that the individual may be more adept at enlisting compensatory mechanisms to maintain function. Thus the question of the ethical implications of identifying those who may be at risk of AD with cumulative positive biomarkers but who in their lifetime may never in fact develop AD.

Disease-modifying drugs: battling the slings and arrows of outrageous fortune

Currently there are no disease-modifying agents available for AD. The results of prior trial treatments aimed at cure remain disappointing for the millions of people living with dementia and their families. Some failures are attributed to targeting the disease process too late in the sequence of neuropathological change [38]. The case for early diagnosis may thus be made from a dual perspective – if the neuropathological processes are to be identified early enough to intervene, diagnosis must be made early. Here we discuss just some of the past disappointments and still newer agents hopeful of future success.

Anti-amyloid approaches

The majority of AD therapeutic strategies aim to reduce the accumulation of amyloid. The amyloid theory however has its detractors who can readily cite the failure of multiple preclinical successes to translate to the human phase trials. Even when there has been a reduction in the amyloid burden there has not always been amelioration in cognition. In the amyloid cascade hypothesis, Aβ plays an upstream and pivotal role in the pathogenesis of the disease. Two proteases β-secretase and γ-secretase which act on APP in a sequential manner to produce Aβ42, have long been considered prime targets for drug development [39].

A phase III trial which involved the compound Semagacestat that targeted γ-secretase was stopped prematurely due to significant decrements in cognitive function in the treatment group and poor selectivity of the compound (including inhibition of the systemically active Notch enzyme – with an associated increased incidence of skin cancer in the treatment group).

A Europe-wide multicentre phase III clinical trial is currently underway to assess the efficacy of Nilvadipine. This antihypertensive (a 1,4-dihydropyridine L-type calcium channel blocker) reduced the risk of developing AD in large population-based observational studies [40]. Nilvadipine has since been shown to be well tolerated and to stabilize cognition, albeit as yet in small cohorts [41, 42]. Rather than simply being a selective anti-amyloid approach, transgenic mouse models hint at an ability to hit many of the hypothesised pressure points: blood flow, anti-amyloid, anti-tau and anti-inflammatory [43]. This multimodal mechanism of action is in some ways analogous to clozapine in schizophrenia, indeed perhaps just as clozapine can lead to improvements in refractory psychosis via numerous receptor pathways, Nilvadipine may work especially well in late-onset AD given that there are likely many overlapping pathologies at work.

Targeting the immune response

Inflammation is known to accompany the neuropathological processes of AD – whether this is a consequence or a driver of the disease is yet to be determined. Many remain proponents of the pivotal role of an abnormal neuroinflammatory response despite the failure of trials involving anti-inflammatory compounds. With epidemiological evidence pointing to a 50% reduction in incidence of AD in those with chronic NSAID use, again it is considered that anti-inflammatory agents may need to be trialled earlier to have an impact [44].

Immunisation – harnessing the immune response rather than preventing it – in theory is capable of targeting production, aggregation and deposition of amyloid [45]. A tantalising trio of the most pursued anti-amyloid mechanisms of actions. This therapeutic strategy however has been disappointing – including recent results from trials involving the compound Bapineuzumab and another monoclonal antibody, Solanezumab which failed to live up to the promise of earlier phase studies. Subanalysis of the effects on those with milder forms of AD however, does suggest some cognitive improvement – perhaps adding wind to the sails of the early interventionists [46].

The year 2013 sees the possibility of three trials commencing in asymptomatic individuals, finally truly putting the early intervention hypothesis to test [46]. The best known of these will use the compound Crenezumab (again a monoclonal antibody) in approximately 300 *pre*symptomatic members of a Colombian family each of whom has a dominantly inherited form of early-onset AD. This trial is set to last 5 years.

Tau late?

Strategies targeting tau, which is widely accepted to be a process downstream of Aβ accumulation is another possible modifiable part of the amyloid hypothesis. Tau may therefore represent the intervention point of choice in those in whom clinical features are already manifested. Two possible therapeutic compounds include lithium and methylthioninium chloride, thought to act by inhibition of tau phosphorylation and aggregation respectively [45].

The future
Improving research in Alzheimer's disease

Both therapeutic and observational AD trials to date have had numerous widely cited limitations. Principle among these perhaps, is the heterogeneity of cohorts where participant selection has been necessarily reliant on subjective report and consensus-based clinical diagnosis [35]. Furthermore, the move towards multisite trials has brought with it the problems of variation in training, instrumentation and analysis. Biomarkers may now help dictate selection of participants for both disease-modifying clinical trials and longitudinal observational studies.

Research has also been hampered by lack of a definitive animal model. The advent of recombinant DNA and the discovery of the genes coding for dominantly inherited AD lead to the production of murine models of AD and Aβ accumulation. Critics suggest that this is not an accurate reflection of the human neuropathology – mice do not live long enough to naturally develop AD and the levels of amyloid present in murine models far outweigh those produced in the human brain [47]. This may explain why findings in basic science have not been replicated in humans.

For some, improving the quality of research is not enough – the scope must also be broadened. It has been proposed that there is a need to think beyond the accepted confines of the amyloid hypothesis in order to find new therapeutic targets and accompanying therapeutic success. Herrup, for example envisages a weakened neuron which has been made vulnerable via ageing and an 'initiating injury', be that head trauma or less well-defined insults such as depression or grief [25]. Such theories may explain why specific psychiatric diagnoses have been suggested to relate intimately to cognitive decline, in some cases representing perhaps the earliest indicators of dementia and transition from MCI. Inevitably, such 'injuries' accumulate over one's lifetime thus increasing risk of AD.

Ethical considerations

The ethical implications of identifying individuals at risk for AD but not currently displaying symptoms, is leading to significant ethical and moral debate in the internationally recognised leading research centres focused on AD [48]. In a recently published study focusing on familial forms of AD with specific genetic mutations (cited previously in this chapter), no information regarding the participant's carrier status was given [19]. Furthermore, the published results were carefully screened so as to prevent inadvertent identification of participants.

The results of any test confirming AD risk has of course potentially huge implications, particularly in the ongoing absence of successful disease-modifying therapies and the lack of clear delineation of the prognostic implications of presumptive biomarkers [49]. Communicating such uncertainty to patients, their families, friends, and potentially their insurance companies is laden with potentially life-altering repercussions.

Despite clear ethical pitfalls, the overarching goal remains ethically sound: to improve the diagnosis and treatment of AD, a debilitating, terminal neurodegenerative disorder set to reach epidemic proportions. Attaining this goal is closer than ever before. As the detection of the early stages of the disease becomes feasible in a standard clinical setting there will be ever greater opportunity for therapeutic intervention – to delay progression and perhaps even to arrest the disease process in its tracks.

Futurology

With recent research indicating that cognitive decline begins as early as the third decade, the need for further collaboration with colleagues specialising in mid-life mental health (and potentially even younger) is greater than ever before. It is imperative for all those working in every mental health discipline to increase their knowledge of the key concepts of maintaining cognitive and mental health throughout life.

While we await the next bold therapeutic strategy in AD, be that lifelong prevention or late-onset cure, it is incumbent upon all of those working in the field to view each novel investigative and treatment modality with cautionary optimism. Staging and early intervention in AD will help prepare the patient and their family for the next steps, allow informed choice, increase hope and perhaps eventually enable every patient not just to live well with Alzheimer's disease, but potentially never to develop Alzheimer's *dementia* at all.

Box 10.1   *Seven Secrets on How to Keep Yourself Mentally Sharp*

Although we may not yet be in a position to provide a clear programme for primary prevention, based on the evidence that is available, we present our 'top tips' on how to empower each patient to maintain their emotional and cognitive health as they age.

1. Exercise: 30 minutes of exercise, five times per week can improve brain function and keep you sharp

2. Mental stimulation: doing crosswords, Sudoku can improve mental sharpness

3. Exposing yourself to new experiences: reading, art, music theatre can enrich your brain connections

4. Social engagement: keeping active with people and organizations outside the home has been proven to improve your life expectancy and may protect brain cells

5. Reduce stress if possible: relaxation and meditation can increase control and lower stress. Stress is bad for your brain and your memory

6. A good diet: eat fruit, dark vegetable and fish if you can as there may be a protective effect for your brain

7. Think young: do not focus on your age and what you cannot do. Think young and focus on what you can do!

© Mercer's Institute for Successful Ageing, Hospital 4 Top Floor, St. James's Hospital, Dublin 8

References

1. McGorry PD, Killackey E and Yung A. (2008). Early intervention in psychosis: concepts, evidence and future directions. *World Psychiatry* **7**: 148–156.
2. Connolly M. (2012). Futurology and mental health services: are we ready for the demographic transition? *The Psychiatrist* **36**: 161–164.
3. Alzheimer's Association. (2012). 2012 Alzheimer's disease facts and figures. *Alzheimer's & Dementia: The Journal of the Alzheimer's Association* **8**: 131–168.
4. Banerjee S. (2010). Living well with dementia—development of the national dementia strategy for England. *International Journal of Geriatric Psychiatry* **25**: 917–922.
5. Wimo A and Prince MJ. (2010). *World Alzheimer Report 2010: The Global Economic Impact of Dementia*. Alzheimer's Disease International.
6. Sanchez N. Dramatic variation in dementia diagnosis across UK. http://www.alzheimers.org.uk/site/scripts/news_article.php?newsID=1463
7. Getsios D, Blume S, Ishak KJ, Maclaine G and Hernández L. (2012). An economic evaluation of early assessment for Alzheimer's disease in the United Kingdom. *Alzheimer's & Dementia: The Journal of the Alzheimer's Association* **8**: 22–30.
8. Snowden JS, Thompson JC, Stopford CL, et al. (2011). The clinical diagnosis of early-onset dementias: Diagnostic accuracy and clinicopathological relationships. *Brain* **134**: 2478–2492.
9. Ahmad S, Orrell M, Iliffe S and Gracie A. (2010). GPs' attitudes, awareness, and practice regarding early diagnosis of dementia. *British Journal of General Practice* **60**: e360–e365.
10. Albert MS, DeKosky ST, Dickson D, et al. (2011). The diagnosis of mild cognitive impairment due to Alzheimer's disease: recommendations from the National Institute on Aging-Alzheimer's Association workgroups on diagnostic guidelines for Alzheimer's disease. *Alzheimer's & Dementia: The Journal of the Alzheimer's Association* **7**: 270–279.
11. Glodzik L, Galvin J, Pirraglia E and de Leon M. (2012). Ordering of Alzheimer disease biomarkers. *Archives of Neurology* **69**: 414; author reply 414–415.
12. Hardy J and Allsop D. (1991). Amyloid deposition as the central event in the aetiology of Alzheimer's disease. *Trends in Pharmacological Sciences* **12**: 383–388.
13. Jack CR Jr, Vemuri P, Wiste HJ, et al. (2011). Evidence for ordering of Alzheimer disease biomarkers. *Archives of Neurology* **68**: 1526–1535.
14. Sperling RA, Aisen PS, Beckett LA, et al. (2011). Toward defining the preclinical stages of Alzheimer's disease: recommendations from the National Institute on Aging-Alzheimer's Association workgroups on diagnostic guidelines for Alzheimer's disease. *Alzheimer's & Dementia: The Journal of the Alzheimer's Association* **7**: 280–292.

15. Hughes TF, Snitz BE and Ganguli M. (2011). Should mild cognitive impairment be subtyped? *Current Opinion in Psychiatry* **24**: 237–242.

16. Koepsell TD and Monsell SE. (2012). Reversion from mild cognitive impairment to normal or near-normal cognition: risk factors and prognosis. *Neurology* **79**: 1591–1598.

17. Jack CR Jr. (2012). Alzheimer disease: new concepts on its neurobiology and the clinical role imaging will play. *Radiology* **263**: 344–361.

18. Chandra V and Pandav R. (1998). Gene-environment interaction in Alzheimer's disease: a potential role for cholesterol. *Neuroepidemiology* **17**: 225–232.

19. Bateman RJ, Xiong C, Benzinger TL, et al.; Dominantly Inherited Alzheimer Network. (2012). Clinical and biomarker changes in dominantly inherited Alzheimer's disease. *New England Journal of Medicine* http://www.nejm.org/doi/full/10.1056/NEJMoa1202753

20. Parra MA, Sala SD, Abrahams S, et al. (2011). Specific deficit of colour-colour short-term memory binding in sporadic and familial Alzheimer's disease. *Neuropsychologia* **49**: 1943–1952.

21. Caraci F, Leggio GM, Drago F and Salomone S. (2012). Epigenetic drugs for Alzheimer's Disease: hopes and challenges. *British Journal of Clinical Pharmacology* **75**: 1154–1155. doi:10.1111/j.1365-2125.2012.04443.x

22. Jonsson T, Atwal JK, Steinberg S, et al. (2012). A mutation in APP protects against Alzheimer's disease and age-related cognitive decline. *Nature* **488**: 96–99.

23. Salthouse TA. (2009). When does age-related cognitive decline begin? *Neurobiology of Aging* **30**: 507–514.

24. Singh-Manoux A, Kivimaki M, Glymour MM, et al. (2012). Timing of onset of cognitive decline: results from Whitehall II prospective cohort study. *BMJ* **344**: d7622.

25. Herrup K. (2010). Reimagining Alzheimer's disease — an age-based hypothesis. *Journal of Neuroscience* **30**: 16755–16762.

26. Rovio S, Kåreholt I, Helkala EL, et al. (2005). Leisure-time physical activity at midlife and the risk of dementia and Alzheimer's disease. *The Lancet Neurology* **4**: 705–711.

27. Cacioppo JT and Hawkley LC. (2009). Perceived social isolation and cognition. *Trends in Cognitive Sciences* **13**: 447–454.

28. Wilson RS, Krueger KR, Arnold SE, et al. (2007). Loneliness and risk of Alzheimer disease. *Archives of General Psychiatry* **64**: 234–240.

29. Fratiglioni L, Winblad B and von Strauss E. (2007). Prevention of Alzheimer's disease and dementia. Major findings from the Kungsholmen Project. *Physiology and Behaviour* **92**: 98–104.

30. Okamoto Y, Yamamoto T, Kalaria RN, et al. (2012). Cerebral hypoperfusion accelerates cerebral amyloid angiopathy and promotes cortical microinfarcts. *Acta Neuropathologica* **123**: 381–394.

31. Sonnen JA, Larson EB, Crane PK, et al. (2007). Pathological correlates of dementia in a longitudinal, population-based sample of aging. *Annals of Neurology* **62**: 406–413.

32. Fried LP, Tangen CM, Walston J, et al. (2001). Frailty in older adults: evidence for a phenotype. *The Journals of Gerontology Series A: Biological Sciences and Medical Sciences* **56**: M146–M157.

33. Buchman AS, Schneider JA, Leurgans S and Bennett DA. (2008): Physical frailty in older persons is associated with Alzheimer disease pathology. *Neurology* **71**: 499–504.

34. Mhaoláin AMN, Gallagher D, Crosby L, et al. (2012). Frailty and quality of life for people with Alzheimer's dementia and mild cognitive impairment. *American Journal of Alzheimer's Disease and Other Dementias* **27**: 48–54.

35. Hampel H. (2012). Current insights into the pathophysiology of Alzheimer's disease: selecting targets for early therapeutic intervention. *International Psychogeriatrics* **24** (Suppl 1): S10–17.

36. Knopman DS, Parisi JE, Salviati A, et al. (2003). Neuropathology of cognitively normal elderly. *Journal of Neuropathology & Experimental Neurology* **62**: 1087–1095.

37. Singh-Manoux A, Marmot MG, Glymour M, et al. (2011). Does cognitive reserve shape cognitive decline? *Annals of Neurology* **70**: 296–304.

38. Karran E, Mercken M and De Strooper B. (2011). The amyloid cascade hypothesis for Alzheimer's disease: an appraisal for the development of therapeutics. *Nature Reviews Drug Discovery* **10**: 698–712.

39. De Strooper B, Vassar R and Golde T. (2010). The secretases: enzymes with therapeutic potential in Alzheimer disease. *Nature Reviews. Neurology* **6**: 99–107.

40. Khachaturian AS, Zandi PP, Lyketsos CG, et al. (2006). Antihypertensive medication use and incident Alzheimer disease: the Cache County Study. *Archives of Neurology* **63**: 686–692.

41. Kennelly S, Abdullah L, Kenny RA, et al. (2012). Apolipoprotein E genotype-specific short-term cognitive benefits of treatment with the antihypertensive nilvadipine in Alzheimer's patients—an open-label trial. *International Journal of Geriatric Psychiatry* **27**: 415–422.

42. Kennelly SP, Abdullah L, Paris D, et al. (2011). Demonstration of safety in Alzheimer's patients for intervention with an anti-hypertensive drug Nilvadipine: results from a 6-week open label study. *International Journal of Geriatric Psychiatry* **26**: 1038–1045.

43. Mullan M, Bachmeier C, Ait-Ghezala G, et al. (2011). Mechanism of action of new Alzheimer's therapeutic in phase III clinical trials. *Alzheimer's & Dementia: The Journal of the Alzheimer's Association* **7**: e61.

44. Gorelick PB. (2010). Role of inflammation in cognitive impairment: results of observational epidemiological studies and clinical trials. *Annals of New York Academy of Sciences* **1207**: 155–162.

45. Salomone S, Caraci F, Leggio GM, Fedotova J and Drago F. (2012). New pharmacological strategies for treatment of Alzheimer's disease: focus on disease modifying drugs. *British Journal of Clinical Pharmacology* **73**: 504–517.

46. Callaway E. (2012). Alzheimer's drugs take a new tack. *Nature* **489**: 13–14.

47. Marchesi VT. (2012). Alzheimer's disease 2012: the great amyloid gamble. *American Journal of Pathology* **180**: 1762–1767.

48. Naylor MD, Karlawish JH, Arnold SE, et al. (2012). Advancing Alzheimer's disease diagnosis, treatment, and care: recommendations from the Ware Invitational Summit. *Alzheimer's & Dementia: The Journal of the Alzheimer's Association* **8**: 445–452.

49. Peters KR, Lynn Beattie B, Feldman HH and Illes J. (2013). A conceptual framework and ethics analysis for prevention trials of Alzheimer disease. *Progress in Neurobiology*. doi:10.1016/j.pneurobio.2012.12.001

III
Early Intervention in Specific Settings

11

Primary Prevention of Mental Disorders

Inge Petersen[1], Arvin Bhana[1], Crick Lund[2] and Helen Herrman[3]

[1]School of Applied Human Sciences, Howard College, University of KwaZulu-Natal, Durban, South Africa
[2]Department of Psychiatry and Mental Health, University of Cape Town, Rondebosch, Cape Town, South Africa
[3]Collaborating Centre for Mental Health, University of Melbourne, Parkville, Melbourne, Victoria, Australia

Introduction

In the context of the growing burden of mental disorders, there is increasing concern over the cost and capacity of societies worldwide to provide treatment services. Increasing evidence of the effectiveness of mental disorder prevention, as well as economic evaluation studies showing a substantial return on investment, particularly for interventions early in the lifespan [1, 2], make the case for increased investment in prevention of mental disorders.

Using an integrated measure of disability adjusted life-years (DALYs)[1] which combines years lived with disability (YLD) with years of life lost (YLL), the Global Burden of Disease (GBD) Report 2004 indicates that neuropsychiatric disorders account for 13% of the GBD. The burden varies according to country income levels, accounting for 25% of the total burden in high-income countries, 16.6% in middle-income countries and 8.8% in low-income countries [3]. Globally, unipolar depression is the third leading overall burden and the leading burden amongst women (15–44 years). It is predicted to rise to the overall leading GBD by 2030 [4].

---

[1] DALYs combines years lived with disability (YLD) with years of life lost (YLL).

Early Intervention in Psychiatry: EI of nearly everything for better mental health, First Edition.
Edited by Peter Byrne and Alan Rosen.
© 2014 John Wiley & Sons, Ltd. Published 2014 by John Wiley & Sons, Ltd.

Definition of primary prevention

The *prevention* of mental disorders follows the public health understanding of prevention, occurring at three levels, namely, primary, secondary and tertiary [5]. *Primary prevention* aims to reduce the onset of mental disorders, thus reducing incidence. Secondary and tertiary prevention do not reduce incidence, but seek to lower the prevalence of established cases. *Secondary prevention* is concerned with early detection and treatment of mental disorders and *tertiary prevention* aims to reduce relapse and disability as well as enhance rehabilitation and morbidity. Secondary and tertiary prevention thus do not aim to reduce incidence, but together with primary prevention and treatment, share the common goal of reducing the burden of mental disorders [6].

Mental health *promotion* overlaps with primary prevention and is essentially concerned with promoting optimal mental and behavioural health and psycho-physiological development [7, 8]. Both mental health promotion and primary prevention aim to reduce risk factors for mental ill health as well as strengthen protective factors for mental well-being. They are thus interrelated. Promoting mental health may have an effect on reducing the incidence of mental disorders, as positive mental health is protective against mental disorders. Mental disorder prevention may use mental health promotion strategies. Both concepts may thus be present in the same intervention, but have different and complementary outcomes [9].

The scope of this chapter is limited to *primary* prevention, although the relationship between mental health promotion, the different levels of prevention and with treatment is often blurred. For example, treatment of depression in adults may prevent the onset of mental disorders in their children, and treatment of childhood depression can help to prevent depression in adulthood [6].

Primary prevention interventions can be universal, selective or indicated. *Universal* interventions target the whole population, with the assumption that the intervention is likely to benefit the entire population. *Selective* interventions target individuals or groups whose risk of developing a mental disorder is elevated as a result of biological, social or psychological risk factors. *Indicated* prevention programmes target individuals having preclinical minimum but detectable signs of mental illness that do not warrant a diagnosis of a mental disorder. Selective and indicated interventions are likely to show more focused benefits, given the elevated risk among the target groups for the development of disorders. Gordon [10] understands primary prevention as being aimed at people who do not show any suffering, discomfort or disability from the disorder to be prevented. Consequently, it has been suggested that indicated primary prevention overlaps with secondary prevention or early intervention for symptoms that may be part of the initial or prodromal phase of a disorder [11]. The importance of indicated prevention is, however, underscored by findings that the longer the duration of a disorder, the more difficult it is to treat [12]. Thus, even if it is considered early intervention, indicated prevention is likely to have better outcomes than delayed treatment.

Primary prevention interventions are essentially concerned with reducing risk and strengthening protective factors for the development of mental disorders. Risk factors refer to conditions that increase the probability of onset of a mental disorder, as well as greater severity and duration of the disorder. By contrast, protective factors serve to improve a person's resilience to risk factors through modifying, mediating, ameliorating or altering conditions to promote more adaptive responses to environmental stressors [13].

Recent evidence from advances in developmental neuroscience

The recent surge in evidence from developmental neuroscience and life course development and epidemiological studies provide evidence of malleable social and environmental risk factors that are associated with the development of mental disorders.

While family and gene association studies have demonstrated a genetic susceptibility to mental disorders, such as autism, schizophrenia, addiction and bipolar disorder; evidence from advances in developmental neuroscience indicate that the onset of most mental disorders is determined by an interaction of multiple interacting genetic and environmental factors as well as life experiences. The impact of environmental factors and life experience on the development of a mental disorder is mediated by genetic vulnerability. In turn, the impact of genetic vulnerability is mediated by environmental factors and life experiences [6].

Developmental neuroscience also provides biological evidence of, *inter alia*: (i) The neural plasticity of the human brain – how physiological processes, environmental factors and life experiences affect basic neurodevelopmental processes such as neuronal migration, synaptogenesis, synaptic pruning and myelination, all of which can effect neurocognitive and socio-emotional functioning; (ii) The epigenetic modification of genes to the environment that has enduring effects and can even be transmitted to the next generation. Early exposure to stress, for example, can result in epigenetic modifications in a person's stress response which influences reactivity to stress later in life; and (iii) There are also sensitive periods in brain development where environmental influences can affect specific developmental processes. The most sensitive period is during prenatal development and infancy, although plasticity does persist into adulthood. In adults, this is thought to underpin the mechanisms by which the brain can compensate or recover from a mental disorder. For example, through cognitive reappraisal, adults can improve self-regulatory control of thoughts, emotions and behaviour, learning to reassign different emotional labels to stimuli that previously evoked unpleasant emotions. This is a technique used in cognitive behavioural therapy (CBT), commonly used to treat anxiety and depressive disorders in adolescents and adults [6].

These advances in developmental neuroscience, together with epidemiological and life course development studies, have resulted in an emerging body of evidence that highlights specific opportunities for strengthening protective factors and reducing risk factors at critical developmental stages when the effect of such interventions are likely to be most beneficial.

The emerging evidence on the role played by social determinants (discussed in the Section 'Risk factors for mental disorders across the lifespan') and their interaction with genetic influences in the onset of mental disorders suggests that mental disorders can be prevented by reducing environmental risk factors and negative life experiences and enhancing protective factors. Given particular developmental vulnerabilities across the lifespan, the need for a developmental approach which is sensitive to this is indicated. The multifaceted nature of risk influences also demands a multifaceted response. This supports the adoption of an *ecological developmental* approach such as that provided by Bronfenbrenner [14] three decades ago.

An ecological developmental approach

An ecological developmental approach provides a framework for addressing the multiple risk and protective factors that interact in the development of mental disorders, as well as being sensitive to particular developmental vulnerabilities associated with lifespan development. As indicated in the Section 'Recent evidence from advances in developmental neuroscience', the most sensitive period in the life of a human being is during prenatal development and infancy. Environmental exposure and life experiences during this period lay the foundation for future development and well-being. The preschool years (3–5 years), middle childhood (6–12 years) and adolescence are all associated with specific developmental vulnerabilities that interact with environmental factors and life experiences to affect the development of adult competencies, which in turn can impact on the development and health of the next generation.

As indicated, risk and protective factors for the development of mental disorders are also multifaceted. They range from individual level factors, that include genetic influences, personality and physical health; proximal interpersonal and immediate factors related to family, peer, school and community factors; to more distal factors related to societal structural and cultural factors, that provide the context for exposure to environmental influences and life experiences. Mental ill health generally results from the interplay of multiple risk factors within the context of a paucity of protective factors, having a cumulative effect on the development of mental disorders.

In view of the emerging evidence on social determinants of mental disorders, there is a need for distal societal and population level interventions to reduce risk factors that result from upstream social determinants. These include gender and socio-economic policies that promote inequities resulting in marginalized populations being more vulnerable to risk factors for mental disorders. Addressing distal gender and economic policy level factors are key public health endeavours that overlap with many initiatives aimed at combating socio-economic inequities and promoting human and socio-economic development globally. They are not unique to the prevention of mental disorders.

In the main, interventions that are unique to the prevention of mental disorders operate at the individual and proximal levels, strengthening protective factors to moderate or mediate the impact of risk factors, building resilience in the face of exposure to risk. With moderation, the outcome of exposure to a risk factor is moderated by protective factors that interact with a risk factor. For example, a supportive warm relationship with an existing caregiver can moderate the impact of loss of an attachment figure in a child's life. With respect to mediation, the effect of a protective factor operates independently from a risk factor, compensating for the negative outcome of the risk factor. For example, the impact of early loss of a caregiver can be compensated for by the introduction of another attachment figure following the loss [6, 15]. The most successful examples of primary prevention programmes are those that target strengthening multiple protective factors. For example, a review of the determinants of family resilience in low- and middle-income countries

(LMICs) emphasised the dynamic transactions and relationships between the individual, the community and the dominant culture. Social support and community ties were noted to be particularly important in promoting resilience in LMICs [16].

Risk factors for mental disorders across the lifespan
Prenatal development and infancy

As indicated in the Section 'Recent evidence from advances in developmental neuroscience', developmental neural plasticity is most prominent during prenatal development and early infancy. During this period, the brain develops rapidly and environmental influences can affect basic neurodevelopmental processes such as neuronal migration, synaptogenesis, synaptic pruning and myelination. Together with epidemiological and life course studies, there is an emerging body of evidence on the impact of the following risk factors on these neurodevelopmental processes.

Prenatally, *micronutrient deficiencies*, especially low vitamin folic acid and iodine can affect brain development causing irreversible neurocognitive deficits [17, 18]. Vitamin folic acid deficiency has been associated with disorders in the formation of the neural tube [6]. Iron deficiency can also cause neurocognitive deficits and poor socio-emotional development in children [17, 18]. Epidemiological studies indicate increased risk of schizophrenia in children born during famines. This is thought to be a result of deprivation of essential micronutrients causing disruptions in brain development [19]. *Prenatal exposure to infectious diseases* such influenza, rubella and toxoplasmosis can also affect neural developmental processes increasing risk for mental retardation, schizophrenia and autism [6].

Prenatal and postnatal exposure to environmental toxins such as lead, arsenic, pesticides, tobacco smoke and alcohol also negatively affects the developing brain, placing the developing foetus and infant at risk for neurocognitive deficits. For example, alcohol prenatally can result in foetal alcohol syndrome (FAS) associated with facial anomalies, growth retardation and abnormalities in the central nervous system, which can cause neurocognitive and social deficits in children, as well as substance abuse in adulthood [20, 21]. Prenatal and postnatal exposure to lead and prenatal exposure to tobacco smoke can result in attention deficit and conduct disorder in school-going children [22, 23]. *Premature birth and low birth weight* are also risk factors for a number of disorders including schizophrenia, autism and learning disabilities [6]. Anoxia as a consequence of *birth trauma,* is associated with brain malfunction, which can cause a range of mental and physical disabilities [20].

Postnatally, the development of a secure attachment relationship between an infant and his/her caregiver is essential for healthy development [20]. *Disturbances in early infant–caregiver relationships* such as loss of primary attachment figures, caregiver depression, as well as abuse and neglect can result in disturbances in social and emotional development and interpersonal attachments later in life in the form of behavioural disorders, anxiety, depression and attention problems [20]. This is thought to be a result of the development of abnormalities in stress-response hormone production [6]. *Deprivation in cognitive and psychosocial stimulation during infancy* has also been found to be associated with cognitive and socio-emotional impairment [20]. The development of synapses or connections between neurons reaches its peak during infancy; the synapse being the primary site of information transfer in the nervous system. Cognitive and socio-emotional impairment during this period is thought to be as a result of synaptic pruning, whereby some synaptic connections that are unused as a result of lack of environmental stimulation are pruned. Given plasticity persists throughout childhood and adulthood, regeneration of neurons and synapses is possible, but is contingent on environmental stimulation [6].

Many of these risk factors during prenatal development and infancy are more prevalent in scarce-resourced contexts. Iron deficiency anaemia is widespread in LMICs, and associated with dietary deficiency as well as helminthic infestations, malaria and diarrheal disease [17]. A third of children in LMICs under the age of 5 years have stunted growth for their age, a measure of chronic under-nutrition [17]. LMICs also have a much higher rate of infectious diseases such as HIV/AIDS and malaria that can result in neurocognitive deficits if untreated [4]. Raised lead exposure affects about 40% of children in LMICs [17].

Childhood and adolescence

Preschool children (3–5 years) begin to start regulating their attention, emotions, motor behavior and cognitions, developing a sense of a distinct self-identity [20]. They begin to be exposed to influences beyond the family and the development of social relatedness and self-regulatory control, which form the building blocks for healthy cognitive and social competence, are important developmental tasks. Exposure to undue stress such as child maltreatment, family conflict/violence or parental loss/separation can interfere with the emerging self-regulatory processes, resulting in regressive behaviours such as bed-wetting and anxiety in preschool children.

In school-going children, these same undue stressors as well as bullying are also risk factors for behavioural disorders as well as anxiety and depression. In addition, preexisting neurocognitive and socio-emotional deficits can predispose school-going children to developing disruptive (conduct disorder, oppositional defiant disorder) and substance use disorders, through a cascading process. Upon entering school, high-risk children may experience social rejection, academic failure and conflict with teachers, leading to a defensive approach to dealing with the social world, and withdrawal from peers and school activities. Parental withdrawal may also occur, resulting in lower monitoring and control. As these children grow older they may also be at greater risk of gravitating toward deviant peer groups, which increases risk of antisocial behavior [24].

From a review of more than 50 community surveys worldwide published in the last 15 years, the National Research Council in the United States estimated that about 20% of children will have had at least one DSM-IV disorder in the past 3 months. Most prominent were any anxiety disorder (8%); [generalised anxiety disorder, separation anxiety disorder, social phobia, specific phobia, panic and post-traumatic stress disorder (PTSD)], unipolar depression (5.2%), any disruptive behaviour disorder (6.1%); (conduct disorder, and oppositional defiant disorder), and attention deficit hyperactivity disorder (ADHD) (4.5%) [6]. Comorbidity of disorders is widespread with clear patterns from early childhood. Externalizing disorders – ADHD, disruptive behaviour disorders and substance use disorders tend to co-occur (predominantly among males), while internalizing disorders – depression and anxiety disorders are often comorbid conditions (predominantly among females) [25].

Adulthood

Many adult mental disorders have their roots in genetic vulnerabilities and exposure to environmental risk influences and earlier negative life experiences. Twenty-five percent of adult mental disorders begin before the age of 8 years, and 50% by adolescence [26]. Prevention of many adult mental disorders thus requires interventions earlier in the lifespan.

There are, however, also a number of social risk factors that operate independently or interact with preexisting vulnerabilities in the onset of mental disorders. Evidence from a recent review of the social determinants of depression, which is more prevalent in young adults and females, indicates an association with gender inequity, stressful life events, including exposure to violence and other crimes, conflict and disasters; and chronic physical ill health. There are also increased rates of depression amongst low-socio-economic sectors of society and where there are high levels of income inequality [27]. Exposure to traumatic events has also been associated with PTSD, other anxiety disorders and substance abuse [27]. There is empirical support for certain poverty-related conditions being associated with common mental disorders (CMDs) in LMICs, namely, low education, food insecurity and financial stress [28]. While the precise causal relationships are difficult to establish, stress and stigma associated with low-socio-economic status as well as disempowerment, marginalization and lack of access to health services are some of the mechanisms hypothesized to increase risk for depression [27].

Work stress job strain resulting from high demand and low control as well as effort–reward imbalance, organizational injustice, undesirable work events, and bullying are also associated with increased risk for CMDs [29] as is job loss and unemployment [30]. Substance misuse, especially alcohol, is also associated with depression and shares many of the social determinants associated with depression [27].

Primary prevention interventions
Distal interventions

Distal interventions generally overlap with other public health efforts and socio-economic development initiatives. Evidence of the impact of such efforts on the prevention of mental disorders specifically is difficult to ascertain, given the lack of controlled trials. Evidence of risk factors for mental disorders do, however, indicate that the following interventions will ultimately have an impact on preventing mental disorders.

During prenatal development and infancy, reducing exposure to environmental risk factors such as toxins and micronutrient deficiencies during prenatal development and infancy and improving public health services to prevent/treat communicable diseases and improve obstetric health and prevent birth complications are indicated.

From childhood through to adulthood, many social and environmental risk factors aggregate in poorer communities. Policies to provide upgrading of infrastructure and services to these communities, particularly schools, recreational facilities, health and social services are thus important. In addition, alcohol and substance disorder legislation to limit and regulate access to alcohol; economic policies that promote greater socio-economic equality; labour policies promoting employment security and improved working conditions; and welfare policies that provide social protection to the sick, disabled and unemployed should have a positive impact across all ages and overlap with many poverty alleviation strategies [27].

Individual and proximal interventions

Documenting evidence for universal primary prevention interventions is constrained by the lack of statistical power, with very large numbers of subjects being required, particularly for disorders that have low incidence rates, although there have been some universal programmes that have produced fairly robust evidence (see Section 'Disruptive disorders'). Selective and indicated prevention interventions have, however, been shown to have better effect sizes [11, 12]. Other limitations include that the majority of prevention trials measure changes in protective factors or severity of symptoms. Very few measure whether interventions are capable of reducing the incidence of new cases [12].

There is, however, fairly robust evidence for the primary prevention of *disruptive disorders* (conduct disorder and oppositional defiant disorder) in children and *depression* in both children and adults. Depression poses a large burden on society, as noted in the introduction. Disruptive disorders, especially conduct disorders, also pose a large burden on society, particularly the criminal justice system. While investment in the prevention of conduct disorders in children may be borne by the educational and health and social care sectors; the return, is likely to accrue mostly to the criminal justice system [1]. We review briefly the evidence for both.

Disruptive disorders (conduct disorder, oppositional defiant disorder)   Prevention of the development of disruptive disorders has been extensively studied in relation to both home-based and school-based programmes. On the home front, the focus has been on strengthening protective home environments and parent training to create positive parent–child interactions through increasing emotional communication skills and parenting consistency [31]. Successful school-based programmes have concentrated on improving academic capacities and socio-emotional coping skills in children as well as creating a more protective school environment. A review of randomized control trials of programmes to prevent behavioural disorders in children in infancy, the preschool years and school-going children up to 8 years revealed 32 effective trials worldwide; 9 having a moderate risk of bias and 23 having a high risk of bias, the latter meaning that they did not report correct concealed randomization procedures, had a large loss to follow-up, and/or analyzed only outcomes for families who attended the whole programme [32].

There were two effective programmes during infancy with moderate bias. Both were selective home visitation programmes: *The Nurse Home Visitation Programme* in the United States [33] and the *Early Start Programme* in New Zealand [34]. The *Nurse Home Visitation* programme demonstrates longterm impacts on reductions in symptoms associated with disruptive disorders. It involved nurses conducting pre- and postnatal home visits of vulnerable low-income women who were pregnant with their first children. The nurses focused on improving prenatal health, including using health promotion techniques to reduce prenatal high-risk behaviours such as smoking and alcohol misuse; promoting more sensitive and competent postnatal childcare, including the importance of maternal responsiveness and child stimulation to promote bonding and attachment; as well as helping mothers plan future pregnancies, and providing support to complete their education and find work. As such, this intervention addressed multiple prenatal and postnatal risk influences to promote a healthier home and community environment that provides more health enhancing opportunities for the developing child. Three randomized control trials over 27 years found that the programme was effective in reducing low birth weight, preterm delivery, emergency visits and child abuse in beneficiaries of the programme. Long-term benefits showed that child beneficiaries of the programme evidenced fewer arrests, convictions, substance abuse or promiscuous sexual behavior than control participants [33].

During the preschool years there were two effective programmes with moderate bias. These were the *Family Check Up* programme in the USA, and the *Brief Psycho-educational parenting* programme in Canada [35]. The former screened for family risk in children aged 2–3 years and provided a family support programme to improve parenting for families at risk [36]. The latter provided psychoeducational groups for parents with preschoolers with behavioural problems. Both programmes were found to be effective in preventing preschool behavioural problems. *The Perry Preschool Project* in the United States is an example of an effective programme with high bias but which demonstrates long-term impact. The programme was an intensive well-resourced programme facilitated by trained teachers for disadvantaged preschool children. It involved classes focusing on problem-solving and task persistence and aimed to promote self-esteem and independence in children. Teachers also conducted weekly home visits. At 21 years, lifetime arrests of participants of the programme were half that of the control groups. Intervention participants also demonstrated lowered rates of teenage pregnancy, higher rates of high school graduation, home ownership and lower dependency on social benefits [37].

Several effective programmes with moderate bias were identified for school-aged children. These include the *John Hopkins Prevention Programme* in the United States [38], a universal classroom-centred and family–school partnership intervention for first graders which demonstrated short-term improvements in behaviours for those at greatest risk; the *Good Behaviour Game* in the United States and Netherlands [39], a universal classroom-based programme that rewards positive group as opposed to individual behaviour and was shown to have lasting effects on reducing aggression and substance abuse, especially among boys; The *Fast Track Prevention Programme* in the United States [40], described in greater detail in the following paragraph; the *Montreal Longitudinal Study of Disruptive Boys* in Canada [41], a selective programme involving parent training and social skill training of disruptive boys which showed improvements in behaviour 3 years post the intervention; and the *Brief Family Intervention* in the United States, a selective family strengthening trial focused on family communication and conflict management that showed positive short-term outcomes.

The *Fast Track Prevention Programme* arguably provides the best long-term evidence of the effectiveness of a multicomponent programme in preventing lifetime prevalence of all externalizing disorders. This 10-year programme for vulnerable children from Grade 1–10 addressed a cluster of risk factors for the development of antisocial behaviour, including poor parental behaviour management, deficient child cognitive and socio-emotional coping skills, poor peer relations, weak academic skills and disruptive and rejecting classroom environments, poor parental monitoring and supervision and poor home–school relations. A randomized control trial found significant reductions in psychiatric diagnoses of conduct disorder, oppositional defiant disorder, attention deficit hyperactivity disorder and any other externalizing disorder amongst those at highest-initial risk over multiple assessments over 10 years including 2 years after the intervention ceased [40].

While there have not been any trials in LMICs that have examined the long-term impact of primary prevention interventions on reducing the incidence of disruptive symptoms/disorders, there are examples of successful school-based programmes that provide reasonably robust evidence of positive effects on pupils' emotional and social well-being, and on pupils' school adjustment [42]. Zippy's Friends, is a well-known example of a school-based programme for promoting socio-emotional competencies and adaptive coping skills in pre- and elementary-school-aged children (5–7 years) in Lithuania [43]. There are also a few examples of family strengthening programmes in LMICs [44]. They generally aim, however, to reduce risk behaviour related to HIV infection and demonstrate short-term impact in relation to improved parent–child communication and monitoring and control. The need for long-term impact studies focused on family strengthening to reduce disruptive disorders in LMIC is thus indicated.

Depression   Some of the programmes described under the section on preventing disruptive behaviours also demonstrated reductions in symptoms of internalizing disorders in children. These include the Early Start Programme [34], the Brief Psycho-educational parenting programme [35]. Interventions that have shown definitive success in preventing the onset of depression have used CBT or interpersonal therapy (IPT) with selected or indicated groups. CBT as a prevention strategy moderates responses through 'unlearning' of responses that may have been adaptive to stressors earlier in life, but which are no longer adaptive. IPT is useful for moderating and mediating the impact of existing problems and high-risk situations that increase vulnerability to the development of mental disorders through social support and problem management strategies [12].

Interventions targeted at preventing depression among children and adolescents have been shown to reduce the incidence of depressive disorders by 23% [11]. A review of 42 randomised control trials relating to 28 school-based programmes for the prevention of depression in school-going children and adolescents revealed that the majority of successful programmes were based on CBT and delivered by a mental health professional or graduate student over 8–12 sessions. Indicated interventions targeting students with high levels of depressive symptoms showed the greatest effect sizes [45]. The Clarke Cognitive-Behavioural Prevention intervention [46] targeting adolescents has proved effective for preventing future depression in several randomised trials [6]. In adults, two meta-analyses of proximal primary prevention interventions in high-income countries (HICs) indicate that selective and indicated primary prevention interventions can reduce the incidence of depressive disorders using CBT and IPT by up to 22% in the intervention arms compared to the controls [11, 12].

While similar intervention research is not as extensive in developing country contexts, interventions with adolescents and adults employing cognitive behavioural techniques as well as IPT groups, suggest that these intervention approaches can positively influence outcomes for adolescents and adults in these contexts as well [47–50]. While fairly resource intensive, these approaches have been found to be successfully delivered within a task-shifting approach using trained community members [47–50].

Implications for the practice of primary prevention

There has been significant progress in our understanding of the causes of mental disorders from the recent advances in developmental neuroscience, epidemiological studies and life course development studies. While effective prevention in this and other fields does not depend only on a full understanding of causal mechanisms, this body of evidence highlights the interaction between developmental vulnerabilities and genetic and social determinants in the development of mental disorders, reinforcing the need for an ecological developmental approach to primary prevention science. The evidence-base on effective primary prevention interventions has also progressed rapidly in the last couple of decades. There is now evidence that the incidence of some mental disorders, notably disruptive disorders in children and depression in both children and adults, can be reduced through primary prevention interventions. Economic evaluation studies also provide evidence that investment in primary prevention interventions, particularly with children and adolescents, can provide substantial savings to society across a range of sectors [1, 2, 51].

Implications for the practice of primary prevention include the following:

1. The most crucial period for primary prevention interventions is during prenatal development and infancy, when the developing brain in most vulnerable and when negative environmental influences such as exposure to toxins, micronutrient deficiencies, infectious diseases and obstetric complications can increase risk for a wide range of mental and neurological disorders, as can poor maternal responsiveness and lack of stimulation. Distal and proximal public health efforts to reduce exposure to these risk factors, particularly in LMICs and other scarce resource contexts, need to be high on the global public mental health agenda and overlap with many of the Millennium Development Goals.

2. The relationship between early exposure to risk influences and impact on the development of mental disorders is not a linear one. Multiple risk influences interact with multiple protective influences to moderate and/or mediate the impact on mental health across the lifespan. Primary prevention thus needs to be multifaceted and developmentally timed, occurring across the lifespan, starting with prenatal development. In general, prevention programmes that target multiple domains of family, school or community have better results than single focus interventions. Interventions with children and adolescents demonstrate the greatest long-term return for investment [1, 2].

3. There is evidence that individual and proximal primary prevention interventions are effective in preventing the onset of certain conditions, particularly disruptive disorders in children and depression in children and adults. There is some evidence for the effectiveness of universal interventions in HICs to support healthy development for

all. However, they are resource intensive and evidence of their effectiveness is constrained by the very large numbers of subjects required to obtain statistical power, especially for disorders that have low incidence rates. Selective and indicated interventions may be more resource efficient, especially in LMICs. Screening for risk factors and early symptoms or biomarkers and the implementation of evidence-based interventions for vulnerable groups, is likely to yield greater cost-benefit for countries worldwide and would be especially important in scarce-resource contexts. Primary health care settings, preschool, school and the workplace settings provide opportunities for both screening and interventions.

4. During infancy, home visitation programmes are most effective for selected and indicated vulnerable groups. These can be delivered as part of primary health care programmes to improve, *inter alia*, maternal mental health, parental responsiveness and attachment. These programmes have been delivered largely by professional nurses in HICs. Given the scarcity of professional resources in LMICs, training community care workers to deliver similar interventions should be considered in these contexts. A recent trial of a similar programme delivered by community care workers in South Africa demonstrates the efficacy of this task-shifting approach [52].

5. During childhood, routine screening of children in preschool and school entry for cognitive and socio-emotional difficulties would allow for the identification of 'at risk' children. Wherever possible, multifaceted preschool and school-based programmes should be promoted. Evidence of the long-term impact of programmes for reducing the incidence of disruptive behavioural disorders indicate that multifaceted programmes involving school-based and home-based programmes to enhance, *inter alia*, child academic achievement and social relatedness as well as parental involvement and monitoring and control, are most successful. CBT and IPT interventions have also been shown to be effective in reducing the incidence of depression in vulnerable children and adolescents.

6. Similarly, screening of adults at risk for depression, could be implemented in the workplace and through primary health care settings. These settings also provide possible sites for the provision of CBT and IPT interventions shown to be effective for selective and indicated groups to promote more adaptive functioning and can prevent and/or delay the onset of full-blown depression.

From the abovementioned practice implications, it is evident that the practice of primary prevention is a multisectoral endeavour, requiring the participation of multiple sectors. This presents a challenge for primary prevention practitioners, especially in LMICs where mental health is not a high-public health priority. Harnessing resources for primary prevention of mental disorders will require advocacy and education of policy makers and service providers across multiple sectors as well as the public in general about the need for prevention efforts and the benefits that can accrue.

Acknowledgement

We acknowledge Tasneem Kathree for assisting with literature searches for the review.

References

1. Roberts G and Grimes K. (2011). *Return on Investment: Mental Health Promotion and Mental Illness Prevention*. Canadian Policy Network at the University of Western Ontario: Canadian Institute for Health Information.
2. Knapp M, McDaid D and Parsonage M. (2011). *Mental Health Promotion and Mental Illness Prevention: The Economic Case*. London.
3. World Health Organization. (2008). *The Global Burden of Disease: 2004 Update*. Geneva: World Health Organization.
4. World Health Organization. (2004). *The Global Burden of Disease: 2004 Update*. Geneva: World Health Organization.
5. World Health Organization. (2004). *Prevention of Mental Disorders*. Geneva: World Health Organization.
6. O'Connell ME, Boat T and Warner KE (eds). (2009). *Preventing Mental, Emotional, and Behavioral Disorders Among Young People: Progress and Possibilities*. Washington, DC: National Academies Press.
7. World Health Organization. (2001). *Strengthening Mental Health Promotion. (Fact sheet, No 220)*. Geneva: World Health Organization.
8. World Health Organization. (2004). *Promoting Mental Health. Concepts, Emerging Evidence, Practice. Summary Report*. Geneva: World Health Organization.
9. World Health Organization. (2004). *Prevention of Mental Disorders: Effective Interventions and Policy Options. Summary Report*. Geneva: World Health Organization.
10. Gordon RS Jr. (1983). An operational classification of disease prevention. *Public Health Reports* **98**(2): 107–109. Epub 1983/03/01.
11. Cuijpers P, Van Straten A and Smit F. (2005). Preventing the incidence of new cases of mental disorders: a meta-analytic review. *Journal of Nervous and Mental Disease* **193**(2): 119–125. Epub 2005/02/03.
12. Cuijpers P, van Straten A, Smit F, et al. (2008). Preventing the onset of depressive disorders: a meta-analytic review of psychological interventions. *American Journal of Psychiatry* **165**(10): 1272–1280. Epub 2008/09/04.
13. Saxena S, Jane-Llopis E, and Hosman C. (2006). Prevention of mental and behavioural disorders: implications for policy and practice. *World Psychiatry* **5**(1): 5–14. Epub 2006/06/08.
14. Bronfenbrenner U. (1979). *The Ecology of Human Development: Experiments by Nature and Design*. Cambridge, MA: Harvard University Press.
15. Petersen I and Govender K. (2010). Theoretical considerations. From understanding to intervening. In: Petersen I, Bhana A, Flisher A, Swartz L and Richter L (eds), *Promoting Mental Health in Scarce-Resource Contexts Emerging Evidence and Practice*, pp. 21–48. Cape Town: HSRC Press.
16. Bhana A and Bachoo S. (2011). The determinants of family resilience among families in low- and middle-income contexts: a systematic literature review. *South African Journal of Psychology* **41**(2): 131–139.
17. Walker SP, Wachs TD, Gardner JM, et al. (2007). Child development: risk factors for adverse outcomes in developing countries. *Lancet* **369**(9556): 145–157. Epub 2007/01/16.
18. Durkin M. (2002). The epidemiology of developmental disabilities in low-income countries. *Mental Retardation and Developmental Disabilities Research Reviews* **8**(3): 206–211. Epub 2002/09/07.
19. Brown AS and Susser ES. (2008). Prenatal nutritional deficiency and risk of adult schizophrenia. *Schizophrenia Bulletin* **34**(6): 1054–1063. Epub 2008/08/07.
20. Richter L, Dawes A and de Kadt J. (2010). Early childhood. In: Petersen I, Bhana A, Flisher AJ, Swartz L and Richter L (eds), *Promoting Mental Health in Scarce-Resource Contexts*, pp. 99–123. Cape Town: Human Sciences Research Council Press.

21. Hankin JR. (2002). Fetal alcohol syndrome prevention research. *Alcohol Research Health* **26**(1): 58–65. Epub 2002/08/06.
22. Braun JM, Froehlich TE, Daniels JL, et al. (2008). Association of environmental toxicants and conduct disorder in U.S. children: NHANES 2001–2004. *Environmental Health Perspectives* **116**(7): 956–962. Epub 2008/07/17.
23. Braun JM, Kahn RS, Froehlich T, et al. (2006). Exposures to environmental toxicants and attention deficit hyperactivity disorder in U.S. children. *Environmental Health Perspectives* **114**(12): 1904–1909. Epub 2006/12/23.
24. Dodge KA, Greenberg MT, Malone PS, et al. (2008). Testing an idealized dynamic cascade model of the development of serious violence in adolescence. *Child Development* **79**(6): 1907–1927. Epub 2008/11/29.
25. Egger HL, Erkanli A, Keeler G, et al. (2006). Test-retest reliability of the preschool age psychiatric assessment (PAPA). *Journal of the American Academy of Child and Adolescent Psychiatry* **45**(5): 538–549. Epub 2006/04/08.
26. Flisher A and Gevers A. (2010). Adolescence. In: I Petersen, A Bhana, A Flisher, L Swartz, L Richter (eds), *Promoting Mental Health in Scarce-Resource Contexts Emerging Evidence and Practice*, pp. 143–166. Cape Town: HSRC Press.
27. Patel V, Lund C, Hatherill S, et al. (2010). Mental disorders: equity and social determinants. In: E Blas, and AS Kurup (eds), *Equity, Social Determinants and Public Health Programmes*, pp. 115–134. Geneva: World Health Organization.
28. Lund C, Breen A, Flisher AJ, et al. (2010). Poverty and common mental disorders in low and middle income countries: A systematic review. *Social Science and Medicine* **71**(3): 517–528. Epub 2010/07/14.
29. Bonde JP. Psychosocial factors at work and risk of depression: a systematic review of the epidemiological evidence. *Occupational and Environmental Medicine* **65**(7): 438–445. Epub 2008/04/18.
30. Dooley D, Catalano R and Wilson G. (1994). Depression and unemployment: panel findings from the Epidemiologic Catchment Area study. *American Journal of Community Psychology* **22**(6): 745–765. Epub 1994/12/01.
31. Kaminski JW, Valle LA, Filene JH, et al. (2008). A meta-analytic review of components associated with parent training program effectiveness. *Journal of Abnormal Child Psychology* **36**(4): 567–589. Epub 2008/01/22.
32. Bayer J, Hiscock H, Scalzo K, et al. (2009). Systematic review of preventive interventions for children's mental health: what would work in Australian contexts? *Australian and New Zealand Journal of Psychiatry* **43**(8): 695–710. Epub 2009/07/25.
33. Olds DL. (2006). The nurse–family partnership: An evidence-based preventive intervention. *Infant Mental Health Journal* **27**(1): 5–25.
34. Fergusson DM, Grant H, Horwood LJ, et al. (2005). Randomized trial of the Early Start program of home visitation. *Pediatrics* **116**(6): e803–e809. Epub 2005/12/03.
35. Bradley SJ, Jadaa DA, Brody J, et al. (2003). Brief psychoeducational parenting program: an evaluation and 1-year follow-up. *Journal of the American Academy of Child and Adolescent Psychiatry* **42**(10): 1171–1178. Epub 2003/10/16.
36. Dishion TJ, Shaw D, Connell A, et al. (2008). The family check-up with high-risk indigent families: preventing problem behavior by increasing parents' positive behavior support in early childhood. *Child Development* **79**(5): 1395–1414. Epub 2008/10/02.
37. Schweinhart LJ. (2007). Crime prevention by the High/Scope Perry Preschool Programme. *Victims & Offenders* **2**(2): 141–160.
38. Ialongo NS, Werthamer L, Kellam SG, et al. (1999). Proximal impact of two first-grade preventive interventions on the early risk behaviors for later substance abuse, depression, and antisocial behavior. *American Journal of Community Psychology* **27**(5): 599–641. Epub 2000/02/17.
39. Embry DD. (2002). The Good Behavior Game: a best practice candidate as a universal behavioral vaccine. *Clinical Child and Family psychology review* **5**(4): 273–297. Epub 2002/12/24.

40. Conduct Problems Prevention Research Group. (2011). The effects of the fast track preventive intervention on the development of conduct disorder across childhood. *Child Development* **82**(1): 331–345. Epub 2011/02/05.

41. Tremblay RE, McCord J, Boileau H, et al. (1991). Can disruptive boys be helped to become competent? *Psychiatry* **54**(2): 148–161. Epub 1991/05/01.

42. Barry MM, Clarke AM, Jenkins R, et al. *Rapid Review of the Evidence on the Effectiveness of Mental Health Promotion in low and Middle Income Countries. Mainstreaming Health Promotion: Reviewing the Health Promotion Actions on Priority Public Health Conditions.* Geneva: World Health Organization.

43. Mishara B and Ystgaard M. (2006). Effectiveness of a mental health promotion program ti improve coping skills in young children: Zippy's Friends. *Early Childhood Research Quarterly* **21**: 110–123.

44. World Health Organization; USAID; Family Health International; YouthNet. (2007). *Summaries of Projects in Developing Countries Assisting Parents of Adolescents.* Geneva: WHO.

45. Calear AL and Christensen H. (2010). Systematic review of school-based prevention and early intervention programs for depression. *Journal of Adolescence* **33**(3): 429–438.

46. Clarke GN, Hawkins, W, Murphy, M., et al. (1995). Targeted prevention of unipolar depressive disorder in an at-risk sample of high school adolescents: a randomized trial of a group cognitive intervention. *Journal of the American Academy of Child and Adolescent Psychiatry* **34**(3): 312–321. Epub 1995/03/01.

47. Patel V, Flisher AJ, Nikapota A, et al. (2008). Promoting child and adolescent mental health in low and middle income countries. *Journal of Child Psychology and Psychiatry and Allied Disciplines* **49**(3): 313–334. Epub 2007/12/21.

48. Patel V, Chowdhary N, Rahman A, et al. (2011). Improving access to psychological treatments: Lessons from developing countries. *Behaviour Research and Therapy* **49**(9): 523–528.

49. Petersen I, Swartz L, Bhana A, et al. (2010). Mental health promotion initiatives for children and youth in contexts of poverty: the case of South Africa. *Health Promotion International* **25**(3): 331–341. Epub 2010/04/24.

50. Petersen I, Bhana A, Baillie K, et al. (2011). The Feasibility of adapted group-based interpersonal therapy (IPT) for the treatment of depression by community health workers within the context of task shifting in South Africa. *Community Mental Health Journal* **48**(3): 336–341 Epub 2011/06/21.

51. Zechmeister I, Kilian R, McDaid D, et al. (2008). Is it worth investing in mental health promotion and prevention of mental illness? A systematic review of the evidence from economic evaluations. *BMC Public Health* **8**: 20. Epub 2008/01/24.

52. Cooper PJ, Tomlinson M, Swartz L, et al. (2009). Improving quality of mother-infant relationship and infant attachment in socioeconomically deprived community in South Africa: randomised controlled trial. *BMJ: British Medical Association* **338**: b974. Epub 2009/04/16.

12

Early Intervention in Mental Health Problems: The Role of the Voluntary Sector

Andrew McCulloch, Isabella Goldie and Sophie Bridger

Mental Health Foundation, UK

This chapter attempts to address the role of the voluntary sector [non-government organisations (NGOs) or community managed organisations (CMOs) or sector, private not for profits in the United States] in early intervention in mental health problems.

While acknowledging some very worthy efforts by voluntary organisations elsewhere in the world (e.g. headspace centres in Australia and Headstrong centre in Dublin as consortia partnerships between public and NGO mental health services, drug and alcohol and primary care services to form convenient one stop shops for young people located in their favourite mingling spaces, providing practical help for a wide range of psychosocial disorders), we will concentrate on UK examples as the authors are most familiar with them.

It describes how the voluntary sector in the United Kingdom typically approaches this issue, what sort of solutions and support it offers, what are its strengths and weaknesses, and its future aspirations. The concept of early intervention in the voluntary sector has been fairly widely used since the Melbourne model of early intervention in psychosis was first disseminated in the 1980s by Pat McGorry and others [1]. Whilst most of the teams set up in the United Kingdom have been in the statutory sector, there has been voluntary sector involvement from agencies such as Hafal in Wales and Rethink in England. However, with the currency of the concept of early intervention developing more widely, the use of the term within mental health has become confused and is differently understood to mean:

(a) Early intervention in psychosis following the Australian model;

Early Intervention in Psychiatry: EI of nearly everything for better mental health, First Edition.
Edited by Peter Byrne and Alan Rosen.
© 2014 John Wiley & Sons, Ltd. Published 2014 by John Wiley & Sons, Ltd.

(b)   Early intervention more generally in the course of a disease to prevent it developing, ameliorate it, or cut short its course that is elements of treatment, secondary
and tertiary prevention. It is assumed that *early intervention in the disease process* is
by definition distinct from primary prevention although the content of primary prevention and early intervention services/programmes/interventions might not always
differ. This is where the real scope for confusion arises;

(c)   Early intervention in the life course to prevent mental illness later in life or genera-
tional mental illness cycles as may exist in schizophrenia, for example.

Although early intervention in psychosis services are mainly located within the public
or statutory sector, where they are practiced within the charitable sector, then without
notable exceptions these are operated by specialist mental health organisations. Services
which aim to intervene at an early stage in the development of a mental health problem as
described in point (b) above are also dominated by the specialist mental health voluntary
sector. However, other types of voluntary sector organisations can have a pivotal role to
play, for example, in reducing the incidence of the onset of mental health problems later
in life such as those offering parenting support. Reducing the prevalence of mental health
problems across society may not be an explicit aim of more generic organisations working
with children and young people but none the less actions designed to reduce childhood
poverty may also impact on some very important determinants of mental illness.

There is an evidence and intellectual base for all three types of intervention but the
authors have been able to identify very little literature on early intervention in mental
health that has a specific focus on the voluntary sector's role. We are aware of only one
peer reviewed research study, about a parenting intervention, and this study missed the
opportunity to look at the relevance of the voluntary sector setting for the work [2]. This
chapter has therefore had to be based on anecdotal evidence, grey literature, and systematic information gathered from 11 major charities across the United Kingdom for which
we are most grateful.

After providing some key background, this chapter will attempt to:

(i)   Group or classify voluntary sector work in this area

(ii)   Provide some examples

(iii) Report on the systematic data collected from 11 charities

(iv)   Summarise what the voluntary sector may have to offer

(v)   Draw these threads together and reflect on future directions and challenges.

In doing so we recognise our view is partial and we hope more data will emerge, as early
intervention moves from a concept which is theoretically sound to one with a much more
systematic applied research base.

The voluntary sector and mental health

Briefly, what is the history of voluntary sector in the United States and Australia?

The voluntary sector has a long history of delivery in mental health. The Bethlem was founded in 1247 and many modern mental health charities are over 50-years old [3]. In some ways, the bulk of charitable provision on mental health has remained as it always was – focused on care and support for people with severe mental illness. Most of the £1bn or more charitable spend each year on mental health in the United Kingdom is spent on this group of people and is focused on housing and housing support, employment rehabilitation, day care and other services including inpatient care provided by charitable psychiatric hospital providers. Little of this spend is on any service that could be defined as early intervention, and most of it represents NHS or local authority contracts with, or grants to, charities which are trading as limited companies. The voluntary sector is taken here to imply charitable status and although there are other definitions, for example, including friendly societies and mutuals, this is unlikely to affect the overall analysis offered in this chapter.

How the voluntary sector views early intervention

There continues to be confusion in the sector between early intervention in the disease process and early intervention in the life course – the latter is the way the term is currently most often applied by the UK governments. But in this chapter, we will address all early intervention to prevent, treat or ameliorate mental illness (i.e. primary, secondary and tertiary prevention) regardless of when it comes in the lifespan (pre-birth to old age). Conceptually, age-related definitions of early intervention are not really relevant to many of the risk factors which impact on mental ill health as many are not chronologically determined or may be additive or be involved in dynamic interactions throughout life. Therefore, it makes little sense in this context to regard age three as a cut-off for 'early intervention' and most voluntary organisations in our experience would share this view.

Whilst there is little literature on the subject we would observe that voluntary sector colleagues tend to advance an early intervention model for a number of understandable practical, theoretical and in some cases, evidence based, reasons:

- It is preferable to forestall the development of mental illness for all sorts of reasons – medical, psychological, social and family related – as well as to reduce suffering;

- Economic and presumed economic advantages both generally and in terms of use of specialist services;

- Such interventions can build community and social capital and reduce stigma thereby placing the service user into a more supportive environment;

- Such interventions support recovery and build the user's capacity to survive and thrive;

- They can prevent exit from employment and educational opportunities or facilitate rapid re-engagement;

- They may prevent morbidity, mortality (e.g. from suicide) and comorbidity;

- They are what both service users want and what charities see as fulfilling their missions which often related to disease reduction and mental health improvement as well as just providing support;

- They can combat stigma and discrimination.

- The may prevent or reduce social drift.

There will be others, but it is fair to say that early intervention is generally seen as a presumed good by mental health charities although it is understood that the evidence base is better for some disorders such as schizophrenia and conduct disorder than others; although many would see this simply as the result of a lack of research and service models.

Towards a systematic understanding of early intervention by the voluntary sector

The authors have decided to use Martikainen's model of the generation of health/illness in order to derive the points of leverage at which early intervention might work. His model is presented in Figure 12.1 and using that model we have attempted to classify early intervention by the point of leverage as against the conceptual framework in Table 12.1.

It can immediately be seen that some cells contain interventions which are more amenable to voluntary sector intervention than others, thus there is probably more voluntary sector activity in the last column than the others and more in the row which addresses meso-level factors (factors at community and institutional level) than the rest. This is understandable as most voluntary sector interventions are at a fairly low level in terms of technical content and are often community or setting focused – and none the worse for that, of course. Indeed this is where the greatest gains may be made. The important point however, is that the growth of early intervention by the voluntary sector has been ad hoc and uncoordinated and of course many generic charities do not even see their intervention as primarily mental health relevant.

Case studies

In the following section, we offer some case studies relating to the cells in Table 12.1. where the voluntary sector makes the largest contribution. Arguably these cells are A3, B2, C3, D1 and D2. The types of interventions can be broadly summarised as follows:

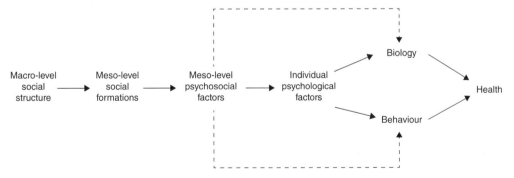

Figure 12.1 The generation of health and illness. After Martikainen et al. (2002). Reproduced with permission of Oxford University Press

Table 12.1 Modalities of early intervention in mental health

	(1) Early intervention in psychosis	(2) Early intervention in the development of mental illness	(3) Early intervention in the life cycle to prevent mental illness and/or improve mental health
(A) Individual biological factors	Proactive medication for psychotic illness	Proactive medication for other illnesses	Physical public health interventions, diet, exercise, maternal health during pregnancy, etc.
(B) Individual psychological factors	Proactive psycho-education	Ditto, also peer support, self-management, relaxation training; coaching, DBT and CBT and related interventions, etc.	Population use of emotional awareness, meditation or cognitive techniques with an emphasis on parents and children
(C) Family-level psychological factors	Pro-active family therapy	Ditto, also other family-level interventions	Parenting education, intergenerational contact interventions
(D) Meso-level factors	Anti-stigma and discrimination initiatives at community level	Settings-based activities e.g. provision of counselling in schools	Wider public mental health interventions in settings – primarily mentally health schools and nurseries, health visiting, family friendly communities
(E) Macro-level factors	Anti-stigma and discrimination initiatives, national policy on early intervention teams	Ditto	Public mental health, tackling inequalities and social drift

Early intervention in the life cycle – individual biological and psychological factors

Typically these interventions are delivered by non-health agencies seeking to implement wider objectives around issues like participation in sport which can deliver a wide range of health and social benefits.

Early intervention in the course of mental illness – individual psychological factors

The voluntary sector has a very specific role here in encouraging, for example, youth work type interventions that build individual self-esteem, peer support and a setting in which care pathways can be accessed early. Offerings like *Right here* contain elements of this approach along with wider elements (case study in Box 12.4). In recent years, mental health and well-being are often an explicit part of such initiatives and mental health care pathways may be available facilitating most specialist early intervention and treatment services. It is hard to distinguish at the margins between targeted prevention and public mental health services, and early intervention services. However, we are not aware of any 'pure' or medically oriented early intervention services run by the voluntary sector although some services run by *rethink mental illness,* especially Uthink (Box 12.1) may come nearest to this. However, voluntary sector services do provide a range of support and rehabilitative/recovery-oriented services which play an important role alongside statutory sector services. These can, of course, only be seen as part of an early intervention model if referrals are made to them or clients access them early in the progression of mental health problems.

Box 12.1   Uthink

The Uthink programme delivers a number of interventions:

1. Recovery learning programmes for 19–25-year olds who have experienced first episode psychosis; regular group sessions facilitated by an experienced team for a given time period.

2. Residential programmes for 19–25-year olds who have experienced first episode psychosis – the only programme of its kind in the country; an intensive activities agenda that introduces young people to new ideas, new experiences and the opportunity to build greater self-esteem and peer support.

3. Modular Emotional Wellbeing programmes for 14–18-year olds who have experience, or are at risk of developing, mental health difficulties; The focus is on raising awareness and prevention of mental illness as well as offering an early intervention for young people demonstrating signs of mental illness.

4. Engagement with schools and colleges by developing and delivering information packs for schools and programmes in educational venues; raising awareness of mental health amongst pupils, teachers and people working within each setting, changing attitudes, tackling stigma and improving access to advice, information and support.

5. Online information and support for young people who have an experience of living with mental illness, carers, siblings and friends; offer advice, information and support and encourage peer to peer support. The information and self-help sheets comprise a guide to good mental health as well as techniques for managing the effects of mental illness, developing support structures and signposting help.

6. Leadership training events; fun interactive day providing skills for public speaking, planning and organising activities and taking part in local forums, etc.

Independent analysis by the University of Central Lancashire shows strong positive outcomes in areas of managing mental health, self-care, daily living skills, development of social networks and relationships, reduced addictive behaviour, improved self-esteem and stronger feelings of trust and hope.

Early intervention in the life cycle – family-level interventions

Many parenting interventions and family support services are offered by the voluntary sector. These may or may not have an explicit mental health content but they are clearly designed as early intervention in the life cycle of the child to support its well-being and resilience. Mellow parenting (case study in Box 12.2) would be a good example.

Box 12.2   Mellow parenting

Mellow parenting is a Scottish Based Organisation delivering high-quality training in its family of evidence-based parenting programmes across Scotland, the United Kingdom and overseas including Germany, Iceland, New Zealand and Russia. Training is delivered to local authority and NHS Staff as well as voluntary agencies working with the most vulnerable families in society.

Mellow Babies and Mellow Parenting are evaluated programmes which have been shown to be effective in engaging hard-to-reach families with children under five and babies under one, and in helping them make changes in their relationships with their children.

Evaluation has shown that compared with other parenting programmes run in family centres, Mellow's programmes improve:

- mother–child interaction

- child behaviour problems

- mother's well-being

- mother's effectiveness and confidence in parenting.

- Mellow Babies research has shown improvement in maternal depression, parent–infant interaction and a reduction in the need for Child Protection Registration and measures of care.

A new antenatal programme, Mellow Bumps, for mums-to-be with additional health and social care needs has recently been added to our family of parenting programmes, and preliminary results indicate significant reductions in self-reported anxiety, and outwards-directed irritability, depression and inwards-directed irritability within the mums-to-be attending the groups.

Sure Start Children's Centre Practice Guidelines recommend Mellow Parenting as an effective evaluated programme, Mellow Parenting meets the criteria recognised by the National Institute for Clinical Excellence (NICE) guidelines for effective parenting programmes and was on the National Academy for Parenting Practitioner's Commissioning Toolkit of Parenting Programmes.

Early intervention in psychosis – community-level interventions

These are initiatives, such as anti-stigma activities, which act as facilitators allowing early intervention to be effective, but do not themselves constitute early intervention. It is the wallpaper which allows people to identify themselves or communities to be more supportive of those receiving such services. An example would be the Brighton site of *Right Here* which works against stigma as well as providing other elements detailed in Box 12.4.

Early intervention in mental illness – community-level interventions

This is an important area for work by the voluntary sector. There is of course a spectrum of interventions ranging from universal to highly targeted. Many interventions which are targeted but open to all can legitimately be regarded both as public mental health and prevention/early intervention initiatives. In practice, this depends on how opportunities with vulnerable individuals are used and what pathways are established. The voluntary sector can have a specific role in this particular area of practice because it can be viewed as operating a range of non-stigmatising services for particular groups that can be fertile territory for early intervention. In some cases, there is a specific early intervention agenda. An example of the latter which has proved successful is the delivery of parenting interventions to reduce child conduct problems [2]. Two examples of voluntary sector initiatives falling under this heading can be found in Boxes 12.3 and 12.4: Grouchy Old Men and Right Here.

Box 12.3   Grouchy old men

Grouchy old men project – This project explored new ways of improving the mental health and well-being of older men, particularly those at risk of isolation, depression and possible suicide. It was a 2 year project that began in April 2008 and was funded by the Department of Health. The Mental Health Foundation met with groups of older men to find out what works and doesn't work in terms of providing them with support around their mental health, as well as looking at evidence from work done elsewhere. We assisted a number of health and social care organisations to consider how they can develop their services to make them more accessible for older men and we successfully piloted a training course on older men's mental health. A 'how to' guide to help organisations and services better meet the needs of older men with mental health issues was published in October 2010. For more information go to http://www.mentalhealth.org.uk/our-work/training-and-development/past-training-dev/grouchy-old-men/?view=Standard.

Box 12.4   Right here

Right here – Right here is a 5-year action research initiative, encouraging partnerships between young people, the voluntary and statutory sectors, to deliver preventative and early intervention activities for 16–25-year olds in four pilot areas (Count Fermanagh in Northern Ireland, Brighton and Hove, Newham, and Sheffield) over 5 years (2008–2013). The pilots are delivering a range of interventions for young people, targeted at young people at risk of developing mental health problems, but open to everyone. These include:

Participatory interventions: young people working with voluntary organisations through youth panels and other mechanisms to design, deliver and commission activities for other 16–25-year olds.

Resilience-building and early intervention activities designed by young people and principally aimed at target groups at risk of developing mental health issues, including:

- In Brighton and Hove (target groups include lesbian, gay, bisexual and transgender (LGBT) and homeless young people): Rock-climbing, music production, anger management and chill-out classes

- In Newham (target group: black and minority ethnic young people (BAME) young people): peer-support delivered through Well-Being Champions, working in generic settings, such as the local sixth form college

- In Sheffield (target groups include young parents and BAME young people): Walk and Talk outdoors group counselling, yoga and relaxation classes and counselling in schools and community groups

- In Fermanagh (target groups include LGBT young people, young men and young women suffering from the legacy of the Troubles): Fishing and drama activities, gender-based group work around mental health in a rural context.

Public Mental Health and Anti-Stigma initiatives in universal settings:

- In Brighton and Hove: young People's Well-being campaign, including well-being scripts, developed by and for 16–25-year olds, and a GP Quality Mark, to measure how well GPs are looking after young people's mental health needs

- In Newham: raising awareness of mental health and the project's offers through outreach to young people in community settings (e.g. barber shops and hairdressers) and "street-bleaching" campaigns, promoting positive mental health messages

- In Sheffield: anti-stigma campaigns through community radio stations and an anti-stigma DVD and Board Game, designed by the project's Youth Panel

- In Fermanagh: mental health awareness campaigns at rock concerts and drama workshops, and a positive mental health text messaging service.

Right Here is being independently evaluated by the Tavistock Institute of Human Relations and early findings are demonstrating the benefits to participants' mental health including: *having more ability to cope with challenges; increased confidence and self-esteem; having a better understanding of mental health issues; gaining new skills and experience; having alternative (and more constructive) leisure activities and the opportunity to make new friends.*

Public mental health interventions

Whilst such services are not usually regarded as "early intervention" they do provide important opportunities to intervene with those participants in programmes who either self-identify as being at risk or are identified by programme workers and are signposted onwards to other interventions. All sorts of voluntary sector interventions could be regarded as having a public mental health component because they address risk factors such as lack of exercise or access to green open space. Others address mental health more directly such as parenting programmes. Generic voluntary organisations, for example Girl Guides which have addressed mental health issues in a number of ways in recent years, offer excellent opportunities for such interventions.

Services offered by the voluntary sector which can contribute to early intervention

In practice, in many areas of the United Kingdom, the voluntary sector will make a peripheral contribution to early intervention by providing services to which people can be rapidly referred or that can support people early in the recovery process (which could be viewed as secondary or tertiary prevention). Typical approaches may include:

(i)   peer support programmes throughout the age range;

(ii) housing support;

(iii) engagement or re-engagement with education;

(iv) awareness and stigma reduction work;

(v)   vocational support;

(vi) employment rehabilitation.

These offers may be stand alone, in which case any early intervention potential will be hit or miss, or part of an explicit or inexplicit hub and spoke or matrix model of partnership, in which case the opportunities for early intervention may be easier to exploit. Many voluntary sector offerings are part of an explicit partnership model, usually with the statutory sector (e.g. NHS, social care and education). Examples so far quoted all have such an element. Another example is Cumbria's explicit partnership in social care which includes early intervention as a fundamental principle [5]. There is also an important intermediary role that the voluntary sector can play in helping people to remain connected with their wider lives and prevent social drift, to lessen the impact of the illness on people's lives but also to see a positive impact on the trajectory of an illness (especially relevant to common mental health problems). A core function for the voluntary sector is arguably about intervening to limit the damage to wider domains of people's lives such as employment or social networks. The sector already have strong links to community life and organisations, but are also most often focused on reconnecting people to employment, housing and education; therefore they could and should have a strong role in helping people within the initial onset of mental illness to remain connected, which is crucial to recovery and continued mental health.

What did the systematic data collection show?

Given the absence of any systematic data in this area, the authors decided to undertake a modest survey of voluntary sector mental health agencies and their approach to early intervention. Seventeen leading mental health charities in England, Scotland and Wales were approached of which 11 replied either via the internet or post to a questionnaire containing a mix of fixed and open response questions. This was considered to be a good response rate in the present pressured environment. Whilst those responding cannot be said to be representative, some of the results are of interest. Eight of the respondents provide direct early intervention services themselves, and three did not but were concerned with campaigning and ensuring such services are developed.

The majority of charities contacted were concerned with adults of working age with a variety of conditions and care pathways, three were concerned with children and adolescents. Eight of them provided their own early intervention services which were funded by a broad range of agencies but local authorities and the NHS were most important funders. Two charities had a high volume of services (£5m+), one was in the range £1–5m and the rest were small (0–500k). Charities had a number of interrelated strands of thinking behind their early intervention approach, but the most common were: 'maximising recovery and reducing disconnection' (all); 'keeping people out of institutional services' (10); 'reducing stigma and labelling' (8) and 'intervening early in the development of problems' (7).

The single fundamental driver for the majority of agencies was to promote recovery and there was generally an illness-based approach probably reflecting an emphasis on early intervention in adults with severe mental illness. Charities were heavily involved in a variety of forms of quality assurance, staff development and user involvement. They were split between those who expected early intervention to grow and those who expected it to remain stable; none thought it would shrink.

Table 12.2 SWOT analysis

Strengths	Weaknesses
Cost efficient	Client confusion and navigation problems
Flexible	Lack of medical and sometimes wider professional
Good community connections	input
Trusted branding (not statutory sector)	Reliance on statutory commissioning both
Can cross bureaucratic boundaries	financially and in terms of understanding
Access especially for hard to reach groups	Variable quality
Sometimes innovation	Governance
Often user input	Management
User friendly style	Vulnerability to external influences
Non-stigmatising	Access to capital
Service user involvement	HR and IT infrastructure
Independent	
Innovative (sometimes)	
Non-medical	
Outcome or solution focused	
Opportunities	Threats
Big society/localism	LA cuts and other spending pressures
Partnership models with local authorities and	Blunt nature of regulation
others	
Importance of economic case for service change	

Charities were asked what their greatest concerns were around early intervention at present. Finance was the overwhelming concern but a lack of understanding of the voluntary sector amongst commissioners and over application of the medical model were also raised. Charities had many ideas on the advantages of the voluntary sector contribution to early intervention. Accessibility, flexibility and lack of stigma were amongst the most common advantages cited. The full set of advantages obtained from the charities has been used to inform the SWOT analysis in Table 12.2.

What does the voluntary sector have to offer?

In considering early intervention by the voluntary sector, together with our previous research on the sector [3], we have come up with the SWOT analysis of the sector's contribution and potential contribution (Table 12.2).

Conclusion

Voluntary organisations have a range of services which are relevant to early intervention and a number of advantages, both perceived and concretely demonstrable, in terms of reaching those who require these services and delivering scalable, relevant and tailored interventions. However, as yet this potential has hardly started to be realised. Voluntary sector mental health services in the United Kingdom are currently turning over well in excess of £1bn but extrapolating from our survey it would appear that the early intervention element of this is only of the order of 1%. In addition, whilst some internal evaluation data are collected there are few independent studies which can inform further developments. Additionally, there are key threats to the voluntary sector at the moment from public sector spending cuts and policy changes across the United Kingdom, and in some cases the infrastructure such as workforce is weak.

Our conclusion is therefore two-edged. Early intervention by the sector has many advantages as it can provide a service with the right style, substance and flexibility to meet the needs of service users and the varied communities in which they live. On the other hand, objectively speaking the sector can hardly be said to be rising to the challenge at present. This is a pity, as we believe the sector can make a major and potentially transformative contribution to early intervention and especially to reaching out to communities and institutional settings in innovative and confidence building ways. The profile of early intervention is being raised within the sector but more clarity is needed about what is meant by the term. We hope that over the next few years the sector will increase the scope of its ambition so that as well as being clear about what it means and wants, it increasingly offers a range of evaluated and effective services. This in turn will require a positive response from commissioners and Government.

Acknowledgements

I thank the voluntary organisations that participated in the survey and colleagues at the Mental Health Foundation for their help and support. The Mental Health Foundation also funded the survey and administrative support required to draft this chapter.

References

1. McGorry P, Yung AR, Phillips LJ, et al. (2002). Randomized controlled trial of interventions designed to reduce the risk of progression to first-episode psychosis in a clinical sample with subthreshold symptoms. *Archives of General Psychiatry* **59**: 921–928.
2. Gardner F, Burton J and Klimes I. (2006). Randomised controlled trial of a parenting intervention in the voluntary sector for reducing child conduct problems: outcomes and mechanisms of change. *Journal of Child Psychology and Psychiatry* **47**(11): 1123–1132.
3. McCulloch A and Howland G. (2009). The role of the voluntary sector. In: C Brooker and J Repper (eds), *Mental health: from policy to practice*. Edinburgh: Churchill Livingstone Elsevier.
4. Martikainen P, Bartley M and Lahelma L. (2002). Psychosocial determinants of health in social epidemiology. *International Journal of Epidemiology* **31**(6): 1091–1093.
5. Cumbria County Council. (2010). *Third Sector Organisations and Adult Social Care – A True Partnership*. Carlisle: Cumbria County Council.

13

Why Primary Care Matters for Early Intervention in Psychiatry

David Shiers[1,2,3] and Helen Lester[4]

[1]National Early Intervention Programme, England
[2]Leek, North Staffordshire, UK
[3]National Mental Health Development Unit, London, UK
[4]Primary Care, School of Health and Population Sciences, University of Birmingham, UK

Introduction

The first challenge in writing for an international readership mainly familiar with psychiatric settings is that primary health care varies from country to country. As two English general practitioners (GPs) attempting to describe how primary care supports the paradigm of early intervention, our views are inevitably UK centric. However, what is universal is the sheer breadth and scale of mental disorder encountered in primary care. This ranges from people struggling with everyday life events to people experiencing often severe and sometimes lifelong conditions such as schizophrenia. It spans all ages from young children experiencing conduct disorder to older people with dementia. It tackles a *real world* in which mental and physical disorders coexist, particularly in more deprived areas [1].

For severe disorders like psychosis, describing how primary care contributes to early intervention appears relatively straightforward. The principles would be similar if we were discussing cancer care or cardiovascular diseases. Steeped in a world of diagnostic uncertainty, GPs are familiar with separating out potentially serious conditions which may present early and in an undifferentiated way. Indeed GPs are frequently consulted in first-episode psychosis and are the most common final referring agency [2] but still only encounter 1–2 patients per year with a suspected psychosis. (Is this still similar to

Early Intervention in Psychiatry: EI of nearly everything for better mental health, First Edition.
Edited by Peter Byrne and Alan Rosen.
© 2014 John Wiley & Sons, Ltd. Published 2014 by John Wiley & Sons, Ltd.

first presentation of juvenile/type I diabetes?) GPs request better collaboration with specialists supported by low-threshold referral services rather than educational programmes to improve their diagnostic ability [3]. However, we believe primary care can contribute to early intervention beyond just detecting psychosis early. Recent research reveals that markers of 'downstream' physical ill health appear within weeks of initiating treatment, emphasising how mental and physical comorbidity can be predicted even at this early stage [4]. This may have important implications for primary care.

For those with milder distress the challenges are different. Contributing significantly to primary care's daily workload, such difficulties have their origins in the complexities of peoples' lives, their relationships with others, and the interactions between their bodies and their minds. Neat categorisation is defied. In terms of prevention and early intervention this is important, given that most serious problems start out as milder ones. Treatment strategies based on formal diagnosis and biomedical solutions offer limited help. Potentially more helpful are holistic and health promoting approaches applied at both individual and community levels. Failure of primary care to contain and respond appropriately may result in entry into formal systems of mental health diagnosis and treatment where the sheer volume would overwhelm specialist services and frustrate clients with ineffectual care.

So, although the ways in which primary care responds to intervene early for someone with a potential psychosis compared to someone with milder distress may be very different, a central theme is that primary care is a major provider of mental health care across this wide spectrum and its distinctive characteristics make it central to an effective care system [5].

The value of primary care

There is enormous international variation in what is meant by the term 'primary care'. According to the Institute of Medicine (1996) in the United States of America, primary care is the:

> '... provision of integrated, accessible healthcare services by clinicians who are accountable for addressing a large majority of personal health needs, developing a sustained partnership with patients, and practicing in the context of the family and community' [6].

Primary care systems can be categorised according to whether they act as gatekeepers to specialist services (as in the United Kingdom), provide free-market services in parallel to specialist services, or function in a complex system containing both free-market and gatekeeper functionality (as in the United States); whether they are free to patients at the point of care delivery; whether they are led by doctors or non-medical personnel; and the degree to which they provide continuity of care.

Barbara Starfield, a respected researcher of primary care across different countries, described primary care as:

> '... the provision of first contact, person-focused, ongoing care over time that meets the health-related needs of people, referring only those too uncommon to maintain competence, and coordinates care when people receive services at other levels of care' [7].

Evidence for the benefits of primary care oriented health systems is robust across a wide variety of different types of studies. In summary, primary health oriented countries:

- Have more equitable resource distributions.

- Have little or no private health insurance.

- Are rated as better by their populations.

- Have primary care that includes a wider range of services and is family oriented.

- Have better health at lower costs.

- Within countries, areas with higher primary care physician availability (but NOT specialist availability) have healthier populations [8, 9].

Primary care as the central provider of mental health services

A common myth runs as follows: *Primary care deals with common and milder mental illnesses and specialist care with rarer and more severe ones.* However, a landmark study by Goldberg and Huxley [10] revealed how primary care dealt with 90% of people with mental ill health, that only 10% required specialist community services and even fewer inpatient hospital care. Mental health problems are the sole basis for 20–25% of consultations and an important feature of around 40% of consultations [10]. Moreover for people with severe mental illness, 30–50% receive their care solely from primary care [11]. Could such levels of need ever be met by specialist services? It is also important to note that many other professions are involved in providing primary care – nurses, receptionists, social workers and pharmacists, often with minimal or no mental health training.

Advantages to providing mental health care in primary care

Primary care offers a low stigma setting close to home; by a health practitioner often with previous knowledge of the person and family, providing holistic treatment and continuity of care for the full range of problems including physical health, and links to local community services for associated social issues. In the United Kingdom, everyone is entitled to register with a GP practice enabling access to medical care free at the point of delivery. However people from disadvantaged groups, such as homeless individuals or those with severe mental illness, are less likely to be registered, increasing their disadvantage. Nevertheless, people with severe mental illness value the care their GP provides describing primary care as the cornerstone of their care [12].

The worried well and primary care

We want to now consider a group of people who frequently attend primary care and where it is often unclear whether their problems reach the level of a formal diagnosis of say anxiety, depression or somatisation. Unkindly parodied as the *worried well*, these groups are as disabled as most sufferers of chronic physical diseases, generating major social and financial burden to families, friends and employers, and consuming scarce health resources [13].

Their problems typically present in vague and ill-defined ways, which shift over time and often elude explanation. An American primary care study reported fewer than 20% of patients presenting persisting symptoms had a diagnosable physical disorder and 10% had a clear psychological disorder [14]. For practitioners and health systems geared to traditional 'disease' approaches, this uncomfortable reality can evoke a tendency to pathologise human distress and experience.

Is this the right direction? Are there alternatives? The sheer scale of human distress seen in primary care, whether overtly described or more subtle in its effects on psychological or (so-called) physical conditions constitutes *business as usual* for its practitioners. We shall now go on to describe how the inherent strengths of primary care can help normalise these experiences without relying on diagnosis and resource-hungry specialist treatments.

Primary care – stronghold of generalism

The question arises 'Are the *worried well* served better through generalism or specialism?' In thinking about this, let us consider some distinctive features of primary care:

- Primary care is delivered by 'specialists in generalism' – defined by James Willis as taking an interest in whatever is of interest to its clients [15]. For a person seeking care for a newly occurring (or newly recurring) problem '*I do not have to have a diagnosis to receive help*'. Primary care bridges the worlds of clients, families, communities and professionals, negotiating meaning around health, illness and disease.

- Effective consultation and continuity: at its heart lies the doctor–patient relationship developed over time. A frequent misconception portrays the GP consultation as a single ten-minute event. Nothing could be further from the reality. Patients see their GPs for short times but over long periods, as and when they want, for all their health-related needs and presenting with undifferentiated mixtures of physical, emotional, family and social problems. An evolving narrative of person-focused (rather than disease-focused) brief interventions over a lifetime, from 'cradle to grave', builds a continuity of relationship and a comprehensiveness of provision that no other health professional can provide.

- A core competency, recognised by the UK Royal College of General Practitioners requires GPs to work in a family-centred and community-orientated way [16]: '*GPs should aim at a holistic approach to the patient and his or her family, where the main focus would be in promoting their health and general wellbeing. GPs are seen to have a responsibility for the individual patient, his or her family and the wider community and need to understand the characteristics of the community including socio-economic, ethnicity and health features*' [16].

- Another core GP competency tolerates uncertainty, exploring patients' own health beliefs, assessing probability and marginalising danger [16]. For someone experiencing mental distress, the GP may need to hold uncertainty, allowing the passage of time to test if the psychological difficulties are transient whilst avoiding a psychiatric stigmatising diagnosis. But of course disorders like psychosis often start off as milder, more common ones, rarely presenting with clear-cut psychotic symptoms. Therefore, tolerance of uncertainty must be balanced with another core function of GPs to detect potentially serious conditions early, when they will offer assessment, treatment, information giving and referral. So alongside tolerance of uncertainty, the GP requires a high index of suspicion.

So in summary, primary care is steeped in a culture of generalism, continuity and holistic practice which makes it distinctively 'person-focused' contrasting the 'disease-focused' nature of specialist care.

In terms of early intervention, our main message here is not about primary care or specialist care being inferior/superior – simply that they are different. It is the degree to which the two systems can successfully integrate that is important to our patients.

Preventing illness and promoting wellness – a wider perspective on primary and secondary prevention

An underpinning principle is that social disadvantage, physical illness and poor mental health are inextricably linked, whether we are discussing relatively mild disorders or more severe ones. In the United Kingdom, the last 10 years have seen average life expectancy improve as a result in part of for major investment in screening/prevention/early intervention for cardiovascular disease and cancer. And yet health inequality widened over the same period. A recent landmark study by Hacking and colleagues found that inequalities in all cause mortality in the north/south divide were severe and persistent over the four decades from 1965 to 2008. The increase in this inequality from 2000 to 2008 was notable and occurred despite the public policy emphasis in England over this period on reducing inequalities in health [17].

However, this is not just an 'impoverished-north'/'more-affluent-south' issue. This study is important because it compares two population blocks of 25 million people. But the principles equally apply to population groups like those with mental ill health, where similar influences play out to create major health inequalities. To better understand this paradox, consider the example of tobacco smoking, the largest cause of preventable deaths in the United Kingdom.

- Increased smoking explains half the difference in survival rates to age 70 between social classes I and V [18].

- Forty-two percent of all tobacco consumed in England is by those with mental disorder (75% with common mental disorders; 25% with severe disorders) [19].

- Despite significant falls in overall United Kingdom smoking prevalence over the past 30 years, this hardly changed among those on low incomes and the least advantaged [20].

Despite major investments, the UK smoking cessation programmes have least benefitted those with mental ill health, the very people at greatest risk of harm. This is despite evidence that their motivation to stop is no different to the general population [21] and that smoking cessation improves mental and physical health [22]. This situation exemplifies the inverse care law where the quality of health care for people with mental ill health is weakest where, on the basis of need, it should be strongest [23].

These disadvantaged groups are left with a sense of fatalism, loss of autonomy and poor resilience. For primary care this means such patients often ignore their health and present late when less can be done, simply reinforcing the negative spiral. Their presentations are typically complex, invariably have a mental health component, but often defy straightforward diagnosis (or are 'sub-threshold' for diagnosis) and clinical intervention. This is an ideal opportunity to build a more preventive and health promoting approach. And even where a person has reached a diagnostic threshold such as depression – this reflects as much a social as a clinical condition. Yet treating the 'clinical condition' is what clinical guidance invariably promotes at the risk of ignoring the social condition.

Furthermore when mental and physical disorders co-exist, for example as commonly happens for older people, the mental disorder may be overlooked [24]. And yet a diagnosis of depression can be uncovered by a simple screening tool [25].

Time for a more biopsychosocial approach?

Holistic care is an accepted part of primary care. But acknowledging that problems like depression reflect as much a social as a clinical condition opens up broader treatment options. While both medication and psychological therapies have a role, social prescribing can strengthen primary care's armoury to respond early and effectively. This can offer advantages such as:

1. Normalises experiences and engages patients in positive mental and physical health promotion.

2. Encourages people to take more responsibility for their health.

3. Acknowledges how social, economic and cultural factors impact on mental health outcomes across the whole spectrum of disorders.

4. Encouraging social prescriptions may reduce reliance on biological ones.

5. Improves access to mainstream services and opportunities for people with long-term mental health problems.

Primary care cannot achieve this alone. It requires active partnership, joint working and cooperation between primary care and a wide range of voluntary and community groups, as well as statutory welfare providers. At a public health level, community development can reduce the incidence of mental disorder/improve community well-being by recognising the importance communities attach to social contact, social activity, opportunities to learn and develop skills, involvement and having a role as positive influences on mental health. This will ensure mental health is integrated within broader strategies for tackling socially disadvantaged communities, closing the opportunity gap and social justice [26].

Physical health of people with psychosis and primary care

Comorbidity is common, and particularly in the socially disadvantaged. Furthermore, the extent of comorbidity is much greater in the youngest age groups, even though there is increasing morbidity with increasing age [27]. This is particularly pertinent for conditions like schizophrenia, where young onset and social disadvantage are norms, and where average life expectancy may be reduced by 25 years [28]. For this group, about three-quarters of premature deaths arise from physical disorders and the remainder from suicide or accidents [29]. These physical disorders include the 'usual suspects' such as diabetes, heart attacks, pulmonary infections and stroke [30]. More shockingly, the mortality gap is widening [30], explained not by suicide but by physical causes, particularly premature cardiovascular deaths [31]. It appears that whilst the general population have benefitted from improved prevention and early intervention for these conditions, those with schizophrenia have been left behind [31].

However, poor physical health is not just experienced through illness or early death. Take the issue of obesity. Antipsychotic medicines are seriously implicated and a recent evidence reappraisal concluded that medication-induced weight gain in first-episode psychosis is three- to fourfold greater than previously realised [32]. Imagine how it feels, aged 19, to gain 10 kilograms in your first year of treatment? How lowering to your self-esteem? How stigmatising *on top* of having a psychiatric illness? How restricting of your fitness and well-being? Should we be surprised when these young people stop their medicines and default clinic attendance only to then run into a cycle of relapsing illness and disillusion with their life ahead? For these young people, this is as much about the impact of diminished well-being as it is about ill health and disease.

Why are these young people at risk of such poor health?

- Social exclusion, impoverished social networks and restricted opportunity emerge quickly from the onset of illness. For instance, they rapidly fall out of education and employment so that within a year approaching 90% have become unemployed (greater than any other disabled group) [33].

- Adverse cardiometabolic risks emerge within weeks of commencing antipsychotic medicines, particularly obesity, glucose dysregulation and hypercholesterolemia [4].

- Notwithstanding metabolic disturbances from antipsychosis medication, these young people often experience other cardiovascular risk factors, including poor nutrition, inadequate exercise, problematic tobacco and substance use [34].

- Tobacco use is a particular concern; 59% of first-episode patients are smokers; they are six times more likely to smoke than their non-psychotic peers [35]; they continue to smoke into adult life [18].

Not only are these young people exposed to potentially modifiable cardiovascular risk but they also receive inferior physical health care, exemplifying again the inverse care law [36]. For instance, despite consulting their GPs more frequently (about 13–14 per year compared with approximately 3 per year for the general population) cardiovascular risk factors, in particular, were less frequently recorded or acted upon [37]. Routine screening for diabetes in psychiatry and primary care appear suboptimal [38]. Fewer routine eye checks and poorer glycaemic and lipid control [39] may explain why those suffering from both diabetes and schizophrenia have 50% poorer survival rates than those with diabetes alone [40].

Where does primary care sit in all of this?

An average GP in the United Kingdom provides care for about 15–20 people with schizophrenia [6]. Many GPs feel that, in contrast with patients with complex diabetes or heart failure, care of such patients is beyond their remit. A study of focus groups with such patients, GPs and practice nurses provides some insights [8]:

> 'I know that I cannot look after people with severe and enduring mental health problems. I do not have the skills or the knowledge. I could not do it well.'

Whereas most of the patients interviewed described primary care as the '*cornerstone*' of their physical and mental health care, for example:

> 'I mean, the GP has to have some understanding of mental health but I do not expect my GP to know all of the issues to do with my illness. I would though expect him or her to refer me to a specialist person. The important thing is that somebody is looking after you so it is not just you on your own.'

Most patients and GPs/practice nurses agreed primary care had a responsibility to continue prescribing drugs initiated in secondary care, monitor side effects and tackle physical health issues. All participants felt that interpersonal and longitudinal continuity was vital for good-quality care. Most patients favoured seeing the same GP for their physical and mental health needs, preferring a continuous doctor–patient relationship and a positive attitude and willingness to learn, rather than seeing a different GP with special expertise in mental health.

What about secondary care?

A UK national study of community-based assertive outreach services found [41]:

- Recorded measurement within the previous year for blood pressure in 26% of patients, obesity in 17%, blood glucose (or HbA1c) in 28% and plasma lipids in 22%, with all four measured in 11%.

- In the total national sample, 6% had documented diabetes, 6% hypertension and 6% dyslipidemia. Extrapolating from established prevalence in similar populations suggests that for every patient known to have diabetes, another was unrecognized, for every known case of hypertension, four were missed, and for every known case of dyslipidemia, seven were missed.

Exploration of the clinical teams' views on obstacles to screening in routine practice found:

- Uncertainty about whose responsibility this was.

- Lack of confidence about interpreting abnormal screening results.

- Limited access to basic equipment.

These results are worrying. These patients are being followed up by these services explicitly because of prior service disengagement. They could hardly be expected to engage primary care well over their physical health care. And despite their acknowledged risks of physical ill health (much derived from their psychiatric medication), many missed out on the most basic level of care.

These findings are not unique to assertive outreach teams. More recently the National Audit of Schizophrenia [42] audited the care of 5,091 people living in England and Wales with a diagnosis of either schizophrenia or schizo-affective disorder in receipt of care from a community-based mental health service over the previous 12 months. Only 29% had an adequate assessment of cardiovascular risk documented (weight or body mass index; smoking status, blood glucose, blood lipid, blood pressure; and family history of premature cardiovascular disease, diabetes, hypertension or hyperlipidaemia). Even a measure as simple as weight went unrecorded in 43%.

Despite a proliferation of articles and editorials exhorting both primary and specialist practitioners to improve the physical health aspects of their clinical practice, these appear to make little difference, indicating system weaknesses rather than isolated poor practice [43]. It seems changing clinical practice will take more than just issuing new guidance. As the EPPIC service in Melbourne has demonstrated, it requires investment in systematic approaches to analysing and understanding the barriers to routine monitoring, organisational commitment to overcoming these, and clinical leadership [44].

A way forward?

We need to acknowledge a group of many thousands of young people in their twenties and thirties with psychosis, at ages not normally considered for active cardiovascular prevention, who are at high risk of dying young. To focus simply on the psychological aspects whilst ignoring the physical precursors of future ill health is to fail these young people. We believe the paradigm of early intervention in primary care for this high-risk population provides the key. Several facets of a potential system solution may already be in place:

- Primary care already provides health promotion and disease management programmes for conditions like heart disease and diabetes – that is the skills and knowledge are already there.

- The population at risk is usually 'known' to specialist services.

- We know that conditions like diabetes and cardiovascular disease can be prevented or delayed by a combination of increased activity, improved diet and weight loss.

- We can identify and track specific modifiable risks (e.g. BMI, lipids, glucose and smoking).

- We know when to target prevention (the early critical phase of illness).

- We know the nature of the lifestyle issues that operate (e.g. tobacco smoking, obesity and lack of exercise).

- We know how to measure health care improvement (e.g. audit; practitioner development and service improvement programmes).

We believe a collaborative approach between primary and specialist care is required to fully address the complex blend of emotional, physical and social factors:

- Provide patients, right from the start of treatment, informed choice and skilled medicines management which acknowledges potential weight gain and metabolic disturbance.

- Get the basics right

  - Address poor housing, poverty and social isolation.

  - Value and support families and other key care-givers as partners in care.

- Guarantee regular physical health screening and early identification and intervention for established risk.

- Address lifestyle issues through health promotion on issues like diet, smoking and physical activity.

Encouragingly the importance of a more preventive approach has been recently highlighted by international consensus, Healthy Active Lives (HeAL) [45]. This coincides with the emergence of systematic screening and treatment programmes which prioritise more integrated primary/specialist care approaches to addressing cardiovascular risk right from the onset of psychosis [44, 46].

Conclusions

The paradigm shift that is early intervention in psychiatry cannot be achieved by specialist care alone. We believe primary care can make a key contribution by bringing its own distinctive characteristics of generalism, continuity, family-centred practice and holism. Moreover, both international comparisons and studies within countries demonstrate the cost-effectiveness of primary care oriented health systems particularly concerning prevention of the progression of illness, and especially at younger ages.

However, primary care may see the challenge of early intervention in psychiatry differently to specialist services. Psychological needs rarely present neatly in primary care. Our two examples – the worried well (more accurately characterised worried sick) and the physically unwell person with schizophrenia – demonstrate how poor emotional resilience, physical ill health and social adversity show a toxic interdependence which operates along the whole spectrum of severity, exerting a spiral of decline. Interrupting the evolution of that spiral is the essence of the early intervention paradigm. The subtle way these factors interact challenges health systems to go beyond an either/or view of diseases; either biomedical or psychosocial, either body or mind, either physical or emotional. This is familiar territory for primary care practitioners where multi-morbidities are to be expected and tolerance of uncertainty is routine.

But familiar territory or not, our systems of health care still fail people with mental and physical comorbidities and social deprivation. For no group is this more apparent than those with severe mental illness exemplifying the law of inverse care. The early intervention paradigm has a real opportunity to challenge the current poor organisation of health services and an ongoing failure by medical doctors in primary and specialist care to agree responsibility [47]. There is a clear mandate for primary and specialist practitioners to collectively engage much earlier and to actively intervene to protect cardiometabolic health. But whilst these arguments over physical health responsibility drag on, these severely mentally ill young patients remain a high-risk population, particularly given the poor physical health care they can expect. For early intervention to be described as a real paradigm shift in psychiatry, then this must embrace both mind and body. For young people with emerging psychosis, delivering this particular both/and will require primary care and specialist care to truly collaborate. Now that would be a paradigm shift.

Acknowledgements

The authors acknowledge co-authors of publications that greatly influenced their work: Dr. Dave Tomson, Dr. Maryanne Freer, Dr. Dick Churchill, Professor Peter Jones, Professor Steve Field, Professor Chris Thompson, Dr. Samantha Callan, Professor Kathy Samaras and Dr. Jackie Curtis.

In special memory of the late Professor Helen Lester:

This chapter would be incomplete without acknowledging the passing on of Helen Lester. In reflecting on our work together over the past 16 years, it feels timely to close our final writing venture with my personal tribute to a wonderful friend and colleague. Her dedication in improving the lives of people and families affected by mental illness has been a beacon to me and many others. I can commend to readers her extraordinary delivery of the James McKenzie Lecture at the Royal College of General Practitioners only months before her death as a perfect accompaniment and fitting close to this chapter [48].

References

1. Venkatapuram S, Bell R and Marmot M. (2010). The right to sutures: social epidemiology, human rights, and social justice. *Health and Human Rights* **12**: 3–16.
2. Skeate A, Jackson C, Birchwood M, et al. (2002). Duration of untreated psychosis and pathways to care in first-episode psychosis: investigation of help-seeking behaviour in primary care. *British Journal of Psychiatry* **181**: 73–77.
3. Simon AE, Lauber C, Ludewig K, et al. (2005). General practitioners and schizophrenia: results from a Swiss survey. *British Journal of Psychiatry* **187**: 274–281.
4. Foley D and Morley KI. (2011). Systematic review of early cardiometabolic outcomes of the first treated episode of psychosis. *Archives of General Psychiatry*. Published online February, doi:10.1001/archgenpsychiatry.2011.2.

5. Starfield B and Shi L. (2002). Policy relevant determinants of health: an international perspective. *Health Policy* **60**: 201–218.
6. Institute of Medicine. (1996). *Primary Care: America's Health in a New Era*. Washington DC: Institute of Medicine.
7. Starfield B. (2008). *The Importance of Primary Health Care in Health Systems*. Qatar-EMRO Primary Health Care Conference, Doha, Qatar.
8. van Doorslaer E, Koolman X and Jones AM. (2004). Explaining income-related inequalities in doctor utilisation in Europe. *Health Economics* **13**(7): 629–647.
9. Shoen C, Osborn R, Hiynh P, et al. (2005). Taking the pulse of health care systems: experiences of patients with health problems in six countries. *Health Affairs* **W5**: 509–525.
10. Goldberg D and Huxley P. (1992). *Common Mental Disorders*. London: Routledge.
11. Kendrick T, Burns T, Garland C, et al. (2000). Are specialist mental health services being targeted on the most needy patients? - the effects of setting up special services in general practice. *British Journal of General Practice* **50**: 121–126.
12. Lester H, Tritter JQ and Sorohan H. (2005). Patients' and health professionals' views on primary care for people with serious mental illness: focus group study. *BMJ: British Medical Association* **330**: 1122.
13. Melzer H, Gill B, Petticrew M, et al. (1995). *OPCS Surveys of Psychiatric Morbidity in Great Britain, Report 1: The Prevalence of Psychiatric Morbidity Among Adults Living in Private Households*. London: HMSO.
14. Kroenke K and Mangelsdorff AD. (1989). Common symptoms in ambulatory care: Incidence, evaluation, therapy and outcome. *American Journal of Medicine* **86**: 262–266.
15. Willis J. (1995). *The Paradox of progress*. Abingdon, Oxon: Radcliffe Medical Press.
16. Royal College of General Practitioners. (2010). *GP Curriculum Statements*, http://www.rcgp-curriculum.org.uk/rcgp_-_gp_curriculum_documents/gp_curriculum_statements.aspx (accessed 14 April 2014).
17. Hacking J, Muller S and Buchan I. (2011). Trends in mortality from 1965 to 2008 across the English north-south divide: comparative observational study. *BMJ: British Medical Association* **342**: 508.
18. Wanless D. (2004). *Securing Good Health for the Whole Population*. London: TSO.
19. McManus S, Meltzer H and Campion J. (2010). Cigarette smoking and mental health in England. Data from the Adult Psychiatric Morbidity Survey. National Centre for Social Research. http://www.natcen.ac.uk/media/21994/smoking-mental-health.pdf (accessed 14 April 2014).
20. Jarvis M and Wardle J. (1999). Social patterning of individual health behaviours: the case of cigarette smoking. In: M Marmot and R Wilkinson (eds), *Social Determinants of Health*, Oxford: Oxford University Press.
21. Siru R, Hulse GK and Tait RJ. (2008). Assessing motivation to quit smoking in people with mental illness: a review. *Addiction* **104**: 719–733.
22. Campion J, Checinski K and Nurse J. (2008). Review of smoking cessation treatments for people with mental illness. *Advances in Psychiatric Treatment* **14**: 208–216.
23. Hart JT. (1971). The inverse care law. *The Lancet* **297**: 405–412.
24. Katon W and Ciechanowski P. (2002). Impact of major depression on chronic medical illness. *Journal of Psychosomatic Research* **53**: 859–863.
25. Arroll B, Khin N and Kerse N. (2003). Two verbally asked questions are simple and valid. *British Medical Journal* **327**: 1144–1146.
26. Friedl L and Watson S. (2004). Social prescribing for mental health: briefing paper. Social Care Institute for Excellence.
27. van den Akker M, Buntinx F, Metsemakers JF, et al. (1998). Multimorbidity in general practice: prevalence, incidence, and determinants of co-occurring chronic and recurrent diseases. *Journal Of Clinical Epidemiology* **51**(5): 367–375.
28. Parks J, Svendsen D, Singer P, et al. (2006). Morbidity and mortality in people with serious mental illness. National Association of State Mental Health Programme Directors, 13th technical report.

29. Nordentoft M, Wahlbeck K, Hällgren, et al. (2013). Excess mortality, causes of death and life expectancy in 270,770 patients with recent onset of mental disorders in Denmark, Finland and Sweden. *PLoS ONE* **8**: e55176. doi:10.1371/journal.pone.0055176.

30. Saha S, Chant D and McGrath J. (2007). A systematic review of mortality in schizophrenia: is the differential mortality gap worsening over time? *Archives of General Psychiatry* **64**: 1123–1131.

31. Brown S, Kim M, Mitchell C, et al. (2010). Twenty-five year mortality of a community cohort with schizophrenia. *British Journal of Psychiatry* **196**: 116–121.

32. Alvarez M, Blanch C, Crespo-Facorro B, et al. (2008). Antipsychotic-induced weight gain in chronic and first-episode psychotic disorders a systematic critical reappraisal. *CNS drugs* **22**(7): 547–562.

33. Killackey EJ, Jackson H J, Gleeson J, et al. (2006). Exciting career opportunity beckons! Early intervention and vocational rehabilitation in first episode psychosis: Employing cautious optimism. *Australian and New Zealand Journal of Psychiatry* **40**: 951–962.

34. Varley K and McClennan J. (2009). Implications of marked weight gain associated with atypical antipsychotic medications in children and adolescents. *Journal of the American Medical Association* **302**: 1811–1882.

35. Myles N, Newall H, Curtis J, et al. (2012). Tobacco use before, at and after first-episode of psychosis – a systematic review and meta-analysis. *Journal of Clinical Psychiatry* **73**(4): 468–475.

36. Newcomer J and Hennekens CH. (2007). Severe mental illness and risk of cardiovascular disease editorial. *The Journal of the American Medical Association* **298**(15): 1794–1796.

37. Kendrick T. (1996). Cardiovascular and respiratory risk factors and symptoms among general practice patients with long-term mental illness. *British Journal of Psychiatry* **169**: 733–739.

38. Frayne SM, Halanych JH, Miller DR, et al. (2005). Disparities in diabetes care: impact of mental illness. *Archives Internationales Medecine* **165**: 2631–2638.

39. Tarrant CJ. (2006). Blood glucose testing for adults prescribed atypical antipsychotics in primary and secondary care. *Psychiatric Bulletin* **30**: 286–288.

40. Vinogradova Y, Coupland C, Hippisley-Cox J, et al. (2010). Severe mental illness and survival in people with diabetes. *The British Journal of Psychiatry* **197**: 272–277.

41. Barnes T, Paton C, Cavanagh M, et al. (2007). A UK audit of screening for the metabolic side effects of antipsychotics in community patients. *Schizophrenia Bulletin* **33**(6): 1397–1403.

42. Royal College of Psychiatrists. (2012). Report of the National Audit of Schizophrenia (NAS) 2012. London: Healthcare Quality Improvement Partnership, www.rcpsych.ac.uk/pdf/NAS%20National%20report%20FINAL.pdf

43. De Hert M, Dekker JM, Wood D, et al. (2009). Cardiovascular disease and diabetes in people with severe mental illness position statement from the European Psychiatric Association (EPA), supported by the European Association for the Study of Diabetes (EASD) and the European Society of Cardiology (ESC). *European Psychiatry* **24**(6): 412–424. http://www.europsy-journal.com/article/S0924-9338%2809%2900017-0/abstract.

44. Hetrick S, Álvarez-Jiménez M and Parker A. (2010). Promoting physical health in youth mental health services: ensuring routine monitoring of weight and metabolic indices in a first episode psychosis clinic. *Australasian Psychiatry* **18**: 451–455.

45. International Physical Health in Youth (iphYs) working group. *Healthy Active Lives (HeAL) consensus statement 2013*. http://www.iphys.org.au.

46. Curtis JE, Newall H and Samaras K. (2012). The heart of the matter: cardiometabolic care in youth with psychosis. *Early Intervention in Psychiatry* **6**: 347–353.

47. Tiihonen J, Lönnqvist J, Wahlbeck K, et al. (2011). No mental health without physical health. *The Lancet* **377**: 611.

48. Lester HE. (2013). Being bothered about Billy. RCGP James McKenzie Lecture 2012. *Brit J of Gen Practice* **608**. http://www.youtube.com/watch?v=tqyACm5OQOM.

14
Early Intervention in the General Hospital

Peter Byrne[1,2] and Iyas Assalman[3]
[1] Homerton University Hospital, London
[2] Royal College of Psychiatrists, UK
[3] Newham Centre for Mental Health, London and East London Foundation NHS Trust

Modern general hospitals cannot function effectively without on-site psychiatric assessment and treatment. This goes beyond the management of delirium (Chapter 19) and the safe evaluation of self-harm (Chapter 20) – respectively, the commonest complication of general hospital admission and the top cause of general hospital presentations among young people. With an ageing population, most admissions comprise people over 65, two thirds of whom will have mental health problems, with about half the population over 70 showing objective evidence of cognitive impairment [1]: Chapter 10. A major component of our work in East London has been the evaluation of drug/alcohol misuse and dependence: we will not revisit the early intervention evidence set out in Chapter 17. On-site mental health personnel also address the high prevalence of common mental disorders in medical and surgical inpatients. Holistic care must include psychological evaluation and appropriate support for inpatients, whose resilience is overwhelmed by physical morbidity: adjustment disorders may develop into depression and/or personality traits may become exaggerated such that they interfere with the business of recovery. Psychiatrists who work in general hospitals treat every type of psychiatric disorder: presentation to and/or frequent use of the emergency department along with hospital admission provide excellent opportunities for early intervention to improve mental and physical well-being. Although functional psychosis has a relatively low incidence in acute care inpatients, people with established schizophrenia and bipolar disorders frequently deteriorate around general hospital admission, where physical ill health is a precipitant (life event) for relapse. As a consequence of the premature morbidity and mortality of people with any mental illness [2], in general hospital psychiatry at least 11% of their referrals comprise people

Early Intervention in Psychiatry: EI of nearly everything for better mental health, First Edition.
Edited by Peter Byrne and Alan Rosen.
© 2014 John Wiley & Sons, Ltd. Published 2014 by John Wiley & Sons, Ltd.

with severe mental illness (SMI). In this chapter, we will set out the evidence for timely interventions in three groups: (i) people with SMI who develop (predictable) physical ill health, including cancer, (ii) patients who are admitted with stroke (cerebrovascular accident) and develop depression and (iii) patients across primary care and specialist services with medically unexplained symptoms (MUS).

A brief note on terminology first. Many US and European centres use the term consultation liaison psychiatry, abbreviated to liaison psychiatry in the United Kingdom. Some US colleagues prefer the term general hospital psychiatry, and this includes emergency psychiatry (e.g. assessing self-harm or risk of harm to others), coincident physical and mental ill health and the range of presentations of people with somatoform disorders. The latter conditions, currently the subject of much debate in both ICD-11 and DSM-V reclassifications, led to many European specialists' description of their work as psychosomatics. The heterogeneity of the patients seen by liaison psychiatrists makes it at once an interesting speciality with a high turnover, but also a challenging area to evaluate, and therefore relatively less well-funded than other branches of psychiatry. If during the 1990s, had we rebranded the speciality 'early intervention psychiatry in general hospitals', this may not have been the case. At time of writing, the United Kingdom has seen a resurgence of interest in liaison psychiatric teams due to the work of Professor George Tadros and others in Birmingham. He and his team demonstrated the health and economic benefits of resourcing a single team to achieve early intervention across all age groups, the Rapid Assessment and Discharge (RAID) Team [3]. Their ethos is rapid, early assessment by senior clinicians through a single point of referral of everything (not 'nearly everything'), with a low threshold to accept cases for assessment: no arguments that the alcohol is 'causing' the depression and only an abstinent patient can be assessed, or that dementia/delirium is 'not psychiatric'. This is clearly the way forward, given that doctors, our primary referrers, will have left medical school with lots of experiences of treatment-resistant schizophrenia but without the skills to accurately differentiate depression from unhappiness or dysthymia from 'whatever'.

The physical health of people with severe mental illness

All scientific studies that examine excess mortality and premature death (by natural and unnatural causes) confirm the same grim findings of the meta-analysis of Harris and Barraclough [2]. Hippisley-Cox et al. [4] record substantially higher rates of illness in populations of SMI of the common physical diseases of coronary heart disease, cerebrovascular accident, chronic obstructive pulmonary disease and diabetes. More striking are the age-adjusted death rates at 5 years from diagnosis, when compared to the general population with the same four diseases respectively, 22% vs. 8% (general population), 28% vs. 12%, 28% vs. 15% and 22% vs. 15%. Overall, the 5-year survival for people with SMI is less than half the expected survival for coronary, cerebrovascular and obstructive lung diseases, and broadly we expect one in five of 'psychiatric patients' to die within 5 years of diagnosis of any of the 4 diseases. We know of several confounders here – factors that will lead to higher rates of both mental illness and to physical morbidities/mortalities:

• low birth weight

• low income (low-income family, recipient of benefits and low educational status)

- poor housing (state housing, institutional care and homelessness) and

- lifestyle factors (poor nutrition, obesity, less exercise, smoking and drug misuse).

It is worth noting that every one of these factors is modifiable by early intervention programmes. Lawrence and Kisely [5] have identified inequalities of the access and delivery to physical health care as possible causes for higher morbidities and mortality of people with SMI, in particular:

- separation of physical health services from mental health services

- health care provider issues, including the stigma of mental illness

- direct consequences of mental illness (itself a risk factor for lower income, poorer housing, poorer nutrition, more sedentary lifestyle etc.) and

- as a direct result of the side effects of psychiatric medication.

While we await integrated public mental health programmes to address the upstream causes of poor health, mental and physical, such as low birth weight and poverty, these latter four categories are a useful focus for all liaison psychiatrists. On-site liaison psychiatry allows near full integration of the liaison team into the general hospital team. We assess and manage patients alongside our medical, nursing and surgical colleagues. Physicians may be nervous around people with the negative symptoms of schizophrenia, and our role is to prompt timely, appropriate physical investigation and management. Diagnostic overshadowing, first described in the learning disability literature 30 years ago, describes how physicians (including psychiatrists) are likely to ascribe physical symptoms to an underlying mental disorder, and thereby less likely to investigate and treat symptoms of physical illness [6]. Recently, a medical registrar asked our team if psychosis could cause a high temperature. The patient was delirious (see Chapter 19) and once the medical cause was identified and treated, septicaemia from a lung infection, he recovered fully. Diagnostic overshadowing preferences assumptions over the methodical search for facts, and is closely related to the therapeutic nihilism some medical and surgical colleagues hold about people with SMI. This leads to less treatment, in some cases denial of life-saving treatments such as organ transplantation [7]. One of us encountered a 45-year-old man with schizophrenia who denied a renal transplant on the basis that his future adherence would be unreliable. Evidence was produced that he had missed one monthly depot antipsychotic injection in 11 years with psychiatric services, and he got his transplant. Embedded in general hospitals and clinics, liaison psychiatrists are ideally placed to persuade, engage and train their hospital colleagues to reverse the adverse effects of stigma and discrimination (see Chapter 26).

Cancer is worth examining in this context. There is convincing evidence that the incidence of cancer in people with SMI is no greater than that of the general population [8, 9], but that SMI populations will get cancer at younger ages than case-matched controls [8]. This does not mean we ignore unhealthy lifestyles (poor diet, obesity and lower rates of exercise) in people with mental health problems, and the most unhealthy lifestyle choice of all – cigarette smoking. Lung cancer is overrepresented in people with SMI, with women:

odds ratio (OR), 1.57; 95% CI, 1.13–2.19; men: OR, 1.52; 95% CI, 1.09–2.12, due to disproportionate high rates of smoking [8]. Smoking cessation programmes in psychiatric inpatients are just as effective as in other populations [10] and we should not allow low expectations/therapeutic nihilism to prevent timely referral. There are two major differences in cancer progression between people with SMI and the general population. Firstly, late presentation is more likely in the former group, with 7.1% having metastases at time of diagnoses, compared to 6.1% of the general population [9]. Secondly, the SMI groups are less likely to receive specialist interventions (surgery, radiotherapy) that prolong life. These combine to explain the 30% higher case fatality rate, all cancers, in people with SMI [9]. The most recent meta-analysis in this area (8 studies comprising 1,448 cancer patients in multiple international centres, where all patients were assessed with the same validated diagnostic instrument) estimated a prevalence of mental disorder in 32% (95% CI 27% to 37%): this reflects high psychosocial morbidity in cancer patients, only a proportion of which are people with mental health problems that predated their cancer diagnosis [11]. Liaison psychiatrists have a low threshold to assess these patients, though many (adjustment disorder, anxiety syndromes and mild depression) will not require medication. Psychosocial interventions for the core disorders work, but these should take place in the context of assessment of carers of referred patients, one quarter of whom will also meet criteria for a diagnosable mental disorder, though in one study less than half received any help for their distress [12]. Early intervention and predictive strategies are established in this patient group [13].

In relation to the physical health consequences of mental illness and its treatment, there are multiple opportunities to intervene. Our good fortune as the treating psychiatrists of a general hospital inpatient with SMI is to be able to access past psychiatric records and speak with the treating team. Simple strategies include repeating what worked before, reading or negotiating advanced directives/known patient preferences, inviting the patient's care coordinator to visit the ward, and enlisting the help of significant others. Medical colleagues might be surprised to learn that their patient requests a smoking cessation programme. We can renegotiate a care package that maximises income and improves diet, housing, activity levels and social networks inter alia to take account of the individual's physical health problems. By contrast, an overweight housebound patient with diabetes is likely to have low/no exercise levels, choose convenience foods over a balanced diet, and social isolation may directly lead to less glycaemic monitoring as well as indirectly increasing solitary alcohol consumption – all to the detriment of physical and mental well-being. Just as personalised packages of integrated care can ameliorate the worst effects of poverty and isolation, medication charts can be collaboratively rewritten to maximise adherence and minimise medications' side effects.

In summary then, liaison psychiatrists rarely diagnose physical health conditions but play a key role in coordinating early intervention for new onset coronary, cerebrovascular, respiratory and diabetic conditions. As a speciality, we can advocate that patients with mental health problems are proactively investigated for treatable and remediable physical disorders (cancer), and where illness is detected, that they receive the same treatment as comparable patients who do not have known mental health problems. In a recent, important victory in the United Kingdom, the Royal College of Psychiatrists achieved statutory recognition of parity of esteem for people with mental disorders: see Chapter 1.

Post-stroke depression

Post-stroke depression (PSD) is among the most common emotional disorders affecting stroke sufferers. Approximately, one third of stroke survivors experience an early or later onset of depression and the diagnosis of PSD is challenging in the acute and chronic aftermath [14] as cognitive, language and functional impairment complicates the recognition of PSD [15]. The interaction between depression and stroke is very complex and the pathophysiological mechanisms have not as yet been fully elucidated, although an interaction between anatomical and psychosocial factors may be important in PSD development [14].

Risk factors correlated significantly with PSD are: a history of previous stroke, a history of previous depression, female gender, living alone and social distress pre stroke [16]. A recent systematic review confirmed these factors and added cognitive impairment and anxiety [17]. PSD impedes the rehabilitation and recovery process, jeopardizes quality of life and increases mortality [14]. Early effective treatment of depression may have a positive effect not only on depressive symptoms but also on the rehabilitation outcome of stroke patients [18].

Different strategies were used to prevent PSD with different outcomes. This includes very early mobilisation after stroke [19], integrated model of care [20, 21] and long-term treatment of post-stroke survivors with folic acid, B6 and B12 [22]. Hackett et al.'s [23] Cochrane review concluded that there was inadequate evidence to support the routine use of antidepressants, psychostimulants or other drugs to prevent depression and improve recovery after stroke. The small positive benefit of psychological strategies probably endorses the use of more structured approaches. However, the amount of evidence to support the routine use of psychological approaches in stroke rehabilitation was limited.

Structured clinical examination of most of stroke patients by a liaison (general hospital) psychiatry service early in their hospital stay should identify anxiety symptoms, presence of depressive symptoms, history of either or other psychosocial difficulties, the degree of cognitive impairment and current disability in the context of current psychosocial difficulties including support post-hospital. Stroke units have developed their own procedures for early rehabilitation and we advocate that appropriate detection of anxiety and anxiety management be written into every aspect of stroke care. Practical obstacles to reducing anxiety are many: degree of disability; cognitive impairment; language impairment (post-stroke) and language barriers and actual/perceived lack of social support post discharge. However, if reducing anxiety had equal priority to (say) reducing blood pressure after stroke, we believe that much morbidity, principally depression, would be avoided. The early treatment of PSD with the antidepressant fluoxetine has some positive effect not only on the depressive symptoms but also on the neurological function, functional ability and cognitive ability [24, 25]. There are effective treatments when PSD is diagnosed; this can be pharmacological and non-pharmacological. Antidepressants are effective treatment but these agents should be used with caution in those with a persistent depressive disorder after stroke, as little is known about the risks, especially of seizures, falls and delirium [26]. Different psychological treatments were tried but with conflicting results [26–28]. It is interesting that there is good evidence to suggest the use of acupuncture for treatment of depression in patients post stroke [29, 30]. Herbal medicine was also tried and showed good efficacy, safety and tolerability in PSD patients [31].

Medically unexplained symptoms

Medically unexplained symptoms (MUS) was a term first coined by Professor David Goldberg in the early 1990s, though he has recently described regret he ever used the phrase due to clinician confusion and its unacceptability to patients (Goldberg 2013, personal communication). It comprises many familiar functional somatic syndromes (irritable bowel syndrome, functional headaches, chronic fatigue syndrome, mechanical back pain, etc.) and the somatoform disorders that prove even harder to define and treat. As an extension of our liaison service, we expanded a primary-care-based pilot to accept and treat MUS patients alongside patients with other long-term conditions (LTCs), principally diabetes, obstructive lung disease and heart failure. We worked with primary case colleagues in our local improved access to psychological therapies (IAPT) service, principally personal well-being practitioners and psychologists to devise a care pathway (Figure 14.1). This compromises the following.

Optimal pathway – our model complements the existing IAPT adherent service provision by adding specific evidence–based low- and high-intensity interventions targeting MUS/LTC, together with enhancement of the assessment and review procedures with collection of sessional MUS/LTC outcome measures. These comprise direct referrals from GPs and case finder-determined cases.

Competency and training – the model provides specific training and protocol-driven supervision of currently employed IAPT therapists to triage primary care referrals of LTC/MUS patients.

Early intervention – Our GP colleagues share our enthusiasm to intervene early with low-intensity treatments, and where needed, more experienced clinicians are consulted to improve the treatment plan and maximise medications, if necessary. Informational materials, translated as necessary, will help overcome some patients' resistance to attend therapies: nonverbal therapies are offered too.

Clinical Competency (1) Low-intensity treatment – we define IAPT workers' core competencies in low-intensity treatments as graded exercise therapy (GET) and cognitive behavioural therapy (CBT) for anxiety and depression, with high intensity comprising specialised CBT: see Figure 14.1. (2) High-intensity treatment – experienced clinicians (psychologist/psychiatrist) will reassess patients who fail to improve with standard treatment for suitability for high-intensity interventions, and (for some) onward referral to existing services for intractable MUS patients. Regular dialogue between therapists, supervisors, trainers and GPs will drive the application of additional resources in treatment-resistant cases.

Efficiency – We adhere to relevant NICE Guidelines (www.nice.org.uk) and manage patients using a stepped, collaborative care model.

Cost Effective Model – Our model adheres closely to proven cost effective models in these patients [32]. Living with any LTC places a significant burden on individuals and families in terms of morbidity, reduced quality of life for the individual and their families and early mortality.

Although some nomenclature and classification differences remain, we already know the breadth of MUS across all the major specialities [33]. We know pervasive patterns of symptom attribution and illness behaviours begin in early childhood and most cases will have an early primary care footprint. The more MUS a person acquires at presentation,

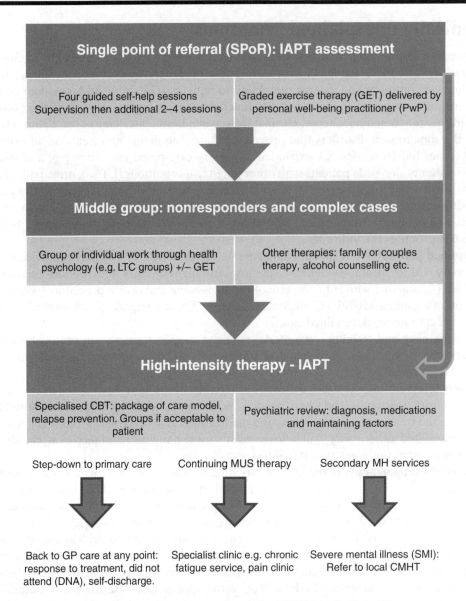

Figure 14.1   Agreed care pathways for MUS/LTC in Newham, UK

or subsequently though mutually frustrating medical consultations, the more psychiatric morbidity will complement the MUS [33]. As a rule, CBT (especially reattribution therapy, but personalised to address the constellation of symptoms) and antidepressant medication are the two most effective treatments. This is true even for pain conditions that will have had very high health service utilisation prior to specialist referral [34]. The application of effective treatments is patchy due to late or disputed diagnoses, and (sadly) the reluctance of MUS patients to undergo 'psychiatric' treatments like CBT, or worse again, antidepressants. Early intervention does not yet have the body of evidence that it prevents chronicity but the argument is made even in the most challenging primary care patients.

Less helpful terms within primary care have described three MUS populations: *frequent fliers, fat filers* or *heartsinkers*. The evidence supports that even in advanced moderate-to-severe symptoms, we can improve symptoms and function in low back pain [35], fibromyalgia [36] and chronic fatigue syndrome [37]. Along with the two latter examples, our work in MUS has added GET to the CBT/medication approach. This is an acceptable, low side effect, nonverbal therapy that is at once practical and a major source of behavioural activation. The challenge is to time these interventions earlier and away from the general hospital, where investigations, waiting times and inconclusive consultations will convert someone with a few functional symptoms into a severe MUS disorder.

References

1. Goldberg SE, Whittamore KH, Harwood RH, et al. (2012). The prevalence of mental health problems among older adults admitted as an emergency to a general hospital. *Age and Ageing* **41**: 80–86.
2. Harris EC and Barraclough B. (1998). Excess mortality of mental disorder. *British Journal of Psychiatry* **173**: 11–53.
3. Tadros G, Salama RA, Kingston P, et al. (2013). Impact of an integrated rapid response psychiatric liaison team on quality improvement and cost savings: the Birmingham RAID model. *The Psychiatric Bulletin* **37**: 4–10.
4. Hippisley-Cox J. et al. (2006). A comparison of survival rates for people with mental health problems and the remaining population with specific conditions. Disability Rights Commission, UK.
5. Lawrence D and Kisely S. (2010). Inequalities in healthcare provision for people with severe mental illness. *Journal of Psychopharmacology* **24**(11) Supplement 4: 61–68.
6. Jones S, Howard L and Thornicroft G. (2008). 'Diagnostic overshadowing': worse physical health care for people with mental illness. *Acta Psychiatrica Scandinavica* **118**: 169–171.
7. Byrne P. (2000). Organ transplantation and discrimination. *British Medical Journal* **320**: 1600.
8. Carney CP, Woolson RF, Jones L, et al. (2004). Occurrence of cancer among people with mental health claims in an insured population. *Psychosomatic Medicine* **66**: 735–743.
9. Kisely S, Crowe E, Lawrence, et al. (2013). Cancer-related mortality in people with mental illness. *Journal of the American Medical Association Psychiatry* **70**: 209–217.
10. Robson D, Cole F, Jalasi S, et al. (2013). Smoking cessation and serious mental illness: a service evaluation of a drop-in stop smoking clinic on an acute in-patient unit. *Journal of Clinical Nursing* **22**: 405–413.
11. Singer S, Das-Munshi J, Brähler E, et al. (2010). Prevalence of mental health conditions in cancer patients in acute care—a meta-analysis. *Annals of Oncology* **21**: 925–930.
12. Vanderwerker LC, Laff RE, Kadan-Lottick NS, et al. (2005). Psychiatric disorders and mental health service use among caregivers of advanced cancer patients. *Journal of Clinical Oncology* **23**: 6899–6907.
13. Harison J and Maguire P. (1994). Predictors of psychiatric morbidity in cancer patients. *British Journal of Psychiatry* **165**: 593–598.
14. Gaete JM and Bogousslavsky J. (2008). Post-stroke depression. *Expert Review of Neurotherapeutics* **8**(1): 75–92.
15. Gupta A, Pansari K and Shetty H. (2002). Post-stroke depression. *International Journal of Clinical Practice* **56**(7): 531–537.
16. Andersen G, Vestergaard K, Ingemann-Nielsen M, et al. (1995). Risk factors for post-stroke depression. *Acta Psychiatrica Scandinavica* **92**(3): 193–198.
17. Ayerbe L, Ayis S, Wolfe CDA, et al. (2013). Natural history, predictors and outcomes of depression after stroke: systematic review and meta-analysis. *British Journal of Psychiatry* **202**: 14–21.

18. Lenzi GL, Altieri M and Maestrini I. (2008). Post-stroke depression. *Revue Neurologique (Paris)* **164**(10): 837–840.

19. Cumming TB, Collier J, Thrift AG, et al. (2008). The effect of very early mobilisation after stroke on psychological well-being. *Journal of Rehabilitation Medicine: Official Journal of the UEMS European Board of Physical and Rehabilitation Medicine* **40**(8): 609–614.

20. Joubert J, Reid C, Joubert L, et al. (2006). Risk factor management and depression post-stroke: the value of an integrated model of care. *Journal of Clinical Neuroscience: Official Journal of the Neurosurgical Society of Australasia.* **13**(1): 84–90.

21. Joubert J, Joubert L, Reid C, et al. (2008). The positive effect of integrated care on depressive symptoms in stroke survivors. *Cerebrovascular Diseases* **26**(2): 199–205.

22. Almeida OP, Marsh K, Alfonso H, et al. (2010). B-vitamins reduce the long-term risk of depression after stroke: The VITATOPS-DEP trial. *Annals of Neurology* **68**(4): 503–510.

23. Hackett ML, Anderson CS, House A, et al. (2008). Interventions for preventing depression after stroke. *Cochrane Database of Systematic Reviews.* Issue 3. Art. No.: CD003689.

24. González-Torrecillas JL, Mendlewicz J and Lobo A. (1995). Effects of early treatment of poststroke depression on neuropsychological rehabilitation. *International Psychogeriatrics* **7**(4): 547–560.

25. Jia W, Zhang X-L, Zhang D-B, et al. (2005). Effect of early intervention on recovery of motor function and recurrent stroke in patients with post-stroke depression. *Zhongguo Linchuang Kangfu* **9**(12): 4–5.

26. Hackett ML, House A, Xia J, et al. (2008). Interventions for treating depression after stroke. *Cochrane Database of Systematic Reviews.* Issue 4. Art. No.: CD003437.

27. Mitchell PH, Veith RC, Becker KJ, et al. (2009). Brief psychosocial-behavioral intervention with antidepressant reduces poststroke depression significantly more than usual care with antidepressant: living well with stroke: randomized, controlled trial. *Stroke: A Journal of Cerebral Circulation* **40**(9): 3073–3078.

28. Zhou C-X, Su X-L, Yang X-Z, et al. (2004). Effect of psychological nursing on the rehabilitation of post-stroke depression. *Zhongguo Linchuang Kangfu* **8**(16): 3008–3009.

29. Li HJ, Zhong BL, Fan YP, et al. (2011). Acupuncture for post-stroke depression: a randomized controlled trial. *Zhongguo Zhen Jiu* **31**(1): 3–6.

30. Wu JP. (2010). Clinical observation on acupuncture treatment of 150 cases of post-stroke depression according to syndrome differentiation. *Zhen Ci Yan Jiu* **35**(4): 303–306.

31. Li LT, Wang SH, Ge HY, et al. (2008). The beneficial effects of the herbal medicine Free and Easy Wanderer Plus (FEWP) and fluoxetine on post-stroke depression. *Journal of Alternative and Complementary Medicine* **14**(7): 841–846.

32. McDaid D, Parsonage M and Park A. (2011). Tackling medically unexplained symptoms. In: M Knapp, D McDaid and M Parsonage (eds), *Mental Health Promotion and Prevention: the Economic Case.* Department of Health.

33. Nimnuan C, Hotopf M and Wessely S. (2001). Medically unexplained symptoms: an epidemiological study in seven specialities. *Journal of Psychosomatic Research* **51**: 361–367.

34. McBeth J, Lovell K, Hanniford P, et al. (2012). Cognitive behavioural therapy or exercise or both for treating chronic widespread pain. *Archives of Internal Medicine* **172**: 48–57.

35. Lamb SE, Mistry D, Lall R, et al. (2012). Group cognitive behavioural interventions for low back pain in primary care: extended follow-up of the Back Skills Training Trial (ISRCTN54717854). *Pain* **153**: 494–501.

36. Jones KD, Adams D, Winters-Stone K, et al. (2006). A comprehensive review of 46 exercise treatment studies in fibromyalgia (1988–2005). *Health and Quality of Life Outcomes* **4**: 67.

37. White PD, Goldsmith KA, Johnson AL, et al. on behalf of the PACE trial management group. (2011). Comparison of adaptive pacing therapy, cognitive behaviour therapy, graded exercise therapy, and specialist medical care for chronic fatigue syndrome (PACE): a randomised trial. *Lancet* **377**: 823–836.

15

Early Intervention Services versus Generic Community Mental Health Services: A Paradigm Shift

Marco Armando[1,2], Franco De Crescenzo[1] and Maximilian Birchwood[3]

[1]*Child and Adolescence Neuropsychiatry Unit, Department of Neuroscience, Children Hospital Bambino Gesù, Rome, Italy*
[2]*School of Psychology, University of Birmingham, Edgbaston, Birmingham, UK*
[3]*YouthSpace; University of Warwick, UK*

Since the beginning of the twentieth century, several authors called attention to the need for early diagnosis and intervention in psychosis [1]. Ultimately, the early intervention model and subsequent early intervention services (EISs) in the first episode of psychosis (FEP) and in ultrahigh-risk states (UHR), were actually developed and put into practice between the end of the 1980s and the beginning of the 1990s. During these years this movement grew theoretically, methodologically and as an increasingly widely applied clinical experience. Indeed, starting from the 1990s, we see the birth of EIS specialised in management of FEP and UHR. Starting in Finland [2], almost simultaneously in England [3] and Australia [4], studies of these services spread to the United States, Asia and many other European nations.

The progressive increase of EIS, alongside of a world-wide state of imbalance between available resources and therapeutic interventions [5], slowly led to a progressive modification in community mental health services (CMHSs), with a strong development of the EIS model specialised in different psychiatric disorders, especially for FEP [6], instead of the generic CMHS model.

Early Intervention in Psychiatry: EI of nearly everything for better mental health, First Edition.
Edited by Peter Byrne and Alan Rosen.
© 2014 John Wiley & Sons, Ltd. Published 2014 by John Wiley & Sons, Ltd.

This progressive shifting can be explained by evidence showing that CMHSs are characterised by a delay in taking charge of individuals with psychotic onset [7], a feeling of demoralization and shock on the part of individuals causing a higher drop-out rate, and a major focus on tertiary prevention rather than secondary and primary prevention [6]. Moreover, the effectiveness of EIS has been demonstrated by a recent systematic review and meta-analysis of randomized clinical trials (RCTs) [8]. It is already in current guidelines (e.g. www.nice.org.uk), and it has been proved to reduce costs and thus to be cost-effective [9].

Even though this unambiguously strong international evidence of both the persistent effectiveness and the economic advantages of the EIS model, several authors [10, 11] argue against a further development of EIS, mainly because of concerns about the continuity of care and the need to engage some individuals in long-term therapeutic relationships. Notwithstanding, they provide no evidence in support of retaining the CMHS alone.

Taking off from these discordant opinions, this chapter seeks to provide a clear description of the worldwide discussion regarding the desirability of a further development of EIS as against CMHS. In particular, the aim of this chapter is the following.

(a)   Describe the historical background of the development of EIS;

(b)   Compare the efficacy of EIS and CMHS concerning treatment and prevention of FEP.

Historical background
The origins of psychosis prevention

Early intervention in psychosis (EIP) is not a recent idea and delaying/preventing young people from psychosis has always been an aspiration.

Indeed, throughout during the twentieth century the prospect and practicality of identifying subjects in the prodromal phase of schizophrenia was debated. The prodromal symptoms and signs were pointed out, but they were extremely non-specific and not useful from a clinical point of view. For example, E. Bleuler (1911) [12] maintained that it was not possible to talk about prodromes, because nearly every symptom can be a forerunner of schizophrenia and at the beginning, when the symptom appears, it is impossible to predict accurately the future evolution of the disease. Nevertheless, Bleuler himself, and many other psychiatrists of the past century, thought early intervention offered the only possibility to improve the outcome of psychotic disorders, even though individual symptoms were not specific enough.

Many other authors (i.e. [1, 13–19]) agreed that psychotic onset should be considered a culmination of an evolving illness. In this chorus of unanimous voices, two eminent psychiatrists struck a discordant note. Schneider and Jaspers in fact, thought that schizophrenia was independent of a premorbid personality, and that it was impossible to detect a pattern of prodromal symptoms. This was the prevailing position during the 1960s, also due to a widespread transition taking place from qualitative to quantitative studies in psychiatry. With the attempt to align psychiatry to other medical disciplines [20] and the consequent development of DSM-III [21], American psychiatry progressively lost interest in conditions with minimal symptomatic expressions and prodromal stages. The limited space reserved for prodromal symptoms in schizophrenia in the DSM-III, disappears completely in the DSM-IV [22], where the possibility of prodromal phases subsists only for cluster A personality disorders.

Classic psychopathologists' research was eclipsed by the pressing need for a valid and widely shared diagnostic system, which can unify and enable comprehension of professionals worldwide. The return to a Kraepelinian model, which requires clear and evident psychotic signs and symptoms exhibited for an extended period before a formal diagnosis, closed the debate on prodromal forms of schizophrenia.

In the 1960s, two research areas developed, both proving to be extremely useful for an evaluation of prodromal phase and schizophrenia prevention: the work of James Chapman et al. [23] on psychotic-like experiences (PLEs) in the United States and the research of Gerd Huber [16] on basic symptoms in Germany.

Regarding PLEs, Chapman [23] and other colleagues like Gillies [24], Meehl [25], etc. hypothesised a continuum in the disease, which evolves progressively from the initial phases to frank psychosis. Huber [16], instead, supported the idea of the existence of 'basic' symptoms, which are mild subclinical and subjective symptoms involving instincts, affect, stress tolerance, thought, language, perception and motility.

A paradigm shift

What is new in the last 20 years is the attempt to find subjects at risk and to treat them at an earlier stage of the disorder. This paradigm shift entails a new approach to mental illness, particularly schizophrenia. At the beginning of the 1990s, as we highlighted in the previous paragraph, the Kraepelinian model, which had dominated during the century and established the basis for the new psychiatric nosology (DSM), was contested.

The neo-Kraepelinian model fallacy, McGorry says, is to posit a double bond between the disorder and its effects, the symptoms and signs and the diagnosis and prognosis, whereas psychosis psychopathology, in fact, is more fluid [26]. The connection between signs and symptoms, diagnosis and prognosis is much weaker and this opens the possibility for a secondary prevention of psychosis that is considered impossible or implausible in the neo-Kraepelinian model.

The birth of EIS

Within this paradigm shift, in the last decade researchers have tried to identify subjects 'at risk' and to intervene early in psychotic disorders [27].

Indeed, the poor predictability of prodromal symptoms has led to the application of a technique, which aims to refine diagnostic capacities and is already widely used in general medicine: the so-called 'close-in' strategy. This strategy consists in identifying the co-presence of many prodromal symptoms, a state–trait model that permits us to better identify cases at risk with a subsequent reduction of false positives. This type of evaluation method, first theorised and applied in Australia and the United Kingdom [27, 28], has also been utilised by many other research groups [29–32] in order to be able to offer a quick and specific response to the first signs or symptoms of the disease and to delay/prevent the psychotic onset [33]. The problem of early symptoms of psychosis is also very important because most young people who need help do not turn spontaneously to a CMHS [34].

Following and in coherence with the paradigm shift described above, an EIS specialised in management of FEP and UHR began to develop in the 1990s. These services developed roughly in parallel in England [3] and Australia [4], and spread to many other European nations, the United States of America, Canada, Singapore, Hong Kong and Japan. This model shift has become increasingly popular and has been applied in a number of countries. The main reason for this 'success' is the perception of the need for EIS instead of CMHS, since CMHSs were not structured to effectively engage and respond to the special needs of young individuals at their psychotic onset.

In the following paragraph we will describe the most important targets on which early intervention focuses and how EIS try to address their interventions specifically to these targets.

The rationale behind EIS

EIP is now facing an urgent problem that is paradigmatic with psychiatry and all medicine. Is it better to adopt a specialised service which can be more focused on a specific disorder, or is it perhaps better not to divert precious money from generalist services? To assess this, it is very important to study the effectiveness of treatment – rather than merely the efficacy – and its cost-effectiveness.

In accordance with evidence from several studies [2, 4, 27] (see Table 15.1), in the late 1990s, specific EIS for FEP were developed mainly to offer a more effective answer to three key elements which strongly influence the outcome of psychotic disorders and which were not adequately addressed by CMHS [35]:

1. Early detection of individuals with at-risk mental state

2. Early treatment of first-episode psychosis

3. Interventions directed to the initial psychotic phase (critical period, [27])

In this paragraph we focus our attention on the above-mentioned three key elements. In the following paragraphs, we will then describe the results of the main trials conducted to date aimed at investigating which of the two models (i.e. EIS vs. CMHS) is more effective and sustainable in preventing/reducing the burden caused by psychotic disorders. Finally, in this period of limited resources available for mental health, we will briefly describe the available evidence regarding cost comparison between EIS and CMHS.

Table 15.1   How deep are early intervention service roots? Core evidence for the development of EIS

Psychotic onsets invariably present with a prodromal phase of functional decline. [Evidence type B]
Shortening duration of untreated psychosis (DUP) correlates with better outcome. [Evidence type A]
Disability sets in early: peaks or plateaus within 3 years from the onset. [Evidence type B]
The outcome at 3 years predicts the outcome in the longer term. [Evidence type A]
Higher suicide risk during the first 5 years after psychotic onset. [Evidence type B]

Evidence A: RCT or cohort study; Evidence B: Retrospective Cohort, Exploratory Cohort or case-control study; Evidence C: Case-series study; Evidence D: Expert opinion.

Early detection of individuals with UHR state

If we detect early signs and symptoms we may hope to delay, or even totally prevent, the development of a full-blown psychosis. This surely represents the most alluring and promising, although controversial, aspect of the field. Intervening in the prodromal phase means intercepting the subject in the period in which signs and symptoms of distress are present, without a real experience of psychotic rupture having taken place. However, since prodromal symptoms are nonspecific, the diagnosis is particularly difficult and the number of false positives is high and remains high [36], even though sensitive criteria have been developed to measure a condition at high risk of transition to psychotic onset. In the European Prediction of Psychosis Study (EPOS), a European, multicenter and prospective study, the combination of attenuated psychotic symptoms (APS) and cognitive basic symptoms (COGDIS) showed the best indication of risk to develop a psychosis in the following 18 months, with 48% of evolution rate [37]. Nevertheless, this means that in half of the at-risk subjects, psychosis does not emerge in the following 18 months. A recent meta-analysis [36] shows that the risk to develop a psychotic episode in a cohort of UHR subjects is 18% at 6 months, 22% at 1 year, 29% at 2 years and 32% at 3 years.

Guidelines for interventions in prodromal phases [35] support evaluating and taking charge of individuals with at-risk mental states, who ask for help. They should be followed over time. They should be offered psychological support together with treatment for specific symptoms such as depression, anxiety and substance abuse and should be assisted with eventual interpersonal, family and professional difficulties. Psychoeducational interventions are useful to develop coping strategies regarding subthreshold psychotic symptoms, together with supportive interventions and family psychoeducation. Treatment with antipsychosis medication at low doses is not indicated with the exception of people at high risk of suicide, rapid psychosocial deterioration or aggressive behaviours. When indicated and effective in the first 6 weeks, with the individual's consent, pharmacological treatment can be continued for 6 months to 2 years. A gradual dosage reduction up to the minimum effective dose is recommended or, in some cases, an interruption of pharmacological treatment after 2 years in a consenting and responsive patient. When an antipsychosis medication is not effective, the administration of a different, second generation one is recommended. When the subject does not ask for help spontaneously, it is possible to get in touch with family and friends.

Evidence that these interventions are effective in reducing transition to frank psychosis is preliminary for now [38]. Further studies are needed to document the effectiveness of these interventions on the course of the illness.

Indeed, the risk/benefit ratio of early intervention in UHR is still unclear and the hypothesis of introducing a 'psychosis risk syndrome' (PRS) in the next DSM-V [39] stimulated a wide debate. At the present time, many researchers believe that introducing a PRS diagnosis in the DSM-V would be premature, mainly because of the significant heterogeneity of UHR subjects, their different clinical needs and prognosis [36]. It would be premature also since there is a lack of research confirming the reliability of standardised procedures for diagnosis, and this does not permit diagnostic validity. Biological and neuropsychological parameters should also be taken into consideration as a support to diagnosis. Only once research is able to provide answers to these questions will it be possible to include the diagnosis of PRS in DSM-V [37]. On the other hand, some authors support the inclusion of PRS diagnosis in DSM-V arguing that individuals with UHR are already ill and with poor functioning and are at high risk to worsen [40]. Moreover, DSM-IV diagnostic criteria are not specific for this condition [41]. There is broad agreement though, on the important role of research over the coming years to clarify the matter and to finally identify and treat subjects at-risk of psychosis.

Despite these different positions regarding UHR criteria and PRS, there is sufficient agreement about the desirability of early intervention for UHR. The main issue regards how this early intervention should be provided. Since CMHSs are not focused on prevention, EIS for UHR are more effective in providing the specific multidisciplinary treatments suggested by international guidelines.

Nevertheless, several authors [10, 11] suggest that the EIS model can pathologise normal developmental processes and lead to over-medicalization. This is not a minor question since it is not ethically acceptable to run the risk of treating people who are not really ill. Moreover, we know that PLEs are present in a large percentage of the population [42].

To avoid treating false positives, two main precautions have been developed:

1. People reach EIS for UHR by seeking help. Services do not screen adolescents in school and do not compel them to attend for treatment.

2. UHR criteria have been introduced to avoid this risk. Indeed, these criteria tend to identify people with a higher risk to develop psychosis and with a good response to treatment. They are identified by the presence of subthreshold psychotic symptoms.

In conclusion, EIS is offered only to the help-seeking, distressed individuals whose psychotic symptoms would be considered too mild to be considered 'properly' psychotic.

Early intervention in first-episode psychosis

Timely detection of psychotic onset allows to reduce the duration of untreated psychosis (DUP), that is the time between the onset of positive psychotic symptoms and the initiation of appropriate treatment. Much evidence supports the view that the longer the time in which a person lives in a situation of frank psychosis without being treated, the worse is the progression and prognosis of the illness. DUP reduction is very important for short- and medium-term outcome [43]. A short DUP is linked to a better response to antipsychosis medication treatment [44] and better social and professional functioning [45–47]. As a consequence of the reduction in DUP, individuals have a better response to treatment since they present less severe positive and negative symptoms and better social functioning than cases with long DUP [48].

The relationship between treatment delay and poor outcome has been clearly established [43, 44]. As we will highlight in this chapter, CMHSs are more often related to a consistent treatment delay as compared to EIS [49], and this supports the idea that specialised pathways to care can reduce DUP and consequently improve outcome.

The 'critical period'

The critical period (CP) is the period of time between 3 and 5 years that follows psychotic onset [27]. The years immediately following the psychotic onset are considered crucial in terms of prognosis [27, 50, 51], and what occurs in this phase can determine the following progression and prognosis of the disorder. In fact, during CP a dramatic progression towards a massive deterioration in social and cognitive skills occurs. This deterioration, once established, reduces the effectiveness of interventions. Indeed, the course of psychosis is characterised by a rapid deterioration in the first period, following which it reaches a plateau where it stabilises without any further worsening or improvement. It is necessary, therefore, to intervene as soon as possible to reduce or prevent psychosocial deterioration. As we indicated above, the crucial period is 3 to 5 years after the first psychotic episode [35, 52] and all international guidelines suggest continuous, intensive and assertive interventions during this phase. It is very important to treat the patient on time and continuously, since after the psychotic onset there is a high risk of relapse, severe disability and increased suicide risk. The entire family should be supported by psychoeducational group therapy. Psychological and psychosocial treatments should be the key elements during the CP to reduce positive and negative symptoms, to face eventual comorbidities and to promote social recovery. Treatment with antipsychosis medications must be accurately monitored to achieve the minimum therapeutic dose in order to reduce side effects that prevent recovery (weight gain, sexual dysfunctions and sedation) [35].

If, on the one hand, EISs are specifically developed to provide intensive and assertive intervention focalised in the CP, on the other hand some criticism of this approach has been voiced, since some authors argue that only individuals who fulfil the DSM-IV B (marked social deterioration) and C (duration of illness of at least 6 months) criteria for schizophrenia should be treated with this intensive model [10]. Although the position regarding treatment should be as conservative as possible, we should be aware that those criteria encourage delayed intervention which is harmful to health, especially in a population like this one, at high risk of death by suicide during the CP.

EIS versus CMHS: randomised controlled trials

Bosanac et al. [10] and Lodge [11] among others highlight another disadvantage arguing against a further development of EIS at the expense of CMHS. In accordance with this position, the EIS model still has to confirm its efficacy on long-term outcomes, and problems concerning the modality of discharge and transition to CMHS of individuals previously followed under EIS are noted. More in general, several authors [10, 11] argue that reallocating available resources from community to specialised services will lead to the failure of well-established services that manage a broad range of clients. However, they provide no evidence in support of these arguments.

Conversely, we concur with Killaspy [53]: 'This progressive discipline (psychiatry) must be responsive to its expanding evidence base'. What do RCTs tell us then about these arguments? Here we will briefly describe some of the most significant randomised studies aimed at verifying the efficacy of the EIS model as compared to standard care. Indeed the Lambeth Early Onset (LEO) trial, the OPUS trial and the treatment and intervention in psychosis (TIPS) trial represent the most significant evidence regarding the opportunity of further development of the EIS model. Apart from these three trials, two other trials: Croydon Outreach and Assertive Support Team (COAST) and Optimal Treatment Project (OTP), evaluated standard care versus EIS, finding the latter more effective in all cases. Results have been pooled together in two different meta-analyses [8, 54] and in a Cochrane systematic review [55].

Lambeth early onset

The LEO trial [56] is a randomised clinical trial conducted in the United Kingdom to evaluate the effects, in terms of drop-out and hospitalization rates, of an EIS compared to CMHS during 18 months in individuals with FEP. The main study published by this research group [56], on a population of 144 first admitted individuals with non-affective psychosis (F20-29 for DSM-IV), after 18 months, shows how specialised care is more effective in reducing dropout, hospitalization rate and relapses. Individuals treated by EIS were also better in terms of social and vocational functioning, satisfaction, quality of life and medication adherence (see Table 15.2).

In a second phase of LEO trial, stability of improvement achieved was verified in the long term after discharge from specialised care and readmission in standard care. Data published relative to a 5-year follow-up [57], highlight a progressive loss of improvement after discharge. Markers of efficacy, in fact, seem to decline in the long term after admission in standard care. These data underline the difficulty of services using a generalist intervention model to maintain the same efficacy of early onset teams (see Table 15.2).

OPUS

A larger randomised clinical trial, called OPUS [58], was run in Denmark on 547 individuals with first-episode psychosis. Trial design considered clinical evaluation of the effects (level of reduction of negative and positive symptoms) of specialised care based on the early intervention model in psychotic onset (assertive community Treatment, family care and social skills training), compared with standard care from territory psychiatry.

Specialised care lasted 2 years with assessment after the first and second years. After one year individuals presented a significant reduction of positive (mean difference between groups $= -0.31$; 95% CI $= -0.55\ -0.07$; $p = 0.02$) and negative symptoms (mean difference between groups $= -0.36$; 95% CI $= -0.54\ -0.17$; $p < 0.001$). The same results were confirmed after 2 years. Beyond these primary markers, the experimental group had less comorbidity with substance abuse, better treatment adherence and greater level of satisfaction (see Table 15.2).

As in the LEO trial, also in this case a follow-up after 5 years was carried out [59] to determine the stability of improvement achieved after discharge from specialised care and 3 years of standard care. Results, similar to those of the LEO trial, highlighted a progressive equalization in terms of positive and negative symptoms between the experimental and control groups, although maintaining a lower hospitalization rate and better autonomous, independent living (see Table 15.2).

On the basis of these results, the Copenhagen research group decided to start a second phase of the OPUS II trial [60] that extends specialised care for three further years, to determine whether extension of treatment for the length of the CP [61] allows a stabilization of the improvements achieved.

To date the OPUS trial represents probably the most solid evidence in favour of EIS. Indeed, it was rated as having an overall low risk of bias by the latest Cochrane review [55]. However, it did not provide a blinding of outcome assessment after 2 years, which may have led to an overestimation of effect. OPUS II trial will have less methodological bias than OPUS I, since a blinded outcome assessment is assured [60] and hopefully will address the remaining doubts on EIS effectiveness.

Table 15.2 Main studies comparing early intervention services to community mental health teams

	Study	Randomisation	Participants	Intervention	Results	Follow-up
LEO	Craig 2004 Gafoor 2010	+	144 FEP non-affective psychosis 71 EIS versus 73 CMHT 5 years follow-up	Early intervention service based on principles of assertive outreach including psychosocial interventions versus services offered by local community mental health teams.	Individuals in early intervention service group compared with community mental health teams had significant lower rates of relapse, readmission and drop-out.	Five-year data from the follow-up did not highlight significant differences between groups of treatment.
OPUS	Petersen 2005 Bertelsen 2008	+	547 FEP non-affective psychosis 275 EIS versus 272 CMHT 5-years follow-up	Early intervention service based on assertive community treatment, family intervention and social skills training versus services offered by local community mental health teams.	Significantly fewer people left early by 1 year in the early intervention service group compared with the standard care group (RR 0.59). GAF, SAPS, SANS endpoint scores significantly favored the early intervention service.	Five-year data from the follow-up did not highlight significant differences between groups of treatment.
TIPS	Melle 2004 Melle 2008 Hegelstad 2012	–	281 non-affective psychosis first treatment 141 ED area versus 140 non ED area 2- and 10-years follow-up	Early detection program versus non-early detection program. Same treatment between groups: low dosage second generation antipsychosis medication, individual psychosocial interventions, family psychoeducation.	Duration of untreated psychosis was significantly shorter for individuals in ED areas (median 5 weeks) compared with individuals from non-ED areas (median 16 weeks). At start of treatment the PANSS was better for individuals from the ED area and this result was maintained at 3 months.	A significantly higher percentage of individuals in ED areas had recovered at 2 and 10 years of follow-up and a higher drop-out rate was observed in individuals in non-ED areas.

EIS = early intervention service; CMHT = community mental health team; FEP = first-episode psychosis; ED = early detection; EIS = early intervention service; GAF = global assessment of functioning scale; OR = odds ratio; RR = risk ratio; SAPS = Scale for assessment of positive symptoms; SANS = scale for assessment of negative symptoms; PANSS = positive and negative syndrome scale;

Treatment and intervention in psychosis

The TIPS trial was conducted in Norway and Denmark on 281 individuals [62]. It is not randomised and is slightly different from those already discussed. In fact, both experimental and control groups were under the same treatment (the same algorithm was used for low-dosage second generation antipsychosis medications, individual psychosocial interventions and family psychoeducation). The difference consisted in a massive awareness raising campaign for the entire population, general practitioners, social workers and access to care was easier, thanks to a toll-free number. Initial results showed the efficacy of this intervention: the experimental group had a significant DUP reduction (5 weeks vs. 16 weeks) and a better clinical condition at baseline and after 3 months [62] (see Table 15.2).

The experimental group also maintained a greater reduction for positive, negative and depressive symptoms with a better neurocognitive functioning at follow-up after 2 [63] and 5 years [64]. This study is the only one with a long-term follow-up of about 10 years and the results have recently been published [65]. They highlight how the experimental group remains more effective than the control group for functional recovery, underlining how these data can prove a link between early intervention and prognosis (see Table 15.2).

The TIPS study demonstrates the need for early detection programs and provides a strong rationale for the implementation of EIS, arguing also that a reorganization of the existing CMHS in this direction is very unlikely.

Cost-effectiveness

In the present historical period, in which resources are limited and it is imperative to stick to the budget, it is fundamental to evaluate the economic burden of EIS and compare it with those of the services that are already available. This evaluation should consider all cost variables derived from the illness, which means direct costs (directly attributable to medical care), indirect costs and, where possible, the so-called intangible or psychosocial costs (see [66, 67]).

In this direction some studies have compared specialised care for early psychosis using standard services by cost-effectiveness analysis. McCrone et al. [68] recently published a study on costs and cost-effectiveness regarding the LEO trial. Clinical variables and direct costs were measured relative to care management of individuals at accrual and then after 6 and 18 months. At the same time, information on quality of life and work re-engagement was gathered to evaluate cost-benefit. Relative to total direct costs, no statistically significant difference appeared between individuals in the specialised care branch as compared with those in standard care branch (£11.685 vs. £14.062). Cost-benefit analysis was clearly in favour of specialised care, showing a better clinical outcome with equal costs. In Australia, Mihalopoulos et al. [69] verified a reduction of direct costs in areas where an EIS was instituted, due to reduction of inpatient costs, especially in the medium-long term, after the service is fully operational [70].

Another interesting study highlights a reduction of direct costs and an improvement of the cost-benefit ratio after the institution of EIS for psychosis. Valmaggia et al. [9], in fact, analyzed the costs of their service allocated in south London, showing that costs do not differ from standard care in the first 12 months, but at 18 months a significant reduction begins to appear. Robust evidence of this cost reduction comes from a recent study [71], where it is estimated that over a 3-year period an EIS for FEP saves the NHS £15.862 per person with first-episode psychosis when compared to standard services. That is a potential £119 million saving for the NHS.

In summary, studies published up until now highlight a lack of increase, if not a downright reduction, of direct costs, with an improvement in the cost-benefit ratio.

Discussion: specialist early intervention service teams compared with generic CMHS teams

Since the end of the 1990s, a number of randomised clinical trials that compare the efficacy of early intervention with traditional services have been published. In synthesis we can state that we have enough evidence that EIS, compared to traditional ones, significantly affect several variables (see also Box 15.1):

Reduction of DUP

Reduction of hospitalization rate

Reduction of suicide rate

Reduction of positive symptoms

Increase of functional recovery in the short-medium term

Reduction of direct and indirect costs with improvement of the costs-benefit ratio.

Box 15.1 Advantages and possible limitations of Specific EIS teams compared with CMHT teams:

Advantages:

Reduction of duration of untreated psychosis (TIPS)

Lower rate of relapse (OPUS, LEO)

Lower rate of hospitalization (OPUS, LEO)

Reduction of positive and negative symptoms (OPUS, LEO)

Better adherence to treatment (OPUS, LEO)

Cost efficacy (Andrews et al. 2012)

CMHT's never demonstrated to be effective with Early Intervention (Nice Guidelines)

Possible Limitations:

Results are not maintained at follow up (OPUS, LEO) unless systematic effort with specific EIS type team is continued (i.e. Nordentoft; Linzen; etc.)

Further RCTs needed to demonstrate long term improvement with EIS, if any (waiting for OPUS II).

In line with this evidence and after a deep consultation and exploration of the existing scientific literature, the UK Schizophrenia Commission [72] has recognised the efficacy of the early intervention model. Indeed, the Commission has stated that early intervention is crucial to improving outcomes. The Commission's view is that EIP has been the most positive development in mental health services since the beginning of community care. What is even more significant is the following recommendation: 'We want the values and ethos of EIP to spread across the entire mental health system (...) We recommend that Clinical Commissioning Groups commission services to extend the successful principles of early intervention to support people experiencing second and subsequent episodes of psychosis' [72], pp. 15–16).

Some of the main points which lead the Commission to these conclusions are: (1) CMHS cannot ever devote the time required to deliver all the evidence-based treatments for psychosis in NICE (2012); (2) compared to the early intervention model, there is no evidence for CMHS as a valuable vehicle for the management of schizophrenia during prodromal and first-episode phases.

The value of CMHS may be as a front-of-house coordination hub from which people who meet the criteria for more intensive services are able to rapidly access them, and then move easily and gradually between teams if their needs are then reduced following access to timely more concentrated care [73]. However, as concluded yet again by the National Institute of Clinical Excellence in the United Kingdom [NICE Guidance on managing schizophrenia in adults (CG82, pp. 336)] there is no evidence to support the effectiveness of CMHS per se as a service delivery system or vehicle in comparison to specialist service modules like EIS teams [73].

Nevertheless, the 'first generation' of EIS, although it proved to be more effective on several variables compared to CMHS [74], still need to address several issues (see Box 15.1). Indeed, as we previously described, many problems regarding the EIS model have raised and EIS does not show a strong efficacy on some specific UHR population and on FEP long-term outcomes.

Firstly, we know that not all individuals treated in EIS have the same response to treatment [55]. About 40% of individuals with extremely poor functioning in adolescence and with high disability at EIS entry do not show any significant improvement after 12 months of treatment. According to this evidence, future research should be intensified and focused more on 'non-responders' and on those with major disability at entry to EIS, applying phase-specific interventions on high premorbid disability and on meds discontinuations. Research focused on psychopathology and UHR criteria will be fundamental for better primary care, alongside of the EIS's already excellent integrated specialised psychosis care pathway. Furthermore, in order to be of help in difficult and 'out of the ordinary' situations, assertive outreach aspects need to be as flexible as possible instead of adopting a 'one size fits all' model.

Secondly, clinical improvements achieved with EIS are robust as long as the intervention is provided. Longer-term data show that some of these gains are lost when care is transferred back to CMHS. A reappraisal of generic services and an understanding of the active ingredients of early intervention are needed to be tailored for longer input in individuals with poorer outcome trajectories [75, 76], Rosen A and Byrne P, Concluding chapter).

A third concern regards the continuity of care and the client's transition from EIS to CMHS. Indeed, some individuals need to be engaged in long-term therapeutic relationships. The current model tries to address this issue by having a generic front-end CMHS co-located with primary care where possible and specialised back streams. Indeed, this process still lacks efficacy and we should be aware of the fact that, although it is important to implement EIS, at the same time this implementation should not militate against the already well-established CMHSs which are still fundamental.

Conclusion

Some 15 years have gone by since the first development of EIS and, although there are some unanswered questions that still need to be addressed, ever increasing evidence of the efficacy of the early intervention model has been accumulated. Indeed, the early intervention model and subsequent EIS are now recommended from a clinical point of view as a best practice by several national and international guidelines and at the same time as a fundamental curricula during the training in Psychiatry, as it has been recently stated by the *Committee on Education* of the *World Psychiatric Association* [77]: '...All curricula for the training of psychiatrists and examinations for certification of psychiatrists should include understanding of the theory and practical application of early interventions in first-episode psychosis relevant to psychiatrists and to the functioning of multidisciplinary teams and to the organization of services in and with the local community'.

References

1. Sullivan HS (ed.). (1927). *Schizophrenia as a Human Processs.* New-York-London: W.W. Norton & Company.
2. Tuori T, Lehtinen V, Hakkarainen A, et al. (1998). The Finnish National Schizophrenia Project 1981–1987: 10-year evaluation of its results. *Acta Psychiatrica Scandinavica* **97**: 10–17.
3. Birchwood M and Macmillan F. (1993). Early intervention in schizophrenia. *Australian and New Zealand Journal of Psychiatry* **27**(3): 374–378.
4. McGorry PD, Edwards J, Mihalopoulos C, et al. (1996). EPPIC: an evolving system of early detection and optimal management. *Schizophrenia Bulletin* **22**(2): 305–326.
5. Prince M, Patel V, Saxena S, et al. (2007). No health without mental health. *Lancet* **70**: 859–877.
6. Phillips L, Yung AR, Hearn N, et al. (1999). Preventative mental health care: accessing the target population. *Australian and New Zealand Journal of Psychiatry* **33**(6): 912–917.
7. Norman RMG and Malla AK. (2001). Duration of untreated psychosis: a critical examination of the concept and its importance. *Psychological Medicine* **31**: 381–400.
8. Bird V, Premkumar P, Kendall T, et al. (2010). Early intervention services, cognitive-behavioural therapy and family intervention in early psychosis: systematic review. *British Journal of Psychiatry* **197**(5): 350–356.
9. Valmaggia L, McCrone P, Knapp M, et al. (2009). Economic impact of early intervention in people at high risk of psychosis. *Psychological Medicine* **39**: 1617–1626.
10. Bosanac P, Patton GC and Castle DJ. (2010). Early intervention in psychotic disorders: faith before facts? *Psychological Medicine* **40**(3): 353–358.
11. Lodge G. (2012). How did we let it come to this? A plea for the principle of continuity of care. *The Psychiatrist* **36**: 361–363.
12. Bleuler E. (1991). Dementia Praecox oder Gruppe der Schizophrenien, (Handbuch der Psychiatrie, herausgegeben von Prof. Dr. G. Aschaffenburg, Spez. Teil IV: 1). Deuticke, Leipzig und Wien.
13. Minkowski E (ed.). (1927). *La schizophrénie: Psychopathologie Des schizoides Et Des Schizophrènes.* Paris: Payot.
14. Cameron DE. (1938). Early schizophrenia. *American Journal of Psychiatry* **95**: 567–578.

15. Zilboorg G. (1941). Ambulatory schizophrenia. *Psychiatry* **4**(2): 149–155.

16. Hüber G. (1957). Die coenästhetische schizophrenie. *Fortschritte der Neurologie-Psychiatrie* **25**: 491–520.

17. Blankenburg W. (2001). First steps toward a psychopathology of 'common sense'. *Philosophy, Psychiatry, and Psychology* **8**: 303–315.

18. Kretschmer E. (1921). *Korperbau und Charakter*. Berlin: Springer.

19. Mayer-Gross W. (1932). Die Schizophrenie. In: O Bumke (ed.), *Hanbuch der Geisteskranken-heiten*, vol. IX. Berlin: Springer.

20. Wilson M. (1993). DSM-III and the Transformation of American Psychiatry: a history. *American Journal of Psychiatry* **150**: 399–410.

21. American Psychiatric Association, DSM–III–R. (1987). Washington.

22. American Psychiatric Association, DSM-IV-TR. (2000). Washington.

23. Chapman J. (1966). The early symptoms of schizophrenia. *British Journal Psychiatry* **112**: 225–251.

24. Gillies H. (1958). The clinical diagnosis of early schizophrenia. In: TF Rodger, KM Mowbray and JR Roy (eds), *Topics in Psychiatry*. London: Cassell.

25. Meehl PE. (1962). Schizotaxia, schizotypy, schizophrenia. *American Psychologist* **17**: 827–838.

26. McGorry PD. (1991). Paradigm failure in functional psychosis: review and implications. *Australian and New Zealand Journal of Psychiatry* **25**: 43–55.

27. Birchwood M, McGorry O and Jackson C. (1997). Early intervention in schizophrenia. *British Journal of Psychiatry* **170**: 2–5.

28. Yung AR and McGorry PD. (1996). The prodromal phase of first episode psychosis: past and current conceptualizations. *Schizophrenia Bulletin* **22**: 353–370.

29. Häfner H, Maurer K, Ruhrmann S, et al. (2004). Early detection and secondary prevention of psychosis: facts and visions. *European Archives of Psychiatry and Clinical Neuroscience* **254**(2): 117–128.

30. Miller TJ, McGlashan TH, Rosen JL, et al. (2002). Prospective diagnosis of the initial prodrome for schizophrenia based on the Structured Interview for Prodromal Syndromes: preliminary evidence of interrater reliability and predictive validity. *American Journal of Psychiatry* **159**(5): 863–865.

31. Miller TJ, McGlashan TH, Rosen JL, et al. (2003). Prodromal assessment with the structured interview for prodromal syndromes and the scale of prodromal symptoms: predictive validity, interrater reliability, and training to reliability. *Schizophrenia Bulletin* **29**(4): 703–715.

32. Morrison AP, Nothard S, Bowe SE, et al. (2004). Interpretations of voices in patients with hallucinations and non-patient controls: a comparison and predictors of distress in patients. *Behaviour Research and Therapy* **42**(11): 1315–1323.

33. Schultze-Lutter F, Ruhrmann S and Klosterkötter J. (2006). Can schizophrenia be predicted phenomenologically? In: JO Johannessen, B Martindale and J Cullberg (eds), *Evolving psychosis. Different Stages, Different Treatments*, p. 104–123. London, New York: Routledge.

34. Armando M, Fagioli F, Borra S, et al. (2009). [Mental uneasiness, perceived stress and help-seeking in a non-resident university student sample]. *Epidemiologia e Psichiatria Sociale* **18**(2): 154–160.

35. International Early Psychosis Association Writing Group. (2005). International clinical practice guidelines for early psychosis. *British Journal of Psychiatry* **187**: s120–s124.

36. Fusar-Poli P and Yung AR. (2012). Should attenuated psychosis syndrome be included in DSM-5? *Lancet* **379**(9816): 591–592.

37. Ruhrmann R, Schultze-Lutter F, Salokangas R, et al. (2010). Prediction of psychosis in adolescents and young adults at high risk. results from the prospective european prediction of psychosis study. *Archives of General Psychiatry* **67**(3): 241–251.

38. Preti A, Cella M, Raballo A. (2011). How psychotic-like are unusual subjective experiences? *Psychological Medicine* **41**: 2235–2236.

39. Carpenter WT. (2009). Anticipating DSM-V: Should psychosis risk become a diagnostic class? *Schizophrenia Bulletin* **35**: 841–843.

40. Pérez J. (2013). What if DSM 5 attenuated psychosis syndrome did not refer to risk, but a forme fruste? *Psychopathology* **46**(2): 131–132.

41. Woods S, Walsh B, Saksa J, et al. (2010). The case for including attenuated psychotic symptoms syndrome in DSM-5 as a psychosis risk syndrome. *Schizophrenia Research* **123**: 199–207.

42. Gale CK, Wells JE, McGee MA, et al. (2011). A latent class analysis of psychosis-like experiences in the New Zealand Mental Health Survey. *Acta Psychiatrica Scandinavica* **124**(3): 205–213.

43. Marshall M, Lewis S, Lockwood A, et al. (2005). Association between duration of untreated psychosis and outcome in cohorts of first-episode patients : a systematic review. *Archives of General Psychiatry* **62**: 975–983.

44. Perkins D, Gu H, Boteva K, et al. (2005). Relationship between duration of untreated psychosis and outcome in first-episode schizophrenia: a critical review and meta-analysis. *American Journal of Psychiatry* **162**: 1785–1804.

45. Malla AK, Norman MG, et al. (2004). Determinants of quality of life in first-episode psychosis. *Acta Psychiatrica Scandinavica* **109**: 46–54.

46. Browne S, Clarke M, Gervin M, et al. (2000). Determinants of quality of life at first presentation with schizophrenia. *British Journal of Psychiatry* **176**: 173–176.

47. Larsen TK, McGlashan TH and Moe LC. (1996). First-episode schizophrenia. 1. Early course parameters. *Schizophrenia Bulletin* **22**: 241–256.

48. Joa I, Johannessen J, Auestad B, et al. (2008). The key to reducing duration of untreated first psychosis: information campaigns. *Schizophrenia Bulletin* **34**: 466–472.

49. Norman RM, Malla AK, Verdi MB, et al. (2004). Understanding delay in treatment for first-episode psychosis. *Psychological Medicine* **34**: 255–266.

50. Jackson C and Birchwood M. (1996). Early intervention in psychosis: opportunities for secondary prevention. *British Journal of Clinical Psychology* **35**: 487–502.

51. Crumlish N, Whitty P, Clarke M, et al. (2009). Beyond the critical period: longitudinal study of 8-year outcome in first-episode non-affective psychosis. *British Journal of Psychiatry* **194**(1): 18–24.

52. Birchwood M, Todd P and Jackson C. (1998). Early intervention in psychosis. The critical period hypothesis. *British Journal of Psychiatry. Supplement* **172**: 53–59.

53. Killaspy H. (2012). Importance of specialisation in psychiatric services. Commentary on … How did we let it come to this? *Psychiatrists* **36**: 364–365.

54. Harvey PO, Lepage M and Malla A. (2007). Benefits of enriched intervention compared with standard care for patients with recent-onset psychosis: a metaanalytic approach. *Canadian Journal of Psychiatry. Revue Canadienne De Psychiatrie* **52**(7): 464–472.

55. Marshall M and Rathbone J. (2011). Early intervention for psychosis. *The Cochrane Database of Systematic Reviews* (6): CD004718.

56. Craig T, Garety P, Power P, et al. (2004). The lambeth early onset (LEO) team: randomised controlled trial of the effectiveness of specialised care for early psychosis. *British Medical Journal* **329**: 1067–1072.

57. Gafoor R, Nitsch D, Craig TK, Garety PA, et al. (2010). Effect of early intervention on 5-year outcome in non-affective psychosis. *British Journal of Psychiatry* **196**(5): 372–376.

58. Petersen L, Nordentoft M, Jeppesen P, et al. (2005). Improving 1-year outcome in first-episode psychosis: OPUS trial. *British Journal of Psychiatry* **8**: s98–s103.

59. Bertelsen M, Jeppesen P, Petersen L, et al. (2008). Five-year follow-up of a randomized multi-center trial of intensive early intervention vs standard treatment for patients with a first episode of psychotic illness: the OPUS trial. *Archives of General Psychiatry* **65**(7): 762–771.

60. Melau M, Jeppesen P, Thorup A, et al. (2011). The effect of five years versus two years of specialised assertive intervention for first episode psychosis - OPUS II: study protocol for a randomized controlled trial. *Trials* **12**: 72–80.

61. Edwards J, Harris MG and Bapat S. (2005). Developing services for first-episode psychosis and the critical period. *British Journal of Psychiatry* **187**: s91–s97.
62. Melle I, Larsen TK, Haahr U, et al. (2004). Reducing the duration of untreated first episode psychosis: effects on clinical presentation. *Archives of General Psychiatry* **61**(2): 143–150.
63. Melle I, Larsen TK, Haahr U, et al. (2008). Prevention of negative symptom psychopathologies in first episode schizophrenia: two year effects of reducing the duration of untreated psychosis. *Archives of General Psychiatry* **65**(6): 634–640.
64. Larsen T, Melle I, Auestad B, et al. (2011). Early detection of psychosis: positive effects on 5-year out come. *Psychological Medicine* **41**: 1461–1469.
65. Hegelstad W, Larsen T, Auestad B, et al. (2012). Long-term follow-up of the TIPS early detection in psychosis study: effects on 10-year outcome. *American Journal of Psychiatry* **169**: 374–380.
66. Knapp M. (2003). Schizophrenia costs and treatment cost-effectiveness. *Acta Psychiatrica Scandinavica* **102**: 15–18.
67. McCrone P and Knapp M. (2007). Economic evaluation of early intervention services. *British Journal of Psychiatry* **51**: s19–s22.
68. McCrone P, Craig TK, Power P, Garety PA, et al. (2010). Cost-effectiveness of an early intervention service for people with psychosis. *British Journal of Psychiatry* **196**(5): 377–382.
69. Mihalopoulos C, McGorry PD and Carter RC. (1999). Is phase-specific community orientated treatment of early psychosis an economically viable method for improving outcome? *Acta Psychiatrica Scandinavica* **100**: 47–55.
70. Phillips LJ, Cotton S, Mihalopoulos C, et al. (2009). Cost implications of specific and non-specific treatment for young persons at ultra high risk of developing a first episode of psychosis. *Early Intervention in Psychiatry* **3**: 28–34.
71. Andrews A, Knapp M, Parsonage M, McCrone P, et al. (2012). *Effective Interventions in Schizophrenia; The Economic Case.* London School of Economics and Political Science.
72. Murray R, et al. (2012). The abandoned illness. A report by the Schizophrenia Commission, http://www.schizophreniacommission.org.uk/the-report/
73. Rosen A, Stein L, McGorry P, et al. (2013). Specialist community teams backed by years of quality research. *The Psychiatrist* doi: 10.1192/pb.37.1.38
74. Lester H, Birchwood M, Freemantle N, et al. (2009). REDIRECT: cluster randomised controlled trial of GP training in first-episode psychosis. *British Journal of General Practice* **59**: 183–190.
75. Shiers D, Rosen A and Shiers A. (2009). Beyond early intervention: can we adopt alternative narratives like 'Woodshedding' as pathways to recovery in schizophrenia?. *Early Intervention in Psychiatry* **3**: 163–171.
76. Rosen C, Marvin R, Reilly JL, et al. (2012). Phenomenology of first-episode psychosis in schizophrenia, bipolar disorder, and unipolar depression: a comparative analysis. *Clinical Schizophrenia and Related Psychoses* **6**(3): 145–151.
77. World Psychiatric Association Committee on Education. (2009). First-episode psychoses. recommended roles for the psychiatrist: world psychiatric association committee on education. *Early Intervention in Psychiatry* **4**: 239–242.

IV
Early Intervention in Specific Disorders

16

Prevention and Early Intervention in Depression and Anxiety Disorders

Irwin Nazareth[1] and Tony Kendrick[2]

[1] Department of Primary Care & Population Health, London, UK
[2] Hull York Medical School, University of York, York, UK

Depression and anxiety disorders are common and costly

Reducing the prevalence of depression and anxiety disorders is a public health challenge for the twenty-first century. These mental health disorders affect as many as one in six people in the community. The 2007 Office for National Statistics (ONS) household survey of adult psychiatric morbidity in England found that 16% of working age adults had an anxiety or depressive disorder [1]. Of those, 4.4% were diagnosed with generalised anxiety disorder (GAD), 3% with post-traumatic stress disorder (PTSD), 2.3% with major depression, 1.4% with phobias, 1.1% obsessive–compulsive disorder (OCD) and 1.1% with panic disorder. The most common problem was mixed anxiety and depression, found in 9% of patients [1]. (The total adds to more than 16% because patients can have more than one disorder.)

The high prevalence and relapsing nature of depression and anxiety disorders means that they account for at least 35% of all disability and sick leave days due to mental health problems [2]. Even subclinical depression and anxiety states, which do not reach the threshold for psychiatric diagnostic classification, may have major impacts on quality of life [2, 3]. The commonest disorder, mixed anxiety and depression, causes 20% of days lost from work in Britain [3]. Although there are high indirect costs from the substantial burden of illness, direct treatment costs tend to be relatively low due to low recognition and

Early Intervention in Psychiatry: EI of nearly everything for better mental health, First Edition.
Edited by Peter Byrne and Alan Rosen.
© 2014 John Wiley & Sons, Ltd. Published 2014 by John Wiley & Sons, Ltd.

low rates of treatment [2]. McCrone and colleagues estimated the likely costs of depression over 20 years from 2006 to 2026 to include £1.7–£3 billion in drugs, hospital care and social services, but the projected costs of employment loss and benefits for depression for the same period were up to £9.2 billion [4].

Course and prognosis: opportunities for prevention and early intervention

The onset of common mental disorders is usually in adolescence or early adulthood, and earlier onset disorders tend to have a worse prognosis. The estimated median age of onset for anxiety disorders was 11 years and for depression 30 years in the US National Comorbidity sample – half of all lifetime cases had started by 14 years and three-quarters by the age of 24 [5]. This means efforts to prevent the onset of depression and anxiety disorders need to start in adolescence if possible [6].

The longer the disorders continue before intervention, the worse the prognosis too, which is the rationale for intervention early in any specific episode. More than 50% of people following their first episode of major depression will go on to have at least one more episode and after the second and third episodes, the risk of relapse rises to 70% and 90% respectively [7]. So a past history of depression is an important predictor of future episodes, and interventions which increase resilience against future depression are important in secondary prevention.

Relapse and recurrence is common even among people whose disorders appear for the first time in old age, and elderly people often suffer subclinical symptoms for a period before the disorder becomes apparent, offering the possibility of early intervention to reduce the number of full-blown disorders [8].

Barriers to the presentation of symptoms and the early detection of disorders

Depression and anxiety disorders are even more common among patients attending general practices than they are in the community. The New Zealand Magpie Study of 2006 found a similar prevalence to the ONS study in the community, of 15%, but a higher prevalence, 21%, in primary care [9]. However only 38% of people with disorders in the ONS survey had asked their doctor for help [1], which is one reason why disorders are missed.

There are significant barriers to access to both primary care and secondary care for mental health problems, which particularly affect the elderly, and black and minority ethnic patients, especially those for whom English is not their first language [10]. The stigma attached to a label of depression or anxiety prevents many people from presenting their symptoms and asking for help overtly, especially older people brought up in a time when people were not encouraged to discuss their feelings for fear of appearing weak. Access to care is generally poorer among people of lower social class, those with sensory impairments or learning difficulties, and in particular sociodemographic groups including young men as well as older people.

Even when patients in primary care do present their symptoms of depression or anxiety they are often not diagnosed by their GPs. Kessler and colleagues screened general practice attenders to identify cases of anxiety and depression and followed them up over 3 years, looking whether and when they were diagnosed by their GPs. As many as 30% of the cases of anxiety and depression they found remained undetected by their GPs at 3 years follow-up, of which 14% were severe cases who were disabled by their problems [11].

As a consequence of their reluctance to present their symptoms, and the lack of GP recognition of many common mental health disorders, only a minority of patients get help in primary care. Only 24% of sufferers in the ONS survey were receiving treatment: 14% medication; 5% counselling or therapy; and 5% both [1].

General practitioners vary widely in their ability to recognise common mental health disorders, with some recognising virtually all the patients found to be depressed when independently interviewed by a psychiatrist, and others recognising very few [12]. According to Goldberg, 10 behaviours are associated with greater detection. These include factors such as making eye contact, asking open-ended questions, asking specifically about feelings, and asking about problems at home or at work [12]. Attempts to improve GP detection have met with mixed results [13–15], and interventions often fail to improve patient outcomes, despite changes in doctors' consultation skills [16].

The fact that common mental disorders often go undiagnosed among primary care attenders has led to suggestions that clinicians should systematically screen for hidden disorders [17]. Screening is the presumptive identification of unrecognised disorders by the application of tests which can be applied rapidly. Screening tests attempt to distinguish in a population between a group of people who probably have a condition and the remainder who do not. However, screening is not without costs, in terms not only of the resources needed to mount a screening programme, but also in terms of missing some cases while falsely labelling some people who turn out not to have significant anxiety or depression on further assessment, because no screening test has 100% sensitivity and specificity [18].

Instead of screening, targeted case identification (case finding), which involves screening a smaller group of people known to be at higher risk based on the presence of particular risk factors, may be a more efficient way of improving the recognition of common mental health disorders in primary care. However, a key challenge in prevention and early intervention is to develop a clear understanding of the nature of risk factors for the development of disorders [19].

Predicting the onset of depression and anxiety disorders

Clinical prediction rules for cardiovascular diseases such as the Framingham, Dundee and the European risk scores are now widely used in primary care. These scores have over the last 10 years revolutionised the preventive management of coronary heart diseases and stroke and have allowed the development and delivery of a range of prevention approaches to cardiovascular diseases. Risk scores such as these have now been developed to predict future depression and anxiety disorders too.

We know a great deal about the risk factors for the common mental health disorders. Low socioeconomic status [20–22] and female sex [23] are most consistently identified. Socioeconomic risk factors include low income and financial strain [20], unemployment

[20], work stress [23], social isolation [24], and poor housing [21]. Other factors such as family history of depression play a part [25].

It is important to distinguish between modifiable risk factors and factors that can only function as markers, such as female gender and a positive family history, which are not modifiable. Possible genetic markers have also been identified through research reporting a higher incidence of depression after stressful life events in people with one or two short alleles of the serotonin transporter gene [26]. However, a subsequent meta-analysis [27] found no association between the incidence of depression and the serotonin transporter gene, either alone or in combination with stressful life events.

Negative life events should still be considered a risk factor, regardless of genetic make-up. Additional risk factors identified in general practice populations are poor physical health, poor marital or other interpersonal relationships, a partner or spouse's poor health, and problems with alcohol [28]. Poor social support, loneliness and physical disability are risks for older adults [29–31]. Unfortunately, effective strategies for the prediction of major depression are hindered by a lack of evidence about the *combined* effect of this large number of known risk factors.

Developing an algorithm to predict depression

The predictD algorithm for the onset of major depression in European general practice attenders was developed on people attending general practice in six European countries [32, 33]. The risk model was based on the approach used for creating risk indices for cardio-vascular disease [34], which provide a percentage risk estimate over a given time period. The main outcome measure was DSM-IV major depression. Data were collected on 39 known risk factors in order to construct a risk model for onset of major depression using stepwise logistic regression. The model was then tested in an independent general practice attender population in Chile.

The predictD risk model contained 10 factors.

- Age
- Sex
- Country
- Educational level
- History of depression
- Family history of psychological difficulties
- Physical health (subscale scores on the Short Form 12 generic health measure)
- Mental health (subscale scores on the Short Form 12)
- Unsupported difficulties in paid or unpaid work
- Experiences of discrimination.

Half of the participants who developed major depression also met the criteria for an anxiety disorder. The algorithm demonstrated good discriminative power with a c-index

[35] of 0.790 (95% CI 0.767, 0.813), which compares favourably with c-indices between 0.71 and 0.82 for a risk index for cardiovascular events developed in 12 European cohorts [36]. When predictD was then tested in a second population (in Chile) the c-index was 0.710 (95% CI 0.670, 0.749).

To put this more concretely, GP attenders in the upper quintile of risk (i.e. one in five of all attenders) on the PredictD algorithm in the United Kingdom are two and a half times more likely to develop major depression in the next 12 months than the average attenders [33].

This application of this algorithm for the early identification and prevention of people at risk for depression is now been evaluated in the United Kingdom and Spain in two separate randomised controlled trials.

Extending the algorithm to generalised anxiety and panic

As an extension to the work described above, a further evaluation of the anxiety symptoms was done on the same general practice attender cohort in order to construct a risk model for GAD and panic disorder (predictA) [37].

Similar factors contributed to the final algorithm.

- Sex

- Age

- Country

- Lifetime depression screen

- Family history of psychological difficulties

- Short Form 12 physical health subscale score

- Short form 12 mental health subscale score

- Unsupported difficulties in paid and/or unpaid work.

The discriminative power of this model was as good as predictD. The similarity between the two algorithms may be at least in part due to the close correlation (comorbidity) of depressive and anxiety disorders [38]. Recent calls have been made for not separating these disorders into separate chapters in the DSM/ICD psychiatric classification systems [39]. Moreover, others have suggested that a core psychopathology around neuroticism is common to both anxiety disorders and depression [40].An alternative explanation to comorbidity is the possibility that depressive and anxiety disorders are expressions of a broader latent pathological process [41–44]. In light of the findings for predictA [37], it would be prudent to consider the use of just one of these algorithms for both types of common mental disorders, as this would capture most of the people at risk of depression, GAD and panic disorders.

Improving the identification of disorders in primary care

Once people more at risk of depression have been identified, subsequent targeted case finding needs to be more systematic, to improve the levels of detection of disorders among primary care attenders.

The NICE guidelines on depression in adults (CG90) [45] and depression in people with chronic physical disorders (CG91) [46] recommend that GPs be alert for depression in patients with a past history of depression, and in patients with a chronic physical health problem, and ask them the two 'Whooley' questions to screen for depression.

Whooley and colleagues [47] found that two questions were particularly sensitive in identifying depression.

- *During the last month, have you often been bothered by feeling down, depressed or hopeless?*

- *During the last month, have you often been bothered by having little interest or pleasure in doing things?*

These questions will be familiar to GPs and practice nurses in the United Kingdom who have used them to screen patients with diabetes and coronary heart disease for depression annually, under the terms of the UK general practice quality and outcomes framework [48]. If a patient answers 'yes' to either question, the screen is positive.

If the person screens positive, further follow-up assessments should then be undertaken before reaching a diagnosis. A number of questionnaires have been identified as useful in the further assessment of possible depression. The NICE 2009 depression guideline recommends practitioners consider using measures such as the nine-item Patient Health Questionnaire [49], the depression subscale of the Hospital Anxiety and Depression Scale [50] or the Beck Depression Inventory, second edition [51, 52]. The rationale for using such instruments is that doctors' global assessments of severity do not agree well with valid and reliable self-report measures of severity in terms of cut-off levels for case identification [53, 54], which can result in the overtreatment of mild cases and undertreatment of moderate to severe cases [15, 54].

For case finding in anxiety, the NICE guideline on the identification and pathways to care for common mental health disorders CG123 [55] recommends the two-item generalised anxiety disorder (GAD-2) questionnaire for detecting anxiety [56], which asks:

Over the last 2 weeks, how often have you been bothered by the following problems?

- *Feeling nervous, anxious or on edge?*

- *Being unable to stop or control worrying?*

The GAD-2 is scored as follows, according to the response: *Not at all*: 0, *Several days*: 1, *More than half the days*: 2, *Nearly every day*: 3. If a person scores 3 or more the practitioner should consider a possible anxiety disorder.

In the event of a positive response to the GAD-2 questionnaire, the common mental health disorders guideline [55] recommends considering asking a further five questions which together with the first two make up the GAD-7 questionnaire [57]:
Over the last 2 weeks, how often have you been bothered by:

• *Worrying too much about different things?*

• *Having trouble relaxing?*

• *Being so restless that it is hard to sit still?*

• *Becoming easily annoyed or irritable?*

• *Feeling afraid that something awful might happen?*

All the seven questions (the GAD-7) are scored with the scoring system above, and a total score greater than 8 indicates a possible anxiety disorder [57].

It is important to stress at this point that screening alone cannot improve outcomes by itself [58], and it is crucial that even targeted screening or case finding should only be carried out if effective treatments are in place to offer to those who test positive, which is often not the case [18].There are now well established, effective treatments for depressive and anxiety disorders [59, 60] but even when the disorders are recognised treatment is often not adequately provided due to a lack of systematic, organised care [61]. Collaborative care [62], case management [63], and stepped care [64] for depression and anxiety disorders are underpinned by evidence from randomised controlled trials, and treatment programmes such as these should ideally be in place before screening or case finding is undertaken.

Prevention programmes for common mental disorders

There are well-established clinical systems within general practice in the United Kingdom for conducting systematic or opportunistic assessment of patients for the risk of developing diseases. Existing service models for cardiovascular and diabetes prevention programmes could be applied to depression and anxiety disorders. Strategies for the identification of attenders at risk for common mental disorders and the delivery of preventive care in primary care should be considered. General practice attenders can be opportunistically assessed for their risk of developing major depressive disorders using an algorithm such as predictD. Management strategies focussing on the prevention in people at high risk for developing depression and anxiety disorders can then be applied.

The risk level at which prevention might be offered would depend entirely on the work generated to offer preventive treatment to people at risk. For example the cumulative 12 month incidence of DSM-IV major depression in the European population in the predictD study was 7.7% [33]. This varied from one country to another as follows: United Kingdom, 8.8%; Spain, 15.1%; Slovenia, 4.2%; Portugal, 8.5%; The Netherlands, 5.4%; and Estonia, 5.9% [33]. Those with risk scores indicating a 12-month risk greater than the expected incidence for their country would be the group on whom preventative treatments should be considered.

However, the workload generated by such an approach could be overwhelming and may not prove to be cost-effective. In the absence of cost-effectiveness data, it would be appropriate to define a risk threshold at which the numbers of people falsely identified as at risk of depression (i.e. false positives) is kept to a minimum. This can be determined by establishing the sensitivity and specificity of using different cut offs [33]. In general, intervention offered only to those at a higher level of risk (e.g. 13.9% or more) would offer better specificity and hence minimise the number of false positives, even if this would be at the cost of missing some of those who would go on to develop depression over 12 months (false negatives). However, for preventive interventions which require little input by practitioners (e.g. a self-help leaflet or a web-based self-help prevention package), a lower cut-off could be considered, as the larger number of positives caught in the net could be offered the intervention without substantially increasing the costs to the health service.

Preventive interventions

Recognition of those at high risk of depression in family practice may be helpful when it leads to watchful waiting or active support, such as restarting drug or psychological treatments in patients with a history of depression and anxiety disorders, to prevent recurrence. Prevention of depression with adults in clinical practice [65, 66] may be effective and prevention of depression after serious medical crises, such as stroke, has shown significant effects for antidepressant treatment but not for problem-solving strategies [67]. A Cochrane review of prevention recommended that strategies should be tailored to target populations [68]. Although the studies identified in this review were aimed at younger people, these are important recommendations for the prevention of depression in all age groups.

Advising patients on the nature of depression and anxiety through the delivery of brief cognitive behavioural or problem-solving strategies might also reduce the risk of developing the disorder in the first place. Cognitive behavioural interventions aim to reduce dysfunctional automatic negative thoughts and to increase patients' activity levels. Patients are taught to evaluate, challenge, and modify their dysfunctional beliefs (cognitive restructuring), aiming to change their learnt behaviour patterns. Homework assignments are set between sessions, designed to record situations which bring on symptoms, and to identify and increase the frequency of more rewarding activities. An educational, collaborative approach is used to teach patients new ways of coping with their stressful situations.

Psychological interventions that involve combinations of cognitive behavioural therapy (CBT), education and problem solving can be effective in preventing depression. Promising results have been shown for primary prevention in younger people [68–73], either in schools or by targeting adolescents whose parents have a history of depression, although there is still no final consensus on whether or not they are effective [68, 74].

Among CBT-based interventions, the *Coping with Depression* course developed by Lewinsohn and colleagues is a commonly used preventive intervention. It is usually delivered in group sessions, and participants learn practical skills intended to help them cope with and overcome depressive feelings. These include social skills, cognitive restructuring, and behavioural activation to increase pleasant events (activity scheduling) [75]. The *Coping with Stress* course for the prevention of depression in adolescents has fewer sessions than the treatment version of the Lewinsohn course and focuses on cognitive restructuring [76]. A meta-analysis of six studies examining the success of the *Coping with Depression* programme in preventing depression in adolescents and adults demonstrated a reduction in risk of 38% [77].

Equivocal results have been reported for the prevention of postnatal depression [78] and although a reduction in negative thinking has been shown in low-income single mothers, trials have often been underpowered to detect a change in the incidence of depression. Studies often failed to exclude women already meeting diagnostic criteria for depression at entry and did not necessarily establish the incidence of depression in treatment and control groups according to diagnostic criteria [78].

Scaled-up delivery of interventions

Delivering CBT electronically by CD, DVD or the Internet shows promise for the treatment of anxiety and depression but there is uncertainty about a role for therapist support and there continues to be a need for more primary-care-based research.

In 2006, NICE appraised UK-developed products and recommended *Beating the Blues* and *FearFighter* as computerised packages of CBT that showed evidence of cost-effectiveness in treatment of depression or anxiety disorders [79]. *MoodGYM*, a well-established web-based CBT programme developed in Australia (http://www.moodgym. anu.edu.au/), was not included in the cost-effectiveness appraisal as it was not a UK-based product. The Internet offers easy and economical access to CBT packages of care. It is anonymous, users can obtain treatment at any time, work at their own speed, and go back over things whenever they like.

Internet-based packages also enable monitoring of usage. They also have great potential to be scaled up once shown to be effective and delivered *en masse*, reaching many individuals who may need prevention. When prevention of common disorders is the goal, applications need to be scalable, with capacity to be rolled out immediately. Another advantage is that the database can be used to improve or tailor the programme. In computer dedicated CDs or DVDs the data across individuals cannot readily be pooled, and thus cannot readily be used for evaluation or for tailoring and feedback.

Internet packages have been shown to be effective in treating pain and other physical health problems [80]. They are also moderately effective in the treatment of depression and anxiety, particularly if there is some degree of support using the package. However, little is known about their role in prevention [81].

Early intervention to prevent subthreshold disorders developing

Higher levels of symptoms on questionnaire measures, while below the threshold for diagnosis, nevertheless predict future episodes of depression [82]. Several studies have recruited individuals with subthreshold symptoms to determine the effects of mood management methods on the subsequent incidence of full-blown depressive disorders. Munoz and colleagues recently reviewed a large number of recent studies of prevention programmes aimed at strengthening protective factors, including social skills, problem-solving skills, stress management skills, social behaviour, and social support, using cognitive behavioural methods. They found evidence that such programmes could reduce the risk of subthreshold symptoms developing into full disorders, and that such interventions could be cost-effective [83].

Van't Veer-Tazelaarand and colleagues investigated the effectiveness of a prevention programme for depression and anxiety disorders in patients aged 75years and older, with subthreshold symptom levels of depression or anxiety who did not meet the full diagnostic criteria for the disorders, in 33 primary care practices in The Netherlands [84]. Participants were randomly assigned to a preventive stepped-care programme (n = 86) or to usual care (n = 84). Stepped-care participants received (sequentially) watchful waiting, CBT-based bibliotherapy, CBT-based problem-solving treatment, and medication if required. The intervention halved the 12-month incidence of full-blown depressive and anxiety disorders, from 24% in the usual care group to 12% in the stepped-care group (relative risk, 0.49; 95% confidence interval, 0.24–0.98).

Early intervention for people with subthreshold symptoms also needs to be scaled up, given the even larger numbers of people they affect. Spek and colleagues found a moderate effect size after 12 months for an eight session Internet CBT package in the prevention of full-blown depressive disorder in 300 men and women aged 50 and over who were recruited with subdiagnostic symptoms of depression [85].

The potential shown in these relatively small studies needs to be confirmed in larger studies, and health economic studies need to be carried out to determine whether their costs exceed the benefits they bring. The huge cost to society of the common mental hcalth disorders suggests that early intervention should indeed be cost-effective, especially if Internet-based programmes involving little or no therapist time can work.

Conclusion

During the last 10 years great strides have been made in the investigation of ways of identifying people at a higher risk of depression and anxiety disorders, and in case finding and confirming diagnoses. Research studies have shown great promise for prevention and early intervention through cognitive behavioural approaches delivered individually, through groups, or remotely via the Internet. Further research is needed to confirm the cost-effectiveness of such approaches in the prevention of these common and costly disorders, which if successful have great potential to improve the health of the public.

References

1. McManus S, Meltzer H, Brugha T, et al. (2009). *Adult Psychiatric Morbidity in England, 2007: Results of a Household Survey.* London: NHS Information Centre for Health and Social Care.
2. Andlin-Sobocki P and Wittchen HU (2005). Cost of anxiety disorders in Europe. *European Journal of Neurology* **12**(Suppl 1): 39–44.
3. Das-Munshi J, Goldberg D, Bebbington PE, et al. (2008). Public health significance of mixed anxiety and depression : beyond current classification. *The British Journal of Psychiatry* **192**: 171–177.
4. McCrone P, Dhanasiri S, Knapp M, et al. (2008). *Paying the Price: the Cost of Mental Health Care in England to 2026.* London: King's Fund.
5. Kessler RC, Berglund P, Demler O, et al. (2005). Lifetime prevalence and age of onset distributions of DSM-IV disorders in the national comorbidity survey replication. *Archives of General Psychiatry* **62**: 593–602.

6. Horowitz JL and Garber J. (2006). The prevention of depressive symptoms in children and adolescents: a meta-analytic review. *Journal of Consulting and Clinical Psychology* **74**: 401–415.

7. Kupfer DJ. (1991). Long-term treatment of depression. *Journal of Clinical Psychiatry* **52**: 28–34.

8. van't Veer-Tazelaar N, van Marwijk H, van Oppen P, et al. (2006). Prevention of anxiety and depression in the age group of 75 years and over: a randomised controlled trial testing the feasibility and effectiveness of a generic stepped care programme among elderly community residents at high risk of developing anxiety and depression, versus usual care. *BMC Public Health* **6**: 186.

9. Magpie Research Group. (2003). The nature and prevalence of psychological problems in New Zealand primary healthcare: a report on mental health and general practice investigation (MAGPIE). *New Zealand Medical Journal* **116**: 1171–1185.

10. Dowrick C, Gask L and Edwards S. (2010). Programme to increase equity of access to high quality mental health services in primary care. *Journal of Affective Disorders* **122**: 18–19.

11. Kessler D, Bennewith O, Lewis G, et al. (2002). Detection of depression and anxiety in primary care: follow up study. *British Medical Journal* **325**: 1016–1017.

12. Goldberg DP and Huxley P. (1992). *Common Mental Disorders: A Bio-Social Model*. London, New York: Tavistock/Routledge.

13. Tiemens BG, Ormel J, Jenner JA, et al. (1999). Training primary-care physicians to recognize, diagnose and manage depression: does it improve patient outcomes? *Psychological Medicine* **29**: 833–845.

14. Thompson C, Kinmonth AL, Steven L, et al. (2000). Effects of a clinical-practice guideline and practice-based education on detection and outcome of depression in primary care: Hampshire Depression Project randomized controlled trial. *Lancet* **355**: 50–57.

15. Kendrick T, Stevens L, Bryant A, et al. (2001). Hampshire Depression Project: changes in the process of care and cost consequences. *British Journal of General Practice* **51**: 911–913.

16. Gask L, Dowrick C, Dixon C, et al. (2004). A pragmatic cluster randomised controlled trial of an educational intervention for GPs in the assessment and management of depression. *Psychological Medicine* **34**: 63–72.

17. U.S. Preventive Services Task Force. (2002). Screening for depression: recommendations and rationale. *Annals of Internal Medicine* **136**(10): 760–764.

18. Gilbody S, Sheldon T and Wessely S. (2007). Should we screen for depression? *British Medical Journal* **332**: 1027. doi: 10.1136/bmj.332.7548.1027

19. Schmidt NB and Zvolensky MJ. (2007). Risk factor research and prevention for anxiety disorders : introduction to the special series on risk and prevention of anxiety pathology. *Behavior Modification* **31**: 3–7.

20. Weich S and Lewis G. (1998). Poverty, unemployment, and common mental disorders: population based cohort study. *British Medical Journal* **317**(7151): 115–119.

21. Weich S and Lewis G. (1998). Material standard of living, social class, and the prevalence of the common mental disorders in Great Britain. *Journal of Epidemiology and Community Health* **52**: 8–14.

22. Weich S, Sloggett A and Lewis G. (1998). Social roles and gender difference in the prevalence of common mental disorders. *The British Journal of Psychiatry* **173**: 489–493.

23. Stansfeld SA, Fuhrer R, Shipley MJ and Marmot MG. (1999). Work characteristics predict psychiatric disorder: prospective results from the Whitehall II Study. *Occupational and Environmental Medicine* **56**: 302–307.

24. Bruce ML and Hoff RA (1994). Social and physical health risk factors for first-onset major depressive disorder in a community sample. *Social Psychiatry and Psychiatric Epidemiology* **29**: 65–71.

25. Angst J, Gamma A and Endrass J. (2003). Risk factors for the bipolar and depression spectra. *Acta Psychiatrica Scandinavica. Supplementum* **418**: 15–19.

26. Caspi A, Sugden K, Moffitt TE, et al. (2003). Influence of life stress on depression: moderation by a polymorphism in the 5-HTT gene. *Science* **301**: 386–389.

27. Risch N, Herrell R, Lehner T, et al. (2009). Interaction between the serotonin transporter gene (5-HTTLPR), stressful life events, and risk of depression: a meta-analysis. *The Journal of the American Medical Association* **301**: 2462–2471.

28. Salokangas RKR and Poutanen O. (1998). Risk factors for depression in primary care: Findings of the TADEP project. *Journal of Affective Disorders* **48**: 171–180.

29. Prince MJ, Harwood RH, Blizard RA, et al. (1997). Impairment, disability and handicap as risk factors for depression in old age. The Gospel Oak Project V. *Psychological Medicine* **27**: 311–321.

30. Prince MJ, Harwood RH, Blizard RA, et al. (1997). Social support deficits, loneliness and life events as risk factors for depression in old age. The Gospel Oak Project VI. *Psychological Medicine* **27**: 323–332.

31. Prince MJ, Harwood RH, Thomas A and Mann AH. (1998). A prospective population-based cohort study of the effects of disablement and social milieu on the onset and maintenance of late-life depression. The Gospel Oak Project VII. *Psychological Medicine* **28**: 337–350.

32. King M, Weich S, Torres F, et al. (2006). Prediction of depression in European general practice attenders: the PREDICT study. *BMC Public Health* **6**(1): 6.

33. King M, Walker C, Levy G, et al. (2008). Development and validation of an international risk prediction algorithm for episodes of major depression in general practice attendees: the PredictD study. *Archives of General Psychiatry* **65**(12): 1368–1376.

34. King M, Bottomley C, Bellón-Saameño JA, et al. (2011). An international risk prediction algorithm for the onset of generalized anxiety and panic syndromes in general practice attendees: predictA. *Psychological Medicine* **41**(8): 1625–1639.

35. Anderson KM, Wilson PW, Odell PM and Kannel WB. (1991). An updated coronary risk profile. A statement for health professionals. *Circulation* **83**: 356–362.

36. Pepe MS, Janes H, Longton G, et al. (2004). Limitations of the odds ratio in gauging the performance of a diagnostic, prognostic, or screening marker. *American Journal of Epidemiology* **159**: 882–890.

37. Conroy RM, Pyorala K, Fitzgerald AP, on behalf of the SCORE project group, et al. (2003). Estimation of ten-year risk of fatal cardiovascular disease in Europe: the SCORE project. *European Heart Journal* **24**: 987–1003.

38. Gorman J. (1996). Comorbid anxiety and depression spectrum disorders. *Depression and Anxiety* **4**: 160–168.

39. Goldberg DP, Krueger RF, Andrews G and Hobbs MJ. (2009). Emotional disorders: cluster 4 of the proposed Risk algorithm for anxiety 13 meta-structure for DSM-V and ICD-11. *Psychological Medicine* **39**: 2043–2059.

40. Griffith JW, Zinbarg RE, Craske MG, et al. (2010). Neuroticism as a common dimension in the internalizing disorders. *Psychological Medicine* **40**: 1125–1136.

41. Tyrer P, Seivewright B, Ferguson J and Tyrer J. (1992). The general neurotic syndrome: a coaxial diagnosis of anxiety, depression and personality disorder. *Acta Psychiatrica Scandinavica* **85** 201–206.

42. Mennin DS, Heimberg RG, Fresco DM, and Ritter MR. (2008). Is generalized anxiety disorder an anxiety or mood disorder? Considering multiple factors as we ponder the fate of GAD. *Depression and Anxiety* **25** 289–299.

43. Krueger RF and Markon KE. (2006). Reinterpreting comorbidity : a model-based approach to understanding and classifying psychopathology. *Annual Review of Clinical Psychology* **2**: 111–133.

44. Middeldorp CM, Cath DC, Van Dyck R and Boomsma DI. (2005). The co-morbidity of anxiety and depression in the perspective of genetic epidemiology. A review of twin and family studies. *Psychological Medicine* **35**: 611–624.

45. NICE. (2009). *Depression: the Treatment and Management of Depression in Adults (Update)*. NICE clinical guideline 90. London: NICE. www.nice.org.uk/CG90 (accessed 14 April 2014).

46. NICE. (2009). *Depression in Adults with a Chronic Physical Health Problem: Treatment and Management*. NICE clinical guideline 91. London: NICE. www.nice.org.uk/CG91 (accessed 14 April 2014).

47. Whooley MA, Avins AL, Miranda J and Browner WS. (1997). Case-finding instruments for depression. Two questions are as good as many. *Journal of General Internal Medicine* **12**: 439–445.

48. BMA & NHS Employers. (2011). *Quality and Outcomes Framework Guidance for GMS Contract 2011/2012*. London: BMA.

49. Spitzer RL, Kroenke K and Williams JB. (1999). Patient Health Questionnaire Primary Care Study Group. Validation and utility of a self-report version of PRIME-MD: The PHQ primary care study. *The Journal of the American Medical Association* **282**(18): 1737–1744.

50. Zigmond AS and Snaith RP. (1983). The hospital anxiety and depression rating scale. *Acta Psychiatrica Scandinavica* **67**: 361–370.

51. Beck AT. (1996). *BDI-II, Beck Depression Inventory: Manual*. Boston, MA: Harcourt Brace.

52. Arnau R, Meagher MW, Norris MP, et al. (2001). Psychometric evaluation of the Beck Depression Inventory-II with primary care medical patients. *Health Psychology* **20**: 112–119.

53. Kessler D, Lloyd K, Lewis G, et al. (1999). Cross sectional study of symptom attribution and recognition of depression and anxiety in primary care. *British Medical Journal* **318**: 436–440.

54. Kendrick T, King F, Albertella L, et al. (2005). GP treatment decisions for depression: an observational study. *British Journal of General Practice* **55**: 280–286.

55. NICE. (2011). *Common Mental Health Disorders: Identification and Pathways to Care*. NICE clinical guideline 123. London: NICE. www.nice.org.uk/CG123 (accessed 14 April 2014).

56. Kroenke K, Spitzer RL, Williams JB, et al. (2007). Anxiety disorders in primary care: Prevalence, impairment, comorbidity and detection. *Annals of Internal Medicine* **146**: 317–325.

57. Spitzer RL, Kroenke K, Williams JBW and Löwe B. (2006). A brief measure for assessing generalized anxiety disorder: the GAD-7. *Archives of Internal Medicine* **166**: 1092–1097.

58. Thombs BD, de JP, Coyne JC, et al (2008) Depression screening and patient outcomes in cardiovascular care: a systematic review. *The Journal of the American Medical Association* **300**(18): 2161–2171.

59. Deacon BJ and Abramowitz JS. (2004). Cognitive and behavioural treatments for anxiety disorders : a review of meta-analytic findings. *Journal of Clinical Psychology* **60**: 429–441.

60. van Boeijen CA, van Oppen P, van Balkom AJ, et al. (2005). Treatment of anxiety disorders in primary care practice : a randomised controlled trial. *British Journal of General Practice* **55**: 763–769.

61. Fernandez A, Haro JM, Martinez-Alonso M, et al. (2007). Treatment adequacy for anxiety and depressive disorders in six European countries. *British Journal of Psychiatry* **190**: 172–173.

62. Gilbody S, Bower P, Fletcher J, et al. (2006). Collaborative care for depression: a cumulative meta-analysis and review of longer term outcomes. *Archives of Internal Medicine* **166**: 2314–2321.

63. Gensichen J, Beyer M, Muth C, et al. (2005). Case management to improve major depression in primary health care: a systematic review. *Psychological Medicine* **36**: 7–14.

64. Bower P and Gilbody S. (2005). Stepped care in psychological therapies: access, effectiveness and efficiency: narrative literature review. *British Journal of Psychiatry* **186**: 11–17.

65. Munoz RF, Yu-Wen Y, Bernal G, et al. (2005). Prevention of depression with primary care patients: a randomized controlled trial. *American Journal of Community Psychology* **23**: 199–222.

66. Scott J, Palmer S, Paykel E, et al. (2003). Use of cognitive therapy for relapse prevention in chronic depression Cost-effectiveness study. *The British Journal of Psychiatry* **182**: 221–227.

67. Robinson RG, Jorge RE, Moser D , et al. (2008). Escitalopram and problem-solving therapy for prevention of poststroke depression. A randomized controlled trial. *The Journal of the American Medical Association* **299**: 2391–2400.

68. Merry S, McDowell H, Hetrick S, et al. (2004). Psychological and/or educational interventions for the prevention of depression in children and adolescents. *Cochrane Database of Systematic Reviews* Issue 1. Art. No.: CD003380. doi: 10.1002/14651858.CD003380.pub2

69. Andrews G, Szabo M and Burns J. (2002). Preventing major depression in young people. *The British Journal of Psychiatry* **181**: 460–462.

70. Durlak JA and Wells AM (1997). Primary prevention mental health programs for children and adolescents: a meta-analytic review. *American Journal of Community Psychology* **25**: 115–152.

71. Seligman MEP, Schulman P and Tryon AM. (2007). Group prevention of depression and anxiety symptoms. *Behavior Research and Therapy* **45**: 1111–1126.

72. Calear AL, Christensen H, Mackinnon A, et al. (2009). The YouthMood Project: a cluster randomized controlled trial of an online cognitive behavioral program with adolescents. *Journal of Consulting and Clinical Psychology* **77**: 1021–1032.

73. O'Kearney R, Kang K, Christensen H and Griffiths K. (2009). A controlled trial of a school-based internet program for reducing depressive symptoms in adolescent girls. *Depression and Anxiety* **26**: 65–72.

74. Merry SN. (2007). Prevention and early intervention for depression in young people – a practical possibility? *Current Opinion in Psychiatry* **20**: 325–329.

75. Lewinsohn PM, Munoz R, Youngren MA and Zeiss A. (1992). *Control Your Depression*. New York: Fireside Books.

76. Garber J, Clarke GN, Weersing VR, et al. (2009). Prevention of depression in at-risk adolescents: a randomized controlled trial. *The Journal of the American Medical Association* **301**: 2215–2224.

77. Cuijpers P, van Straten A, Smit F, et al. (2008). Preventing the onset of depressive disorders: a meta-analytic review of psychological interventions. *The American Journal of Psychiatry* **165**: 1272–1280.

78. Dennis CL. (2005). Psychosocial and psychological interventions for prevention of postnatal depression: a systematic review. *Prevention BMJ* **331**: 15. doi:10.1136/bmj.331.7507.15.

79. NICE. (2007). Computerised cognitive behaviour therapy for depression and anxiety (Review of Technology Appraisal 51). http://www.nice.org.uk/TA97 (accessed 14 April 2014).

80. Cuijpers P, van Straten A and Andersson G. (2008). Internet-administered cognitive behavior therapy for health problems: a systematic review. *Journal of Behavioral Medicine* **31**: 169–177.

81. Spek V, Cuijpers P, Nyklicek I, et al. (2007). Internet based cognitive behaviour therapy for symptoms of depression and anxiety: a meta-analysis. *Psychological Medicine* **37**: 319–328.

82. Cuijpers P and Smit F. (2004). Subthreshold depression as a risk indicator for major depressive disorder: a systematic review of prospective studies. *Acta Psychiatrica Scandinavica* **109**: 325–331.

83. Munoz RF, Cuijpers P, Smit F, et al. (2010). Prevention of major depression. *Annual Review of Clinical Psychology* **6**: 181–212.

84. van't Veer-Tazelaar PJ, van Marwijk HWJ, van Oppen P, et al. (2009). Stepped-care prevention of anxiety and depression in late life: a randomized controlled trial. *Archives of General Psychiatry* **66**: 297–304.

85. Spek V, Cuijpers P, Nyklíček I, et al. (2008). One-year follow-up results of a randomized controlled clinical trial of internet-based cognitive behavioural therapy for subthreshold depression in people over 50 years. *Psychological Medicine* **38**: 635–639.

17
Alcohol and Substance Use Prevention and Early Intervention

Nicola C. Newton, Mark Deady and Maree Teesson
National Drug and Alcohol Research Centre, University of New South Wales, Sydney, Australia

Introduction

The high prevalence of alcohol and other drug use by young people clearly highlights the need for effective prevention and early intervention [1–3]. The harms associated with substance use are significant and include accidental injury, disruption to educational and vocational paths and psychological problems [4, 5]. In addition, early initiation to substance use is a strong risk factor for the later development of full-blown substance use disorders [6–8]. To reduce the occurrence of such problems, interventions need to be initiated early before problems begin to cause disability, and vocational, educational and social harms.

What causes substance use problems?

Most adolescents begin to use substances as a result of social influences and rebellious behaviours that typically occur during the teenage years. Adolescence is a time when young people begin to experience increased social, emotional and educational challenges [9], and this developmental progression coincides with periods of enhanced risk for drug use and access to substances [10]. Numerous risk and protective factors have been implicated in the development of substance use and can generally be divided into three main categories: (1) genetic factors (predispositions to drug use), (2) individual (non-genetic) and interpersonal factors (characteristics within individuals and their interpersonal environments) and (3) environmental/contextual factors (broad societal and cultural factors) [11–15]. The risk and protective factors identified below are those which have *strong*

Early Intervention in Psychiatry: EI of nearly everything for better mental health, First Edition.
Edited by Peter Byrne and Alan Rosen.
©2014 John Wiley & Sons, Ltd. Published 2014 by John Wiley & Sons, Ltd.

evidence in the literature to suggest they precede alcohol and drug misuse in adolescence and are based on tables developed by Spooner et al. [16] and Vogl [17].

Genetic factors

Evidence (including twin studies) have shown robust genetic components in alcohol, cannabis, opiate, cocaine and tobacco addictions, suggesting that a genetic predisposition to substance use problems and addictions is probable [13, 16, 18–20]. Not all people who use drugs however will become addicted and it is therefore likely that drug and alcohol problems occur due to an interaction between genetic predisposition and social and environmental factors.

Individual and interpersonal factors

The non-genetic individual and interpersonal factors which influence drug use are associated with personality, attitudes, beliefs and early childhood characteristics [13, 14, 16, 18, 21]. These are outlined in Table 17.1.

Environmental and contextual factors

The major environmental and contextual factors which influence drug use pertain to peers [22, 23], family and society [13, 14, 16, 18]. Social influence is recognized to have a strong effect in determining behaviours in adolescents, including initiation of drug use. In particular, the perception of drug use as a 'normal' behaviour is a good predictor of prevalence

Table 17.1   Individual risk and protective factors for drug use

Risk factors	Protective factors

• Attitudes and beliefs
  – Favourable attitudes to drug use
  – Low perceived risks of drug use
  – Low religiosity
• Personality characteristics which reflect alienation from societal values such as
  – Rebelliousness
  – Nonconformity to traditional values and resistance to traditional authority
  – High tolerance for deviance
  – Strong need for independence
• Other personality characteristics
  – Sensation seeking
  – Adventurous personality
  – Low harm avoidance
• Behavioural and emotional issues
  – Early and persistent aggression
  – Early conduct problems
  – Adolescent delinquency
  – Frequent drug use in late adolescence
	• Easy temperament in childhood
	• Social and emotional competence
	• Religious involvement
	• Shy and cautious temperament
	• Belief in natural order
	• Social problem-solving skills
	• Belief in own self-efficacy

of use. Table 17.2 summarises the risk and protective factors associated with these environmental influences.

Although we know that a greater risk of drug dependence is correlated to a greater number of risk factors that persist and influence an individual over time [13, 18], it is unclear which risk factors or combinations of risk factors are more pertinent in impacting on adolescents' drug use. What we can conclude is that drug use initiation is determined by numerous interacting individual factors and social pressures, and cannot be solved by a single intervention.

In order to develop effective prevention and early intervention, it seems sensible to incorporate a multi-component approach aimed at reducing risks and enhancing protective factors at the individual and societal levels [13, 16]. It is also necessary to determine the appropriate time when programmes should be implemented.

When should we intervene?

The transition to adolescence and young adulthood is a time when individuals move towards independence and autonomy, decrease dependence on families and schools, and place more emphasis on acceptance by peers. For most young people, this progression to adulthood is positive. However, this transition is also the time when risk-taking behaviour is high and vulnerability to substance use disorders is at its peak [24]. Coinciding with these social and emotional influences is the ongoing development of the brain which continues well beyond childhood and adolescence [25, 26]. In particular, the prefrontal cortex (involved in judgment, decision making and control of emotional responses) is one of the last areas of the brain to mature during late adolescence [27]. This can reduce an adolescents' ability to carry out intended and planned choices [28], and can exaggerate the brain's responses to immediate rewards [29].

In light of this research, it is important that prevention and early intervention be introduced in the adolescent years to provide young people with the knowledge and skills they need to make responsible and informed decisions regarding their substance use [30]. There are three periods during early years when the effects of prevention and early intervention can be optimised: the inoculation phase, the early relevance phase and the late relevance phase [31, 32]. The inoculation phase is the phase prior to initial drug experimentation, the early relevance phase occurs when most students are experiencing initial exposure to drugs and the late relevance phase is when the prevalence of drug use increases and the context of use changes. As the goal of prevention is to decrease the uptake of drugs and prevent the establishment of harmful patterns of use, the inoculation phase is considered the most appropriate phase to intervene. Early intervention on the other hand is best implemented during the early relevance and late relevance phases to target youth who have already started to use substances and experiences related harms [33].

The remainder of this chapter will review the evidence around effective prevention and early intervention of substance use in young people.

School-based prevention for substance use

Although prevention is best delivered through school, community and family interventions, such a holistic approach is resource intensive and not easily achievable.

Table 17.2　Environmental risk and protective factors for drug use

Risk factors	Protective factors
PEERS	**PEERS**
• Relationship with peers who are involved in drug use • Perceived support for substance use by peers • Increased perception of friends' use of drugs • Rewards for antisocial behaviour • Gang involvement • Poor peer relationships and peer rejection	• Association with nondrug using peers
SCHOOL	**SCHOOL**
• School failure • Not completing secondary school – evidence is unclear as to whether this may be explained by earlier developmental influences • Low commitment to school	• Opportunities for prosocial involvement • Rewards for prosocial involvement • Antismoking school policies
FAMILY	**FAMILY**

• Attitude and drug behaviour
  – Favourable parental attitudes to drug use
  – Parental alcohol and drug problems
  – Family history of antisocial behaviour
• Poor family management and communication factors
  – Poor family management
  – Parental rules pertaining to drug use
  – Inconsistent discipline strategies
  – High use of harsh discipline
  – High use of physical punishment
  – Negative communication patterns (e.g. blaming and criticism)
• Family bonding and attachment factors
  – Low attachment to parents
  – Low family bonding
  – Family breakdown
  – Child abuse and neglect
  – Parent–adolescent conflict
• Family structure
  – Sole parent families – this factor appears to result from the association with lower economic status and high family conflict
	• Good attachment to family in adolescence – i.e. high in caring and connectedness
	• Good parental supervision – being aware and in charge of what children are doing
	• Sharing of affection and communication with children
	• Parental interest in child activities
	• Minimal parental conflict
	• Opportunities for prosocial involvement
	• Rewards for prosocial involvement

SOCIETY	**SOCIETY**
• Extreme social disadvantage • Disorganisation and chaos in the community structure • Perceived and actual level of community drug use • Availability of drugs in the community • Low involvement in activities with adults in adolescence • Positive media portrayal of drug use • Laws and norms favourable to drug use • Low neighbourhood attachment • Personal transitions and mobility • Community transitions and mobility • Society labelling someone as a substance user after initial use	• Religious involvement • Opportunity for prosocial involvement • Rewards for prosocial involvement

Table 17.3 Effective principles of school-based prevention of substance use

- Be evidence based and theory driven
- Acknowledge and target risk factors for substance use and psychopathology
- Present developmentally appropriate information
- Be implemented before harmful patterns of use are established
- Be part of a comprehensive health education curriculum
- Adopt a social influence or comprehensive approach to prevention; and
  - Provide resistance skills training and
  - Incorporate normative education
- Make content of immediate relevance to students
- Make use of peer leadership, but keep teacher as the central role
- Address values, attitudes and behaviours of the individual and community
- Be sensitive to cultural characteristics of target audience
- Provide adequate initial coverage and continued follow-up in booster sessions
- Employ interactive teaching approaches
- Can be delivered within an overall framework of harm minimization.

School-based drug education is achievable and is the most favoured approach to prevention of substance use due to the advantages it offers. Firstly, school is a location where educators are able to reach large audiences at one time whilst keeping costs low as attendance is a mandatory requirement in most Western countries and young people spend over a quarter of their waking lives at school [34–36]. Not only is school a place where peer interaction (a significant risk factor for drug use) is high, it also coincides with a time when young people are beginning to experiment or are exposed to drugs [37]. Therefore, schools provide a context to deliver preventive interventions before harmful use begins [38].

Historically, approaches to school-based prevention can be divided into four main categories: (1) information dissemination approaches, (2) affective education approaches, (3) social influence approaches and (4) comprehensive approaches [37, 39]. The least effective of these are the information and affective approaches and the most effective appear to be the social influence and comprehensive approaches. As well as the different approaches to school-based prevention, there are certain components that have been identified in the literature as contributing to programme effectiveness. Table 17.3 summarises the principles that have consistently been associated with effective prevention in schools [35, 40–43].

Over the past few decades, the development and evaluation of school-based prevention substance use prevention programmes has significantly increased as has the number of systematic reviews and meta-analyses examining their effectiveness. These reviews have consistently established that school-based prevention can result in significant increases in knowledge about substances and improved attitudes towards substance use [44–48]. However, they have not been able to consistently demonstrate the effectiveness of school-based drug prevention in reducing actual substance use [44]. This is most likely a result of the many barriers or 'obstacles' which can impede on programme effectiveness [49–52]. Arguably, the greatest obstacles to effective school-based drug prevention can be attributed to issues regarding implementation and dissemination of programmes [53].

Disseminating drug prevention programmes into schools is not always entirely successful [36, 37, 44]. For example Ennett et al. [54] found that only 14% of schools in the United States implemented programmes which incorporate the correct content and delivery as identified in the literature as having the largest effect sizes in reducing drug use [48]. It is possible that because evidence-based programmes are rarely designed and packaged in ways that are competitive with commercial programmes and, once funded trials of prevention cease, schools do not have the motivation or sufficient resources to continue using such programmes [35]. It could also be a result of the many challenges that arise when implementing prevention programmes into the classroom. This is known as 'implementation fidelity' which refers to adhering to, and implementing, a programme in the exact way it was designed to be [55]. A study examining the implementation fidelity of substance use prevention programmes indicated that one-fifth of teachers reported not using a curriculum/programme guide at all, and only 15% reported following one very closely [56]. This is of great concern because research shows that programmes delivered with high fidelity lead to superior outcomes for students, and programmes delivered with poor fidelity lead to poorer outcomes for students [51, 55]. In schools, there are a number of potential barriers to fidelity which compromise program efficacy. These relate predominately to inconsistent or incompetent delivery of programmes and include insufficient ongoing teacher training, inadequate resources, problems with adherence to existing guidelines, lack of support for teachers, insufficient time, classroom overcrowding and management, transient student populations and curriculum changes [44, 49, 53, 54, 56]. Internet-based technology offers a way to overcome barriers to implementation and ensure complete and consistent delivery of programmes.

Internet- and computer-based prevention

Internet- and computer-based technology offers many advantages over traditional methods of delivering prevention and are both feasible and scalable to meet the needs of large audiences. Promising research has been conducted into the development and evaluation of interventions delivered by computers or over the internet to reduce substance use in adolescents. From the evidence that exists, it appears that such programmes are both feasible and acceptable. In terms of efficacy, computerised drug prevention programmes for youth have been shown to increase knowledge [17, 57–61], decrease prodrug attitudes [57, 62–64], increase drug resistance [65] and decrease reported intention to use drugs [65, 66]. The evidence for behavioural change is more limited as most studies which have evaluated the efficacy of computer-based drug prevention programmes for youth have failed to collect behavioural measures [57, 65, 66]. From those that have collected measures of behavioural change, the results are promising.

A study conducted by the Body Awareness Resource Network (BARN) group, found their programme to be effective in slowing the progression of drug use from non-use to problem use in a high-risk population [67]. A study by Schinke et al. [62], found youth who completed a 10-session CD-ROM drug prevention programme to have lower monthly rates of alcohol, tobacco and cannabis use than young people who did not receive the intervention up to 3 years following the intervention. A computerised smoking prevention programme for school students was found to be effective in encouraging cessation in existing smokers and delaying onset in non-smokers [68], and the internet-based *Climate Schools* programmes for drug prevention have been found to decrease average alcohol consumption, decrease frequency of binge drinking and decrease frequency of cannabis use up to 2 years following the interventions [59–61, 63].

In summary, research has demonstrated that computerised interventions can give rise to equivalent or even greater changes in desired outcomes than traditional drug intervention programmes can. This coupled with the numerous implementation advantages and high fidelity associated with computers, the internet offers a new and promising delivery method for substance use prevention and potentially early intervention as well.

Early intervention for substance use disorders

Early intervention is a style of therapy aimed at reducing the risk of harm and progression to dependence in 'hazardous users', whose substance use is at an early or mild stage. It seeks to provide a combination of both screening and brief therapy to individuals before they would normally present for treatment [69]. The therapy usually consists of one to three sessions and is focussed around techniques to educate, encourage and motivate at-risk individuals to consider behaviour change to reduce harm associated with substance use [70–73].

Early intervention programmes stem from the assumption that most substance use disorders do not occur immediately upon initial exposure, but rather, abuse and dependence begins with less pathological, but nonetheless, risky patterns of use [74]. Early work undertaken by Kristenson et al. [75] first demonstrated the efficacy of these programmes for problem drinking, subsequent studies have supported these findings [76, 77].

Traditionally, these programmes have focussed primarily on alcohol misuse, therefore, much less is known about the role and effectiveness of early intervention in illicit substance use. Nevertheless, limited findings suggest that such programmes may have similar utility [77–79].

A number of different approaches to early intervention have been trialled, including skill-based programmes, education/information, social norms and personalised-feedback approaches and motivational enhancement using motivational interviewing (MI). MI is a patient-centred interviewing technique with the goal of resolving ambivalence regarding the pros and cons of change, enhancing motivation and encouraging positive changes in behaviour [80]. A number of styles of delivery of these interventions have also been observed, including face-to-face, internet-based and group approaches [81].

Early alcohol interventions in education settings

The onset of drug and alcohol use tends to occur in adolescence and young adulthood, however, despite the high prevalence of disorders and patterns of high-risk behaviour amongst these groups, they rarely seek professional help [82]. As early intervention programmes represent a means of identifying and curtailing behaviours before they become entrenched, a significant portion of these programmes are aimed specifically at young people, with education settings representing a unique opportunity to access these populations. These interventions have demonstrated success in encouraging young people to adopt more moderate and less harmful patterns of use [77, 83, 84].

The majority of primary and high school drug and alcohol education programmes are prevention-based approaches, with less of a focus on intervening post initiation. These are discussed above. Where early intervention programmes exist they are generally targeted prevention interventions [85], aimed at those students viewed as 'high risk' due to other factors such as personality characteristics. Extensive work in this area by Conrod et al. [86–88] has found such programmes to be effective in reducing rates of drinking, rates of binge drinking, quantity consumed and problem drinking behaviours amongst adolescent drinkers.

Generally, basic information/knowledge-based approaches alone have not been shown to be effective in changing alcohol consumption in university samples [89–91]. More successful interventions tend to combine education with additional components such as alcohol skill training [91]. A recent meta-analysis of 14 RCTs examined the effects of single-session personalised-feedback interventions without therapeutic guidance on the reduction of problematic alcohol consumption in young adults [92]. The authors concluded that such interventions were efficacious and cost-effective and recommended the use of internet-based approaches. This reiterated conclusions of an earlier review which claimed that evidence supported the use of interventions that incorporated personalised feedback, either with or without guided support [91]. Similarly, in a systematic review of 22 RCTs of social-norms-based brief interventions, Moreira et al. [93] concluded that both computerised and individual face-to-face sessions appeared to reduce alcohol misuse, but mail-based and group sessions were less effective.

Other early intervention programmes have used CBT and skills-based techniques to stimulate drinking behaviour change. Two recent reviews have found that expectancy challenge interventions were associated with reductions in drinking in heavy-drinking students [91, 94]. Self-monitoring or self-assessment was found to reduce alcohol consumption at 1-month follow-up, but had no effect on drinking outcomes at 12 months [91]. Social skill training has been found to be effective in reducing risky drinking behaviour at 6-month follow-up in university sample [95].

MI-based interventions have also been shown to be effective in reducing high-risk drinking patterns when administered in higher-education settings [96, 97]. Finally, a meta-analysis of brief interventions with substance using adolescents reported the effect size from the eight alcohol interventions ($n = 1075$) to be small but significant [77]. However, despite all studies included being restricted to a specifically adolescent sample, not all occurred in education settings.

Early alcohol interventions in non-education settings

The implementation of early interventions in non-educational settings has also been found to be effective. Primary and specialty medical care settings represent perhaps the most valuable arena in which early substance use intervention can occur. A brief session (5–10 minutes) of advice from a doctor that is directed towards the risks of excessive consumption and strategies to avoid excessive drinking can significantly reduce alcohol use [98].

A recent meta-analysis focussing on patients in primary care concluded that brief (and early) alcohol intervention is effective for both men and women in reducing alcohol consumption at 6 and 12 months [99]. Of these interventions the majority lasted less than 15 minutes, reported accompanying written materials, and the opportunity for the patient to schedule a follow-up visit. In the study with the longest follow-up period, this effect was also reported at 36 and 48 months [100]. These overall findings are consistent with the results of previous systematic reviews that examined the efficacy of these kinds of interventions conducted in primary care and various related settings [101–106].

Despite the positive effects of early interventions, concerns have been raised about the time and resource costs of universal alcohol screening in primary care. In a meta-analysis exploring the effectiveness of screening in early intervention trials conducted in general practice, Beich et al. [107] reported that only 2 or 3 patients per 1000 screened benefited from subsequent interventions. Therefore, considering ways to appropriately target the approach may be most appropriate in this setting.

Early interventions for substances other than alcohol

Although the majority of early intervention programmes have focussed on alcohol misuse, in recent years there has been in increase in the range of programmes available for other substance use. Martin et al. [79] found that two sessions involving individual assessment and personalised feedback in an MI style (with an optional skill-based session) was effective in helping young people (who were not necessarily interested in change) reduce or stop their cannabis use at 3- and 6-month follow-up. However, the lack of a comparison group limits interpretation of these findings.

McCambridge and Strang [108, 109] found a single-session discussion of cannabis use and other risk indicators showed positive results at 3 months, but this effect became non-significant at 12-month follow-up. Recent findings have indicated that MI may be no more effective in moderating use than information alone for young cannabis users [110] or young stimulant users [111]. As MI has been found to be superior to advice across health care settings and professional groups [112], it is possible there are confounding factors. Reasons proposed for the lack of between-group differences in these studies include lack of MI fidelity by inexperienced practitioners [113] and baseline assessment alone being sufficient to elicit change in the control group [114].

Brief CBT-based interventions have also been found to be effective in illicit drug use. Copeland et al. [115] reported that individuals who received one session of CBT were more likely to report abstinence, were significantly less concerned about their control over cannabis use and reported significantly fewer cannabis-related problems than those in a delayed treatment group. Nevertheless, only those receiving six sessions reported significantly reduced levels of cannabis consumption. It could be argued, however, that due to the study's recruitment strategy this represents a brief treatment protocol rather than an example of early intervention, as the participants volunteered to participate and thus had already identified their use as problematic.

Early intervention, by nature, is difficult in less prevalent illicit drug use due to elevated rates of stigma, infrequent screening and identification of users in the early phases of use. Wittchen et al. [116] stress the time window for targeted intervention preventing transition from initiation to abuse to dependence is critically small in substance misusing youth. Brief (though not necessarily early) MI-based interventions have been piloted with out-of-treatment illicit drug users in medical settings and have been shown to have utility [117–119]. In the first large-scale RCT of this type with cocaine and heroin users, a brief face-to-face intervention was tested against screening and written advice and referral amongst cocaine and/or heroin users [99]. The intervention group was more likely to be abstinent than the control group for cocaine alone, heroin alone and both drugs, and displayed reduced mean drug levels for cocaine at 6-months post intervention.

In a multi-substance misusing adolescent sample recruited from community-based clinics, a brief intervention that included MI as well as education and physician advice demonstrated significant reductions (compared to no-treatment controls) in substance use at 1- and 3-month follow-ups [120]. More recently, a brief intervention, treatment and referral programme for substance misuse was found to be associated with reductions in illicit drug use, self-reported improvements in general health, mental health, employment, housing status, and criminal behaviour at 6 months across a range of health care settings and a range of patients [78].

Overall, early interventions have been shown to be effective in curbing substance use across a range of substances and settings. The programmes are economical and positive results have been demonstrated in as little as one 15-minute session. Interventions utilising a combination of MI and personalised/normative feedback or skills training have generally been found to be most effective. The challenge remains, however, as to how to provide the adequate training and financial incentives to make screening and brief interventions for problem substance use routinely implemented across a range of systems [121].

Conclusions

This chapter reviewed the evidence on risk and protective factors for substance use and described when and where prevention and early intervention should occur. Ideally, prevention and early intervention should be introduced in the adolescent years prior to harmful patterns of use being established, so that young people can be provided with the knowledge and skills they need to make responsible and informed decisions regarding their substance use. As outlined, there are a number of evidence-based prevention and early intervention programmes that exist and have shown to be effective in reducing substance use. Despite their existence, there are also a number of obstacles to implementation and dissemination of these programmes. Using computers and the internet to deliver evidence-based programmes offers a way of overcoming these barriers. Such technology can ensure that programmes are implemented with fidelity and have a better chance of reaching young people who are so often reluctant to report or seek help for their substance use.

References

1. Australian Institute of Health and Welfare. (2011). 2010 National Drug Strategy Household Survey report *Drug statistics series no. 25. Cat. no. PHE 145.* Canberra: AIHW.
2. Hibell B, Guttormsson U, Ahlström S, et al. (2007). *The 2007 ESPAD Report: Substance Use Among Students in 35 European Countries.* Stockholm, Sweden: The European School Survey Project on Alcohol and Other Drugs.
3. National Institute on Drug Abuse. (2008). In LD Johnston, PM O'Malley, JG Bachman and J. E. Schulenberg (eds), *Monitoring the Future: National Results on Adolescent Drug Use,* Maryland, MD: National Institutes of Health.
4. Chikritzhs T, and Pascal R. (2004). Under-age drinking among 14–17 year olds and related harms in Australia. *National Alcohol Indicators Bulletin No. 7.* Canberra: Australian Government Department of Health and Ageing.
5. Hall W, Degenhardt L, and Lynskey M. (2001). The health and psychological effects of cannabis use. *Monograph Series No. 44.* Canberra: National Drug Strategy.

6. Anthony JC and Petronis KR. (1995). Early-onset drug use and risk of later drug problems. *Drug and Alcohol Dependence* **40**(1): 9–15.

7. Grant J, Scherrer J, Lynskey M, et al. (2006). Adolescent alcohol use is a risk factor for adult alcohol and drug dependence: Evidence from a twin design. *Psychological Medicine* **36**(1): 109–118.

8. Teesson M, Degenhardt L, Hall W, et al. (2005). Substance use and mental health in longitudinal perspective. In: T Stockwall, P Grueneald, J Toumbourou and W Loxley (eds), *Preventing Harmful Substance Use: The Evidence Base for Policy and Practice*, pp. 43–51. Chichester: John Wiley & Sons, Ltd.

9. Simmons RG and Blyth D. (2008). *Moving into Adolescence: The impact of Pubertal Change and School Context*. New Brunswick: Transaction Publishers.

10. National Institute on Drug Abuse. (2003). Preventing drug abuse among children and adolescents. In: MD Bethesda (ed.), *NIH Publication No. 03-4212B*: National Institutes of Health.

11. Brook JS, Brook DW, Richter L and Whiteman M. (2003). Risk and protective factors of adolescent drug use: implications for prevention programs. In: Z Sloboda and WJ Bukoski (eds), *Handbook of Drug Abuse Prevention: Theory, Science and Practice*. New York: Kluwer Academic/Plenum Publishers.

12. Frisher M, Crome I, Macleod J, et al. (2007). Predictive factor for illicit drug use among young people: A literature review *Home office online report 05/07*. UK: Research Development and Statistics Directorate, Home Office.

13. Hawkins JD, Catalano RF and Miller J. (1992). Risk and protective factors for alcohol and other drug problems in adolescence and early adulthood: implications for substance abuse prevention. *Psychological Bulletin* **112**: 64–105.

14. Stockwell T, Toumbouruo JW, Letcher P, et al. (2004). Risk and protective factors for different intensities of adolescent substance use: When does the prevention paradox apply? *Drug and Alcohol Review* **23**: 67–77.

15. Swadi H. (1999). Individual risk factors for adolescent substance use. *Drug and Alcohol Dependence* **55**: 209–224.

16. Spooner C, Mattick R and Howard J. (1996). The nature and treatment of adolescent substance abuse. *Monograph No. 26*. Sydney: National Drug and Alcohol Research Centre.

17. Vogl L. (2007). *Climate Schools: Alcohol Module: The Feasibility and Efficacy of a Universal School-based Computerised Prevention Program for Alcohol Misuse and Related Harms*. Sydney: Doctor of Philosophy, University of New South Wales.

18. Loxley W, Toumbouruo JW, Stockwell T, et al. (2004). *The Prevention of Substance Use, Risk and Harm in Australia: A Review of the Evidence Monograph*. Canberra: Ministerial Council on Drug Strategy.

19. Lynskey M, Heath AC and Nelson AC. (2002). Genetic and environmental contributions to cannabis dependence in a national young adult twin sample. *Psychological Medicine* **32**: 195–207.

20. Volkow ND and Li TK. (2007). Treating and preventing abuse, addiction, and their medical consequences. In: MY Tsuang, WS Stone and MJ Lyons (eds), *Recognition and Prevention of Major Mental and Substance Use Disorders*. Washington, DC: American Psychiatric Publishing Inc.

21. Scheier LM, Botvin GJ and Baker E. (1997). Risk and protective factors as predictors of adolescent alcohol involvement and transitions in alcohol use: A prospective analysis. *Journal of Studies on Alcohol* **58**: 652–667.

22. Kuntsche E and Delgrande Jordon M. (2006). Adolescent alcohol and cannabis use in relation to peer and school factors: Results of multilevel analyses. *Drug and Alcohol Dependence* **84**: 167–174.

23. Oetting ER and Lynch RS. (2003). Peers and the prevention of adolescent drug use. In: Z Sloboda and WJ Bukoski (eds), *Handbook of Drug Prevention: Theory, Science and Practice*, pp. 101–127. New York: Kluwer Academic/Plenum Publishers.

24. Andrews G, Henderson S and Hall W. (2001). Prevalence, comorbidity, disability and service utilisation. Overview of the Australian National Mental Health Survey. *The British Journal of Psychiatry* **178**: 145–153.

25. Sowell ER, Thompson PM and Toga AW. (2004). Mapping changes in the human cortex throughout the span of life. *Neuroscientist* **10**: 372–392.

26. Tapert SF, Caldwell L and Burke C. (2005). Alcohol and the adolescent brain: Human studies. *Alcohol Research and Health*, **28**(4):205–212.

27. Gogtay N, Giedd JN, Lusk L, et al. (2004). Dynamic mapping of human cortical development during childhood through early adulthood. *Proceedings of the National Academy of Sciences of the United States of America* **101**: 8174–8179.

28. Luna B and Sweeney JA. (2004). The emergence of collaborative brain function: FMRI studies of the development of response inhibition. *Annals of the New York Academy of Sciences* **1021**: 296–309.

29. Galvan A, Hare TA, Parra CE, et al. (2006). Earlier development of the accumbens relative to orbitofrontal cortex might underlie risk-taking behaviour in adolescents. *Journal of Neuroscience* **26**: 6885–6892.

30. Dielman TE. (1995). School-based research on the prevention of adolescent alcohol use and misuse: methodological issues and advances. In: GM. Boyd, J Howard and RA Zucker (eds), *Alcohol Problems Among Adolescents: Current Directions in Prevention Research*, pp. 125–146. Hillsdale: Lawrence Erlbaum Associates.

31. Hawks D, Scott K and McBride N. (2002). *Prevention of Psychoactive Substance Use: A Selected Review of what Works in the Area of Prevention*. Switzerland: WHO.

32. McBride N. (2003). A systematic review of school drug education. *Health Education Research* **18**(6): 729–742.

33. Offord DR. (2000). Selection of levels of prevention. *Addictive Behaviours* **25**(6): 833–842.

34. Botvin GJ. (2000). Preventing drug abuse in schools: social and competence enhancement approaches targeting individual-level etiologic factors. *Addictive Behaviors* **25**(6): 887–897.

35. Cuijpers P. (2002). Effective ingredients of school-based drug prevention programs: A systematic review. *Addictive Behaviors* **27**(6): 1009–1023.

36. Cuijpers P. (2003). Three decades of drug prevention research. *Drugs: Education, Prevention and Policy* **10**(1): 6–20.

37. Botvin GJ and Griffin KW. (2003). Drug abuse prevention curricula in schools. In: Z Sloboda and WJ Bukoski (eds), *Handbook of Drug Abuse Prevention: Theory, Science and Practice*, pp. 45–74. New York: Kluwer Academic/Plenum Publishers.

38. Berkowitz MW and Begun AL. (2003). Designing prevention programs: the developmental perspective. In: Z Sloboda and WJ Bukoski (eds), *Handbook of Drug Abuse Prevention: Theory, Science and Practice*. New York: Kluwer Academic/Plenum Publishers.

39. Botvin GJ. (1999). Prevention in schools. In: RT Ammerman, PJ Ott and RE Tarter (eds), *Prevention and Societal Impact of Drug and Alcohol Abuse*, pp. 281–305. Mahwah: Lawrence Erlbaum Associates Publishers.

40. Ballard R, Gillespie A and Irwin R. (1994). *Principles for Drug Education in Schools: An Initiative of the School Development in Health Education Project*. Canberra: University of Canberra.

41. Dusenbury L and Falco M. (1995). Eleven components of effective drug abuse prevention curricula. *Journal of School Health* **65**(10): 420–425.

42. Meyer L and Cahill H. (2004). *Principles for School Drug Education*. Canberra: Australian Government Department of Education Science and Training.

43. Midford R, Munro G, McBride N, et al. (2002). Principles that underpin effective school-based drug education. *Journal of Drug Education* **32**(4): 363–386.

44. Botvin GJ and Griffin KW. (2007). School-based programmes to prevent alcohol, tobacco and other drug use. *International Review of Psychiatry* **19**(6): 607–615.

45. Faggiano F, Vigna-Taglianti FD, Versino E, et al. (2008). School-based prevention for illicit drugs use: A systematic review. *Preventive Medicine* **46**(5): 385–396.

46. Midford R, Snow P and Lentin S. (2001). School-based illicit drug education programs: A critical review and analysis. *Literature review prepared for the Department of Employment, Training and Youth Affairs*: National Drug Research Institute.

47. Soole DW, Mazerolle L and Rombouts S. (2005). School based drug prevention: A systematic review of the effectiveness on illicit drug use. *Drug Policy Modelling Project, Monograph 07*, Griffith University.

48. Tobler NS, Roona MR, Ochshorn P, et al. (2000). School-based adolescent drug prevention programs: 1998 meta-analysis. *The Journal of Primary Prevention* **20**(4): 275–336.

49. Botvin GJ. (2004). Advancing prevention science and practice: Challenges, critical issues, and future directions. *Prevention Science* **5**(1): 69–72.

50. Dusenbury L and Hansen WB. (2004). Pursuing the course from research to practice. *Prevention Science* **5**(1): 55–59.

51. Elliott DS and Mihalic S. (2004). Issues in disseminating and replicating effective prevention programs. *Prevention Science* **5**(1): 47–53.

52. Kaftarian S, Robinson E, Compton W, et al. (2004). Blending prevention research and practice in schools: critical issues and suggestions. *Prevention Science* **5**(1): 1–3.

53. Cahill H. (2007). Challenges in adopting evidence-based school drug education programmes. *Drug and Alcohol Review* **26**: 673–679.

54. Ennett ST, Ringwalt CL, Thorne J, et al. (2003). A comparison of current practice in school-based substance use prevention programs with meta-analysis findings. *Prevention Science* **4**: 1–14.

55. Dane AV and Schneider BH. (1998). Program integrity in primary and early secondary intervention: are implementation effects out of control? *Clinical Psychology Review* **18**(1): 23–45.

56. Ringwalt C, Ennett S, Johnson R, et al. (2003). Factors associated with fidelity to substance use prevention curriculum guides in the nation's middle schools. *Health Education and Behaviour* **30**(3): 375–391.

57. Gropper M. (2002). Computer integrated drug prevention: combining multi-media and social group work practices to teach inner city Israeli 6th graders how to say no to drugs. *Journal of Technology in Human Services* **20**: 49–65.

58. Marsch LA, Bickel WK and Badger GJ. (2007). Applying computer technology to substance abuse prevention science: results of a preliminary examination. *Journal of Child and Adolescent Substance Abuse* **16**(2): 69–94.

59. Newton N, Teesson M, Vogl L and Andrews G. (2010). Internet-based prevention for alcohol and cannabis use: final results of the Climate Schools course. *Addiction* **105**: 749–759. doi:10.1111/j.1360-0443.2009.02853.x

60. Newton NC, Andrews G, Teesson M and Vogl LE. (2009). Delivering prevention for alcohol and cannabis using the internet: a cluster randomised controlled trial. *Preventive Medicine* **48**: 579–584.

61. Newton NC, Vogl LE, Teesson M and Andrews G. (2009). CLIMATE Schools: alcohol module: cross-validation of a school-based prevention programme for alcohol misuse. *Australian and New Zealand Journal of Psychiatry* **43**: 201–207.

62. Schinke S, Schwinn TM, Noia JD and Cole KC. (2004). Reducing the risks of alcohol use among urban youth: three-year effects of a computer-based intervention with and without parent involvement. *Journal of Studies on Alcohol* **65**: 443–449.

63. Vogl L, Teesson M, Andrews G, et al. (2009). A computerised harm minimisation prevention program for alcohol misuse and related harms: randomised controlled trial. *Addiction* **104**: 564–575.

64. Williams C, Griffin KW, Macaulay AP, et al. (2005). Efficacy of a drug prevention CD-ROM intervention for adolescents. *Substance Use and Misuse* **40**: 869–878.

65. Duncan TE, Duncan SC, Beauchamp N, et al. (2000). Development and evaluation of an interactive CD-ROM refusal skills program to prevent youth substance use: 'refuse to use'. *Journal of Behavioral Medicine* **23**(1): 59–72.

66. Gregor MA, Shope JT, Blow FC, et al. (2003). Feasibility of using an interactive laptop program in the emergency department to prevent alcohol misuse among adolescents. *Annals of Emergency Medicine* **42**(2): 276–284.

67. Bosworth K, Gustafson D and Hawkins R. (1994). The BARN system: use and impact of adolescent health promotion via computers. *Computers in Human Behaviour* **10**(4): 467–482.

68. Ausems M, Mesters I, van Breukelen G and De Vries H. (2002). Short-term effects of a randomised computer-based out-of-school smoking prevention trial aimed at elementary school children. *Preventive Medicine* **34**: 581–589.

69. Saunders JB and Foulds K. (1992). Brief and early intervention: experience from studies of harmful drinking. [Review]. *Australian and New Zealand Journal of Medicine* **22**(2): 224–230.

70. Babor TF and Higgins-Biddle JC. (2001). *Brief Intervention for Hazardous and Harmful Drinking: A Manual for Use in Primary Care.* Geneva: World Health Organization Department of Mental Health and Substance Abuse.

71. Chick J. (1991). Early intervention for hazardous drinking in the general hospital. [Clinical Trial Comparative Study Randomized Controlled Trial]. *Alcohol and Alcoholism. Supplement* **1**: 477–479.

72. Kurz M. (2003). Early intervention strategies in substance abuse. [Review]. *Journal of Neural Transmission, Supplementum* (66): 85–96.

73. Toumbourou JW, Stockwell T, Neighbors C, et al. (2007). Interventions to reduce harm associated with adolescent substance use. *The Lancet* **369**: 1391–1401. doi:10.1016/s0140-6736(07)60369-9

74. Muramoto ML and Leshan L. (1993). Adolescent substance abuse. Recognition and early intervention. [Review]. *Primary Care; Clinics in Office Practice* **20**(1): 141–154.

75. Kristenson H, Ohlin H, Hulter-Nosslin M, et al. (1983). Identification and intervention of heavy drinking in middle-aged men: results and follow-up of 24-60 months of long-term study with randomized controls. *Alcoholism: Clinical and Experimental Research* **7**(2): 203–209.

76. Bertholet N, Daeppen J-B., Wietlisbach V, et al. (2005). Reduction of alcohol consumption by brief alcohol intervention in primary care: Systematic review and meta-analysis. *Archives of Internal Medicine* **165**(9): 986–995. doi:10.1001/archinte.165.9.986

77. Tait R and Hulse G. (2003). A systematic review of the effectiveness of brief interventions with substance using adolescents by type of drug. *Drug and Alcohol Review* **22**: 337–346.

78. Madras BK, Compton WM, Avula D, et al. (2009). Screening, brief interventions, referral to treatment (SBIRT) for illicit drug and alcohol use at multiple healthcare sites: Comparison at intake and 6 months later. *Drug and Alcohol Dependence* **99**(1–3): 280-295. doi:10.1016/j.drugalcdep.2008.08.003

79. Martin G, Copeland J and Swift W. (2005). The adolescent cannabis check-up: feasibility of a brief intervention for young cannabis users. *Journal of Substance Abuse Treatment* **29**: 207–213.

80. Miller WR and Rollnick S. (2002). *Motivational Interviewing: Preparing People to Change Addictive Behaviour*, 2nd edition. New York: Guildford Press.

81. Reavley NJ and Jorm AF. (2010). Prevention and early intervention to improve mental health in higher education students: a review. [Review]. *Early intervention in psychiatry* **4**(2): 132–142.

82. Reavley NJ, Cvetkovski S, Jorm AF and Lubman DI. (2010). Help-seeking for substance use, anxiety and affective disorders among young people: results from the 2007 Australian National Survey of Mental Health and Wellbeing. *Australian and New Zealand Journal of Psychiatry* **44**(8): 729–735. doi:10.3109/00048671003705458

83. McBride N, Farringdon F, Midford R, et al. (2003). Early unsupervised drinking-reducing the risks. The School Health and Alcohol Harm Reduction Project. *Drug and Alcohol Review* **22**: 263–276.

84. Tevyaw T and Monti P. (2004). Motivational enhancement and other brief interventions for adolescent substance abuse: foundations, applications and evaluations. *Addiction* **99**: 63–75.

85. Stewart SH, Conrod PJ, Marlatt GA, et al. (2005). New developments in prevention and early intervention for alcohol abuse in youths. [Congresses]. *Alcoholism: Clinical and Experimental Research* **29**(2): 278–286.

86. Conrod PJ, Castellanos N and Mackie C. (2008). Personality-targeted interventions delay the growth of adolescent drinking and binge drinking. *Journal of Child Psychology and Psychiatry* **49**(2): 181–190.

87. Conrod PJ, Castellanos N and Strang J. (2010). Brief, personality-targeted coping skills interventions prolong survival as a non-drug user over a two-year period during adolescence. *Archives of General Psychiatry* **67**(1): 85–93.

88. Conrod PJ, Stewart SH, Comeau N and Maclean AM. (2006). Efficacy of cognitive–behavioral interventions targeting personality risk factors for youth alcohol misuse. *Journal of Clinical Child and Adolescent Psychology* **35**(4): 550–563.

89. Croom K, Lewis D, Marchell T, et al. (2009). Impact of an online alcohol education course on behavior and harm for incoming first-year college students: short-term evaluation of a randomized trial. *Journal of American College Health* **57**: 445–454.

90. Ichiyama M, Fairlie A, Wood M, et al. (2009). A randomized trial of a parent-based intervention on drinking behavior among incoming college freshmen. *Journal of Studies on Alcohol and Drugs* **16**(Suppl): 67–76.

91. Larimer ME and Cronce JM. (2007). Identification, prevention, and treatment revisited: individual-focused college drinking prevention strategies 1999-2006. *Addictive Behaviors* **32**: 2439–2468.

92. Riper H, van Straten A, Keuken M, et al. (2009). Curbing problem drinking with personalized feedback interventions: a meta-analysis. *American Journal of Preventive Medicine* **36**: 247–255.

93. Moreira M, Smith L and Foxcroft D. (2009). Social norms interventions to reduce alcohol misuse in University or College students. *Cochrane Database of Systematic Reviews* **3**: CD006748.

94. Wood M, Capone C, Laforge R, et al. (2007). Brief motivational intervention and alcohol expectancy challenge with heavy drinking college students: a randomized factorial study. *Addictive Behaviors* **32**: 2509–2528.

95. Caudill B, Luckey B, Crosse S, et al. (2007). Alcohol risk-reduction skills training in a national fraternity: a randomized intervention trial with longitudinal intent-to-treat analysis. *Journal of Studies on Alcohol and Drugs* **68**: 399–409.

96. LaBrie J, Huchting K, Lac A, et al. (2009). Preventing risky drinking in first-year college women: further validation of a female-specific motivational-enhancement group intervention. *Journal of Studies on Alcohol and Drugs. Supplement* **16**: 77–85.

97. Schaus J, Sole M, McCoy T, et al. (2009). Alcohol screening and brief intervention in a college student health center: a randomized controlled trial. *Journal of Studies on Alcohol and Drugs* **16**(Suppl): 131–141.

98. Neighbors C, Larimer M, Lostlutter T and Woods B. (2006). Harm reduction and individually focused alcohol prevention. *International Journal of Drug Policy* **17**: 304–309.

99. Bernstein J, Bernstein E, Tassiopoulos K, et al. (2005). Brief motivational intervention at a clinic visit reduces cocaine and heroin use. *Drug and Alcohol Dependence* **77**(1): 49–59. doi:10.1016/j.drugalcdep.2004.07.006

100. Fleming M, Mundt M, French M, et al. (2002). Brief physician advice for problem drinkers: long-term efficacy and benefit-cost analysis. *Alcoholism: Clinical and Experimental Research* **26**: 36–43.

101. Bien T, Miller W and Tonigan J. (1993). Brief interventions for alcohol problems: a review. *Addiction* **88**: 315–335.

102. D'Onofrio G and Degutis L. (2002). Preventive care in the emergency department: screening and brief intervention for alcohol problems in the emergency department: a systematic review. *Academic Emergency Medicine* **9**: 627–638.

103. Dunn C, Deroo L and Rivara F. (2001). The use of brief interventions adapted from motivational interviewing across behavioral domains: a systematic review. *Addiction* **96**: 1725–1742.

104. Kahan M, Wilson L and Becker L. (1995). Effectiveness of physician-based interventions with problem drinkers: a review. *Canadian Medical Association Journal* **152**: 851–859.

105. Moyer A, Finney J, Swearingen C and Vergun P. (2002). Brief interventions for alcohol problems: a meta-analytic review of controlled investigations in treatment-seeking and non-treatment-seeking populations. *Addiction* **97**: 279–292.

106. Wilk A, Jensen N and Havighurst T. (1997). Meta-analysis of randomized control trials addressing brief interventions in heavy alcohol drinkers. *Journal of General Internal Medicine* **12**: 274–283.

107. Beich A, Thorsen T and Rollnick S. (2003). Screening in brief intervention trials targeting excessive drinkers in general practice: systematic review and meta-analysis. *British Medical Journal* **327**: 536–542.

108. McCambridge J and Strang J. (2004). The efficacy of single-session motivational interviewing in reducing drug consumption and perceptions of drug-related risk and harm among young people. *Addiction* **99**: 39–52.

109. McCambridge J and Strang J. (2005). Deterioration over time in effect of motivational interviewing in reducing drug consumption and related risk among young people. *Addiction* **100**: 470–478.

110. McCambridge J, Slym RL and Strang J. (2008). Randomized controlled trial of motivational interviewing compared with drug information and advice for early intervention among young cannabis users. [Comparative Study Multicenter Study Randomized Controlled Trial Research Support, Non-U.S. Gov't]. *Addiction* **103**(11): 1809–1818.

111. Marsden J, Stillwell G, Barlow H, et al. (2006). An evaluation of a brief motivational intervention among young ecstasy and cocaine users: no effect on substance and alcohol use outcomes. *Addiction* **101**(7): 1014–1026. doi:10.1111/j.1360-0443.2006.01290.x

112. Rubak S, Sandbaek A, Lauritzen T and Christenses B. (2005). Motivational interviewing: a systematic review and meta-analysis. *British Journal of General Practice* **55**: 305–312.

113. Gray E, McCambridge J and Strang J. (2005). The effectiveness of motivational interviewing delivered by youth workers in reducing drinking, cigarette and cannabis smoking among young people: quasi-experimental pilot study. *Alcohol and Alcoholism* **40**: 535–539.

114. Clifford PR and Maisto SAJ. (2000). Subject reactivity effects and alcohol treatment outcome research. *Journal of Studies on Alcohol and Drugs* **61**: 787–793.

115. Copeland J, Swift W, Roffman R and Stephens R. (2001). A randomized controlled trial of brief cognitive–behavioral interventions for cannabis use disorder. *Journal of Substance Abuse Treatment* **21**(2): 55–64. doi:10.1016/s0740-5472(01)00179-9

116. Wittchen HU, Behrendt S, Hofler M, et al. (2008). What are the high risk periods for incident substance use and transitions to abuse and dependence? Implications for early intervention and prevention. [Research Support, Non-U.S. Gov't]. *International Journal of Methods in Psychiatric Research* **17**(Suppl 1) S16–S29.

117. Bernstein E, Bernstein J and Levenson S. (1997). Project ASSERT: an ED-based intervention to increase access to primary care, preventive services, and the substance abuse treatment system. *Annals of Emergency Medicine* **30**: 181–189.

118. Dunn C and Ries R. (1997). Linking substance abuse services with general medical care: Integrated, brief interventions with hospitalized patients. *American Journal of Drug and Alcohol Abuse* **23**: 1–13.

119. Saunders B, Wilkinson C and Phillips M. (1995). The impact of a brief motivational intervention with opiate users attending a methadone programme. *Addiction* **90**: 415–424.
120. Oliansky DM, Wildenhaus KJ, Manlove K, et al. (1997). Effectiveness of brief interventions in reducing substance use among at-risk primary care patients in three community-based clinics. *Substance Abuse* **18**(3): 95–103.
121. Roche A. (2004). Brief interventions: good in theory but weak in practice. *Drug and Alcohol Review* **1**: 11–18.

18
Early Intervention in Childhood Disorders

Rajeev Jairam[1,2] and Garry Walter[3,4]
[1]Gna Ka Lun Adolescent Mental Health Unit, South West Sydney Local Health District, Campbelltown, New South Wales, Australia
[2]School of Medicine, University of New South Wales and University of Western Sydney
[3]Discipline of Psychiatry, University of Sydney
[4]Child and Adolescent Mental Health Services, Northern Sydney Local Health District, New South Wales, Australia

Introduction

Childhood is a fascinating, mystical stage in which many children lead carefree lives without having to worry about the complex gene–environment interplay to which they are constantly subjected. This interplay is the focus of study for a minority of adults, like us, who attempt to discover what makes children 'tick' and what does not, and how one can best assist those that do not. This is particularly important because in children the difference between syndromes and mental health disorders (MHD) can often be blurred. The available navigational maps of the ICD [1] and DSM [2] help only so much in being able to neatly account for all childhood MHD and it is not uncommon in clinical practice to come across children who have a bit of this and a bit of that. As a result, the clinician at the coalface working with children and families with MHD draws on their own professional experience, personal story, and influences around them to make sense of the clinical situation that confronts them and responds accordingly. One disadvantage of this approach is a lack of consistency in the application of evidence-based interventions across different settings. This chapter attempts to negotiate that inconsistency by pointing clinicians towards empirically tested strategies.

In recent decades, the awareness that MHD exist in children has been matched by key epidemiological studies, which estimate that 14–21% of children and adolescents have

Early Intervention in Psychiatry: EI of nearly everything for better mental health, First Edition.
Edited by Peter Byrne and Alan Rosen.
© 2014 John Wiley & Sons, Ltd. Published 2014 by John Wiley & Sons, Ltd.

mental illnesses with associated impairment in functioning [3–5]. This awareness has led to greater early recognition and subsequent attempts at early intervention. Common sense suggests that early intervention for any disorder in anyone should lead to better outcomes! Early-onset mental illness may persist throughout the life span with enduring adverse consequences in the psychological, educational, social and economic domains. Effective primary mental health prevention and early intervention programs are of paramount importance. A recent review of various preventive programs found positive outcomes for anxiety disorders, disruptive behaviour disorders and depressive disorders in children while results for attention-deficit hyperactivity disorder (ADHD) and early-onset schizophrenia were mixed [3].

This chapter examines the techniques of, and evidence for, early intervention in children with MHD. We will first look at early identification, then at individual disorders and examine current evidence for early intervention. We do understand that comorbidity is often the norm and will touch upon it under the relevant sections.

Early identification

An awareness of and ability to identify risk factors and early symptoms of childhood disorders are crucial. Although it would be ideal for parents to have this awareness and promptly bring their children and themselves to the attention of appropriate services, that responsibility generally falls on early childhood clinicians, GPs, paediatricians, child care workers, and preschool and school staff. Early identification can then lead to referral to appropriate services, including child and adolescent mental health services, for intervention which forms the cornerstone of alleviating symptoms, limiting disability and improving function.

Early symptoms of behavioural problems typically precede a mental, emotional or behavioural disorder by 2–4 years [6], and early therapeutic intervention can be highly effective at limiting the severity and/or progression [7].

One factor which continues to be the bane of early identification of mental illness is stigma. Parents are often reluctant to act on the first symptoms owing to a perception that they and their children may be negatively discriminated against at school, among peers and in society in general. Public awareness campaigns are probably the best means to reduce stigma, and further study of stigma affecting young people and their families will better inform such initiatives [8]. At-risk groups for whom higher vigilance is necessary include children of parents with mental illness and substance abuse and children from economically, socially and culturally disadvantaged backgrounds. Average age of onset of different MHD varies. Most developmental disorders (intellectual disability, autistic disorders, ADHD) can be identified very early in life by experienced clinicians. A recent general population study showed that it was possible to identify mental illness in children as young as 1.5 years; risk factors and predictors of mental illness can be identified in the first 10 months of life [5]. Symptoms of childhood anxiety disorders, oppositional defiant disorders (ODD), conduct disorders (CD), depressive disorders, eating disorders, bipolar disorders and psychotic disorders become more evident as the child grows older. Universally, there is a need for mental health screening and intervention in the existing home- and school-based child health surveillance. The choice of instruments (screening, diagnostic, rating scales) will depend not only on their psychometric properties, but also on their ready availability, ease of administration and service setting.

Specific disorders
Intellectual disability

Worldwide, about 780 million children may have some degree of intellectual disability between birth and 5 years of age [9]. There is considerable variance in aetiology of intellectual disability; these include genetic, perinatal (e.g. birth asphyxia) and infectious causes, malnutrition, micronutrient deficiencies, head injuries, lead poisoning, prematurity, low birth weight, malignancies, and potentially the pernicious effects of poverty, child abuse and child neglect [10]. Early intervention studies have largely focused on children with a combination of the above risk factors. A recent comprehensive review of 32 controlled studies reported that efficacious interventions used a combination of specific intervention procedures, including (1) parent involvement in intervention, including ongoing parent coaching that focused both on parental responsivity and sensitivity to child cues and on teaching families to provide the infant interventions, (2) individualization to each infant's developmental profile, (3) focusing on a broad rather than a narrow range of learning targets, and (4) temporal characteristics involving beginning as soon as the risk is detected, and providing greater intensity and duration of the intervention [10]. An earlier comprehensive review of studies in the field found that improvements persisted into late adolescence and adulthood. Early intervention programs that provided more intensive educational services, started earlier and lasted longer appeared to be most beneficial. Similarly, programs that directly targeted the child's everyday experiences, rather than indirectly sought to change this through increasing parental competency or the quality of the child's living conditions, yielded more immediate and greater effects [11]. Overall, there is unequivocal evidence for both the short- and long-term effectiveness of early intervention, with effect sizes in the modest range (from 0.44 to 0.75 SD). It is important to note that most of these results were produced by 'model' programs with considerable resources and highly skilled staff. The extent to which similar outcomes can be achieved by programs embedded within existing community resources remains to be seen [10–12].

Autistic spectrum disorders

Autistic spectrum disorders (ASD) are a heterogeneous group of disorders characterized by a qualitative/quantitative impairment in reciprocal social interaction, a qualitative/quantitative impairment in language and communication and a restricted repertoire of interests/stereotypes together with problems in functional, adaptive and flexible behaviours. Owing to its developmental nature, disability limitation and improving functionality is the mantra. Early intervention focuses on enhancing cognitive, communication and social skills while minimizing core autistic symptoms and other comorbid problem behaviours. Pretreatment variables that seem to predict later outcome are IQ, presence of imitation ability, language, younger age at intervention, severity of symptoms and social responsiveness or 'joint attention' [13].

Among the most thoroughly evaluated are programs involving early intensive home-based behavioural intervention (EIBI), championed by Lovaas (1987) [14], who demonstrated that early intervention with parents as co-therapists works This has been followed by several other types of intervention, all of which have reported varying degrees of success. Most have a mix of developmental, behavioural and educational approaches. Applied behaviour analysis (ABA) forms the basis of behavioural techniques such as EIBI and other approaches such as Pivotal Response Training, Discrete Trial Training and Verbal Behaviour that form part of most early intervention programs for children with autism [15–19]. A recent comprehensive review of literature in the area was undertaken by Howlin and colleagues [20], who compared and contrasted key studies in the field. They report that the interventions based on ABA, particularly those involving home therapy and beginning in the preschool years, have been most comprehensively studied and have the best established evidence base. The EIBI approach is highly prescriptive, with detailed manuals provided to guide and monitor treatment. Learning sessions are provided in a one-to-one discrete trial format, focusing on the systematic teaching of measurable behavioural units, repetitive practice, and structured presentation of tasks from the most simple to the more complex. Alternative approaches have included intensive, parent-directed interventions; reduced intensity EIBI programs; eclectic, public-school-based programs [21]; specialist autism-school-based programs [22] and a mixture of different interventions including those nonintensive ones with a focus on communication and joint social interaction [23]. Most studies have been of 2–6 year durations and demonstrated varying degrees of change in outcome measures, such as improvement of IQ over time, improvement in Vineland Adaptive Behaviour Scale (VABS) [24] scores, improvement of expressive and receptive language skills, reduction in problem behaviours, more positive parental reports and an improvement in school integration following intervention. Early intervention resulted in gains persisting through to adolescence. However, the most substantial gain occurs in the first year of intervention followed by modest gains thereafter.

Asperger's syndrome is part of ASD with a qualitative (not quantitative) impairment in communication and without associated intellectual disability. Owing to this, diagnosis is often delayed, which is unfortunate as the syndrome is often associated with greater psychological and medical comorbidities and significant social impairment. Early intervention strategies focus on (1) developing social skills delivered in the form of a group approach that includes focused instruction on actual target behaviours (such as eye contact), training in social perception, as provided by computer packages such as Let's Face It, or Mind Reading: An Interactive Guide to Human Emotions, and allowing the opportunity to practice skills they learn in varied, naturalistic contexts for generalization and maintenance, (2) encouraging adaptive problem-solving strategies and reducing maladaptive patterns of behaviour, and (3) teaching more effective communication. Early intervention in ASD with psychopharmacological agents for both core symptoms and comorbidities include SSRIs like fluoxetine and low-dose antipsychotic agents such as risperidone [25].

Attention deficit hyperactivity disorder

ADHD is a common neuro-developmental-behavioural disorder of childhood with a 3–6% prevalence rate [26]. Core symptoms include developmentally inappropriate impulsiveness, inattention and hyperactivity which cause significant functional impairment in more than one setting. Eighty percent of all lifetime ADHD begins in the pre/primary school years and symptoms often persist through adolescence and into adulthood, with varying symptom expression and disabilities at different developmental stages [27]. Although there has been some controversy about the validity of the diagnosis, there is very robust evidence for the existence of ADHD and the associated significant disability, including poor self-regulation, planning and execution that impacts across the life span [28, 29]. Comorbidity with learning difficulties, autism spectrum disorders, tics, ODD/CD, mood disorders and substance use later in life is not uncommon. Initial evaluation should involve a full medical, developmental and educational history, including appropriate liaison with preschool/school, exploring ADHD-related symptomatology, comorbidity and its impact on the child's life. Psychological/behavioural intervention is recommended as an initial treatment for preschool children if ADHD symptoms are mild with minimal impairment, the diagnosis of ADHD is uncertain, parents reject medication treatment or there is marked disagreement about the diagnosis between parents or between parents and teachers. In general, parents are involved in 10–20 sessions of 1–2 hours in which they are: (1) given information about the nature of ADHD; (2) taught how to establish a positive relationship with their child through play and child-centred activities; (3) taught to attend more carefully to their child's misbehaviour and when their child complies; (4) able to establish a home token economy including encouraging praise, reward and incentives for appropriate behaviours; (5) given guidance in the use of effective limit setting and clear instruction giving; (6) able to use time out effectively, (7) manage noncompliant behaviours in public settings; (8) use a daily school report card and (9) anticipate future misconduct. Efficacy of the above has been demonstrated in a large study using the 'Incredible Years' parenting program as an early intervention strategy for preschool children with ADHD [30, 31].

Pharmacotherapy consisting of using various short- and long-acting preparations of stimulants (methylphenidate and amphetamines) has the best and most robust evidence of efficacy followed by atomoxetine and clonidine. There is some evidence for the efficacy of stimulants in the preschool years. However, the dose should be titrated more conservatively in preschoolers than in school-age children and lower mean doses may be effective as they metabolize stimulants slower. Evidence is limited with other medications. Appropriate premedication evaluation, parental counselling around effects, side effects, duration of treatment and close monitoring of progress and side effects is vital [28, 31, 32]. The largest intervention trial for ADHD to date was the Multimodal Treatment Study of Children with ADHD [33], which found that while medication was clearly the best intervention for core ADHD symptoms to 24 months; intensive behaviour therapy was associated with improvements in some key associated symptoms such as oppositional behaviour, social skills and family functioning. Responses to multicomponent interventions are better than single-focus therapies.

Left untreated, the long-term prognosis for children with ADHD is poor. They are at a much greater risk of experiencing problems in the educational, personal and social domains and subsequently developing conduct problems, mood disorders, substance abuse and interpersonal and occupational difficulties that can persist into adulthood. Early intervention could possibly mitigate these long-term effects. However, robust evidence for that is currently lacking [28, 30].

Oppositional defiant disorders and conduct disorders

Lifetime prevalence of disruptive behaviour disorders (DBD) in children is about 6.8%, of which ODD makes up about 3% and CD 3–5% [6]. Children who develop a stable pattern of oppositional behaviour during their preschool years are most at risk. They have substantially strained relationships with their parents, teachers and peers, and have high rates of comorbidity with ADHD and mood disorders. They are also at greater risk of developing ODD and CD in later childhood and antisocial personality disorder (ASPD) during adulthood. The need for early intervention is therefore self-explanatory, with parenting programs generally viewed as an essential component. Programs that have demonstrated efficacy in various age groups include the Nurse Home Visitation program in infancy and Family Check Up and Head Start program in the preschool years, which found that positive and proactive parenting skills correlated with changes in child disruptive behaviour and reduction of delinquency. The Triple P (Positive Parenting Program) and Incredible Years parenting series use self-directed, multimedia, parenting and family support strategies to prevent severe behavioural problems in children by enhancing the knowledge, skills and confidence of parents. These programs are most appropriate for parents whose children appear to be in the early stages of emotional and/or behavioural problems. School-based programs that focus on antibullying, antisocial behaviour or peer groups are other effective strategies. Parent Child Interaction Therapy (PCIT) is a promising intervention for CD. Other programs that have shown promise in the field include the Scallywags service, a multicomponent, early intervention scheme, offering support in the educational and home setting of children, aged 3–7 years, and the Fast Track Intervention, a 10-year program (kindergarten to 10 years) addressing parent behaviour management, child social cognitive skills, reading, home visiting, mentoring and classroom curricula. The Fast Track Intervention was the first to demonstrate that long-term intervention can prevent development of CD in high-risk children and the effects can be sustained for at least 2 years after the cessation of the intervention [34–37].

Childhood anxiety disorders

Anxiety disorders typically include selective mutism, phobias, panic disorder, acute and post-traumatic stress disorders and generalized anxiety disorder and can manifest with a variety of symptoms, including separation anxiety and school refusal and are associated with significant disability. Obsessive–compulsive disorder (OCD) is also usually included in this category [38]. One year prevalence of these are 10–20% with higher lifetime prevalence [39]. They commence as early as the preschool years and follow-up studies indicate that they are forerunners to a range of psychiatric disorders in older childhood and adolescence, including other anxiety disorders, panic attacks, CD and ADHD, and may precede the onset of depression in late childhood [40–42]. Early intervention can therefore serve a double purpose of reducing disability due to the disorder itself and potentially preventing the onset of other disorders later in life.

Early detection is very challenging for these disorders as they often go undetected [43]. Screening and assessment are not straightforward as parents often under-report anxiety symptoms. A variety of self-report measures are available to screen and rate anxiety in children, but nothing surpasses a holistic assessment involving the whole family with inputs from school. Intervention would depend on the severity of the disorder, its impact on function and presence of comorbidities.

Early intervention strategies for preschool children with anxiety disorders include the Triple P Program, Parent Education programs, cognitive behavioural therapy (CBT) and play therapy [44]. School- and community-based group programs, such as social effectiveness therapy for children and the 'Cool Kids' program, have demonstrated short- and long-term efficacy [45, 46]. Whole school approaches, coupled with curriculum-based skills building, have also been demonstrated to reduce symptoms of anxiety and depression and further large trials such as Cool Little Kids will only add to our armamentarium of early intervention strategies [47, 48].

In established childhood anxiety disorders, CBT is the first-line option and consists of (1) psychoeducation with child and caregivers about anxiety; (2) somatic education and affective differentiation, that includes self-recognition of affective anxious state and related somatic reactions; (3) somatic management skill training, that includes self-monitoring, muscle relaxation, diaphragmatic breathing and relaxing imagery; (4) cognitive restructuring by identifying and challenging negative thoughts and expectations and modifying self-talk; (5) practicing problem solving by generating several potential solutions for anticipated challenges and generating a realistic action plan ahead of time; (6) exposure methods, including imagined and live exposure with gradual desensitization to feared stimuli; and (7) relapse prevention plans with booster sessions and coordination with parents and school [49]. CBT and selective serotonin reuptake inhibitors (SSRIs), alone and in combination have the best efficacy in all childhood anxiety disorders with OCD usually treated with higher doses of SSRIs [42].

Depressive disorders

Depression becomes increasingly common in later childhood and adolescence, with prevalence rates of 5–14% and female predominance beginning in mid-adolescence and continuing through adulthood [6]. Genetic factors, developmental changes in the neural systems and early adverse experiences together with cognitive and hormonal changes appear to contribute to affect dysregulation and the genesis of depression [50]. Five to ten percent of children have subsyndromal symptoms which can precede the onset of depression and contribute to increased psychosocial impairment, increased risk of developing depression and potentially suicide. Although diagnostic criteria are similar across age groups, children with depression demonstrate mood lability, irritability, low frustration tolerance, temper tantrums, somatic complaints and/or social withdrawal instead of verbalizing feelings of depression. Also, children tend to have fewer melancholic symptoms, delusions and suicide attempts than depressed adults. Depression affects the development of a child's emotional, cognitive and social skills and interferes considerably with family relationships. Sequelae include suicide attempts and completion, and substance abuse and dependence [51]. As with anxiety disorders, evaluation for depression is holistic, involving interview of the child and information from multiple sources including family and school.

Intervention studies in children have largely focused on children at genetic and environmental risk of developing depression. Psychoeducation, as well as cognitive, coping, social skills and family therapies have targeted children who have subsyndromal symptoms, a previous episode of depression and/or a family history of depression. Programs that included populations at-risk were more effective than those targeting general populations (universal studies). Unfortunately, however, the effects of these treatments were small to modest, both immediately post-intervention and at an average follow-up of 6 months [52]. Some group cognitive treatment approaches have shown promise in preventing depression in at-risk adolescents such as the 'coping with stress course' and FRIENDS [37, 45, 53]. It is worth noting the considerable investment in school-based programs enable schools to identify depression (and other mental health problems) and reduce the level of depressive symptoms at an early stage. At face value, these programs have considerable merit [54], but further research is required to ascertain whether such programs make a meaningful impact on the development of the disorder and its features [55]. There are few empirically proven interventions in very young children with depression. One intervention with some promise in preschoolers with depression is 'PCIT' (emotional development module) [56].

Psychoeducation, supportive management and family and school involvement underpins specific intervention for established depression with evidence for the efficacy of both psychotherapeutic (especially CBT and IPT) and psychopharmacological management (fluoxetine and some other SSRIs), alone or in combination [51]. The safety of SSRIs in adolescent depression has generated considerable comment and controversy [57].

Suicide

A devastating tragedy whenever it occurs, completed suicide is relatively uncommon in adolescents (e.g. in Australia in 2008, there were 94 completed suicides in the 15–19 years age group) [58], but self-harm and suicide attempts are frequent. In practice, a variety of strategies are employed in this area, including universal approaches to improving mental health and promoting help-seeking behaviour, and selected and indicated programs (e.g. screening, case-finding and antibullying referral programs). School-based programs are important, although there is a mixed level of evidence about effectiveness. Gatekeeper training is likely to be the most effective and teachers in particular are in a good position to recognize early indicators. While there is, regrettably, a paucity of data to inform practice, a recent multisite study from the United States – the 'Treatment of Adolescent Suicide Attempters' (TASA) study – suggested that, among depressed adolescents who recently attempted suicide, active treatment (SSRI, tailored CBT or the combination) reduces the 6 month rate of reattempts [59]. Other initiatives, including internet-based strategies (e.g. the Reach Out http://au.reachout.com/ and beyondblue websites http://www.youthbeyondblue.com) may be helpful, although there is no firm evidence at this point that they prevent suicide [37]. To organize thinking and potentially services and resources in this area, suicide prevention in Australia has become a federal government priority.

Bipolar disorders

One of the most popular myths in child psychiatry in the second half of the twentieth century was that bipolar disorder did not exist in children and that it was rare in adolescents [60]. Although that has been debunked [61, 62], the low base rate of the disorder in children, its variable clinical presentation, its symptomatic overlap with other disorders and the developmental modulation of symptom expression have made it difficult for clinicians to form a mental template of juvenile bipolar disorder [63]. It also appears that child psychiatrists continually struggle with the current criteria for mania and hypomania in children and adolescents. The majority of symptoms of bipolar disorder are not specific to bipolar illness, but may also be found in other disorders. Consequently, studies on early intervention have been few and far between. Thankfully, some information is beginning to emerge on the response to treatment [64–66].

There are a number of studies that have documented the efficacy of antimanic agents in juvenile bipolar disorder. Mood stabilizers (lithium, valproate, lamotrigine and carbamazepine) and antipsychotic agents (risperidone, olanzapine, quetiapine, aripriprazole and ziprasidone) have been found to be efficacious in treating mania even in young children [64, 67, 68]. There is a lack of literature in prophylaxis of juvenile bipolar disorder, although some studies have commented on the efficacy of lithium in preventing relapse [68, 69]. A larger prospective study found that adherence to medication was associated with rate of recovery and time to recovery, but was not related to the rate of relapse [70]. Psychotherapeutic intervention post-hospitalization was associated with a lower relapse rate and a longer time to relapse [71]. The degree and mechanism by which psychotherapy prevents relapse is worthy of further investigation.

Schizophrenia and related psychotic disorders

Schizophrenia has been identified in children since the early twentieth century. Onset prior to age 13, termed very early-onset schizophrenia (VEOS) is rare, with a prevalence of less than 1 in 30,000 and the disorder in that age group is considered a more severe phenotype [72]. Older studies of children with schizophrenia were complicated by the lack of differentiation between VEOS and autism. Recent research, however, has demonstrated that schizophrenia can be diagnosed reliably in children, and is continuous with the adult disorder [73]. As VEOS is rare, it is important to differentiate it from other disorders such as affective disorders (bipolar disorder and depression with psychotic symptoms), ASD and psychosis related to medical conditions or substance abuse. Taking a careful developmental history and establishing mood congruence of symptoms help in this differentiation. Early identification has focussed on young people deemed ultra high risk (UHR) for psychosis, characterized by attenuated positive symptoms, brief limited intermittent psychotic symptoms, and/or genetic risk factors with functional decompensation [74]. Key clinical features associated with transition to psychosis are ideas of reference, unusual thought content (e.g. magical thinking), perceptual abnormalities (e.g. brief hallucinations), marked and rapid, functional decline and social withdrawal [75] Intervention trials, although ethically controversial, have had mixed results with psychosocial therapies (CBT, supportive therapy and intensive case management), antidepressants and omega 3 fatty acids having a better risk–benefit ratio compared to antipsychotics [76]. Evidence for the application of a clinical staging model for early-onset psychosis, wherein different interventions are applied at different stages of the illness, is gathering traction. These advances have led to service reform with an emphasis on early identification and treatment of first episode psychosis, with the potential for a reduction in long-term disability [77]. Management of established psychosis/schizophrenia involves both pharmacological and psychosocial interventions. Long-term use of antipsychotics remains the best validated treatment, although studies in children are limited. Typical and atypical antipsychotics have been shown to be equally effective in symptom reduction. Clozapine remains the most powerful agent, but is usually third line in children owing to its side-effect profile. Aripriprazole may have a role in clozapine augmentation [78]. There are, however, significant safety concerns, with studies identifying a range of similar side effects as in adults

Table 18.1 Early intervention strategies for specific childhood disorders

Disorders	Early intervention strategies
Intellectual delay/disability [10, 11, 80]	• Beginning as early as the risk is detected and providing greater intensity and duration of the intervention • Parent training focused both on parental responsivity and sensitivity to child cues emphasizing cognitive, linguistic and social development • Individualization to each infant's developmental profile • Focusing on a broad rather than a narrow range of learning targets
Autistic spectrum disorders [20]	Developmental, behavioural and educational approaches: early intensive home-based intervention • One-to-one discrete trial format, focusing on the systematic teaching of measurable behavioural units, repetitive practice and structured presentation of tasks from the most simple to the more complex Specialist autism-school-based program
Attention deficit hyperactivity disorder [30, 31]	• Incredible Years parenting program; parents are involved in 10–20 sessions of 1–2 hours in which they are (1) given information about the nature of ADHD, (2) taught how to establish a positive relationship with their child through play and child-centred activities; (3) taught to attend more carefully to their child's misbehaviour and when their child complies, (4) able to establish a home token economy including encouraging praise, reward and incentives for appropriate behaviours, (5) given guidance in the use of effective limit setting and clear instruction giving, (6) able to use time out effectively, (7) manage noncompliant behaviours in public settings, (8) use a daily school report card, and (9) anticipate future misconduct • Pharmacotherapy including stimulants, atamoxetine and clonidine
Oppositional defiant disorders and conduct disorders [35–37]	In perinatal period • The Nurse Home Visitation program For preschool-aged children • Family check up • Triple P program • Incredible Years • Head Start program • Parent Child Interaction Therapy For school-age children • Fast Track Intervention • The Scallywags service
Anxiety disorders [37, 47, 48]	For preschool children/parents • The Triple P program • The Parent Education program • Cool Little Kids program For older childhood and adolescents • FRIENDS CBT program • Cool Kids program • School approaches – curriculum-based skill building

(continued)

Table 18.1   (*Continued*)

Disorders	Early intervention strategies
Depressive disorders [37, 53, 56]	For preschool-age children • PCIT – emotional development module For school-age children • Coping with stress • FRIENDS Psychopharmacology • SSRIs
Suicide [37, 59]	• Universal approaches to improving mental health and promoting help-seeking behaviour, and selected and indicated programs including school-based programs which focus on suicide awareness, skills training, screening, peer support and gatekeeper training • Systematic treatment of depressed adolescents who have recently attempted suicide with cognitive behavioural therapy, medication or the combination • The use of Reach Out (http://au.reachout.com/) and beyondblue websites (http://www.youthbeyondblue.com/) may be helpful
Bipolar disorders [65, 71]	Scant information on early intervention strategies • Mood stabilizers and atypical antipsychotics have best evidence • Lithium may be effective in relapse prevention • Psychosocial approaches improve treatment adherence, improve functional disability and may help in relapse prevention
Psychotic disorders including schizophrenia [76]	For those at ultra high risk to develop psychosis • Psychosocial therapies (CBT, supportive therapy, intensive case management) • Antidepressants • Omega 3 fatty acids • Low-dose antipsychotics

but these side effects perhaps occur more frequently (especially with polypharmacy) and posing a greater lifetime burden in younger people [79]. Psychosocial interventions include psychoeducation, identifying family supports and, together with the child, families and schools, working towards reducing the developmental impact of the illness. There are, however, no studies that have systematically examined their effectiveness in children [72].

Summary

The field of early intervention is vibrant, generating expectations that systematic, comprehensive, experientially based interventions will alter developmental trajectories and prevent secondary complications [12]. A wide variety of empirically tested early intervention strategies for various childhood disorders have been identified. These are summarized in Table 18.1.

Conclusion

It is an oft repeated quote that children grow up to be who they are despite the influences of their parents and environment. Their resilience is remarkable. Significant genetic and environmental adversity is needed to overcome that protective shield for a psychiatric disorder to manifest. The earlier the first signs of the disorder is identified and attempts to address it implemented, the more likely that enduring disability can be minimised. Interventions (primary and secondary prevention) targeting large groups of at-risk children and families has its place. Once a disorder onsets, interventions must be individualized for each child and family. Furthermore, selecting only one treatment exclusively may hinder progress. The first step is to attempt to identify some of the underlying causes, where possible, and the consequences of the disorder itself (psychological, social, educational and developmental). The next step in successful intervention is to address both the causes and consequences of the disorder, through medication (where indicated), psychotherapy (where indicated), skills training, family intervention, or any other methods needed to assist the child to begin functioning better in all domains – social, academic, work, family and so forth. Such a biopsychosocial approach to treatment of these disorders will likely lead to improvement in the overall outcome.

Strategies to reduce associated stigma and to raise awareness of mental illness should be continued to ensure that parents, care providers and educators respond early to potential mental disturbance in early childhood. The ultimate goal of early intervention is to positively influence children's developmental trajectories so that they achieve successful mental health, academic and social outcomes into adolescence and adult life.

References

1. World Health Organization. (1993). *International Classification of Mental and Behavioural Disorders (ICD-10)*. Geneva: WHO.
2. American Psychiatric Association. (1994). *Diagnostic and Statistical Manual of Mental Disorders*, 4th edition. Washington, DC: American Psychiatric Association.
3. Opler M, Sodhi D, Zaveri D, et al. (2010). Primary psychiatric prevention in children and adolescents. *Annals of Clinical Psychiatry* **22**: 220–340.
4. Sawyer M, Arney F, Baghurst P, et al. (2000). *The Mental Health of Young People in Australia: The Child and Adolescent Component of the National Survey of Mental Health and Wellbeing*. Canberra: Mental Health and Special Programs Branch, Commonwealth Department of Health and Ageing.
5. Skovgaard AM. (2010). Mental health problems and psychopathology in infancy and early childhood. An epidemiological study. *Danish Medical Bulletin* **57**: B4193.
6. O'Connell M, Boat T and Warner K. (2009). *Preventing Mental, Emotional, and Behavioural Disorders among Young People: Progress and Possibilities*. Washington, DC: Board on Children Youth and Families, Institute of Medicine, www.nap.edu (accessed 16 June 2011).
7. Hazel P. (2000). Attention deficit hyperactivity disorder in preschool aged children. In: R Kosky, A O'Hanlon, G Martin and C Davies (eds), *Clinical Approaches to Early Intervention in Child and Adolescent Mental Health*. Adelaide: Australian Early Intervention Network for Mental Health in Young People.
8. Mukolo A, Heflinger CA and Wallston KA. (2010). The stigma of childhood mental disorders: a conceptual framework. *Journal of the American Academy of Child and Adolescent Psychiatry* **49**: 92–103.

9. Olness K. (2003). Effects on brain development leading to cognitive impairment: a worldwide epidemic. *Journal of Developmental and Behavioral Pediatrics* **24**: 120–130.
10. Rogers SJ and Wallace KS. (2010). Intervening in infancy: implications for autism spectrum disorders. *Journal of Child Psychology and Psychiatry and Allied Disciplines* **51**: 1300–1320.
11. Ramey SL and Ramey CT. (1999). Early experience and early intervention for children 'at risk' for developmental delay and mental retardation. *Mental Retardation and Developmental Disabilities Research Reviews* **5**: 1–10.
12. Guralnick MJ. (2005). Early intervention for children with intellectual disabilities: current knowledge and future prospects. *Journal of Applied Research in Intellectual Disabilities* **18**: 313–324.
13. Sallows GO and Graupner TD. (2005). Intensive behavioural treatment for children with autism: four year outcome and predictors. *American Journal of Mental Retardation* **110**: 417–438.
14. Lovaas OI. (1987). Behavioural treatment and normal educational and intellectual functioning in young autistic children. *Journal of Consulting and Clinical Psychology* **55**: 3–9.
15. Dunlap G, Kern-Dunlap L, Clark S, et al. (1991). Functional assessment, curricular revision, and severe problem behaviors. *Journal of Applied Behavior Analysis* **4**: 387–397.
16. Smith IM, Koegel RL, Koegel LK, et al. (2010). Effectiveness of a novel community-based early intervention model for children with autistic spectrum disorder. *American Journal on Intellectual and Developmental Disabilities* **115**: 504–523.
17. Coolican J, Smith IM and Bryson SE. (2010). Brief parent training in pivotal response treatment for preschoolers with autism. *Journal of Child Psychology and Psychiatry and Allied Disciplines* **51**: 1321–1330.
18. Maurice C, Green G and Luce S. (1996). *Behavioral Intervention for Young Children with Autism: A Manual for Parents and Professionals*. Austin, TX: Pro-Ed.
19. Barbera ML and Rasmussen T. (2007). *The Verbal Behavior Approach: How to Teach Children with Autism and Related Disorders*. London: Jessica Kingsley.
20. Howlin P, Magiati I and Charman T. (2009). Systematic review of early behavioural interventions for children with autism. *American Journal on Intellectual and Developmental Disabilities* **114**: 23–41.
21. Eikeseth S, Smith T, Jahr E and Eldevik S. (2007). Outcome for children who began intensive behavioral treatment between ages 4–7: a comparison controlled study. *Behavior Modification* **31**: 264–278.
22. Howard JS, Sparkman CR., Cohen HG, et al. (2005). A comparison of intensive behavior analytic and eclectic treatments for young children with autism. *Research in Developmental Disabilities* **26**: 359–383.
23. Remington B., Hastings RP, Kovshoff H, et al. (2007). Early intensive behavioral intervention: outcomes for children with autism and their parents after two years. *American Journal on Mental Retardation* **112**: 418–438.
24. Sparrow, SS., Balla, D and Cicchetti, DV. (1984). *Vineland Adaptive Behavior Scales*. Circle Pines, MN: American Guidance Service.
25. Woodbury-Smith MR and Volkmar FR. (2009). Asperger syndrome. *European Child and Adolescent Psychiatry* **18**: 2–11.
26. Biederman J and Faraone S. (2005). Attention-deficit hyperactivity disorder. *Lancet* **366**: 237–248.
27. Kessler RC, Amminger GP, Gaxiola SA, et al. (2007). Age of onset of mental disorders: a review of recent literature. *Current Opinion in Psychiatry* **20**: 359–364.
28. Efron D, Hazell P and Anderson V. (2010). Attention deficit hyperactivity disorder. *Journal of Paediatrics and Child Health* no. doi:10.1111/j.1440-1754.2010.01928.x [Epub ahead of print]
29. Rappley M. Attention deficit-hyperactivity disorder. (2005). *The New England Journal of Medicine* **352**: 165–173.

30. Jones K, Daley D, Hutchings J, et al. (2007). Efficacy of the Incredible Years Basic parent training programme as an early intervention for children with conduct problems and ADHD. *Child: Care, Health and Development* **33**: 749–756.

31. Pliszka S. (2007). Practice parameter for the assessment and treatment of children and adolescents with attention-deficit/hyperactivity disorder. *Journal of The American Academy of Child and Adolescent Psychiatry* **46**: 894–921.

32. Greenhill LL, Posner K, Vaughan BS, et al. (2008). Attention deficit hyperactivity disorder in preschool children. *Child and Adolescent Psychiatric Clinics of North America* **17**: 347–366.

33. MTA Cooperative Group. (2004). National institute of mental health multimodal treatment study of ADHD follow-up: 24-month outcomes of treatment strategies for attention-deficit/hyperactivity disorder. *Pediatrics* **113**: 754–761.

34. Burke JD, Loeber R and Birmaher B. (2002). Oppositional defiant disorder and conduct disorder: a review of the past 10 years, part II. *Journal of the American Academy of Child and Adolescent Psychiatry* **41**(11): 1275–1293.

35. Conduct Problems Prevention Research Group. (2011). The effects of the fast track preventive intervention on the development of conduct disorder across childhood. *Child Development.* **82**: 331–345. doi:10.1111/j.1467-8624.2010.01558.x

36. McMenamy J, Sheldrick RC and Perrin EC. (2011). Early intervention in paediatrics offices for emerging disruptive behaviour in toddlers. *Journal of Pediatric Health Care* **25**: 77–86.

37. Royal Australian and New Zealand College of Psychiatrists (2010). Report from the Faculty of Child and Adolescent Psychiatry. Prevention and early intervention of mental illness in infants, childhood and adolescents: Planning strategies for Australia and New Zealand.

38. Woodward LJ and Fergusson DM. (2001). Life course outcomes of young people with anxiety disorders in adolescence. *Journal of the American Academy of Child And Adolescent Psychiatry* **40**: 1086–1093.

39. Costello EJ, Egger HL and Angold A. (2004). Developmental epidemiology of anxiety disorders. In: TH Ollendick and JS March (eds), *Phobic and Anxiety Disorders in Children Curr Psychiatry Rep and Adolescents*, pp. 334–380. New York: Oxford University Press.

40. Egger HL and Angold A. (2006). Common emotional and behavioral disorders in preschool children: presentation, nosology, and epidemiology. *Journal of Child Psychology and Psychiatry and Allied Disciplines* **47**: 313–337.

41. Bittner A, Egger HL, Erkanli A, et al. (2007). What do childhood anxiety disorders predict? *Journal of Child Psychology and Psychiatry and Allied Disciplines* **48**: 1174–1183.

42. Connolly SD, Suarez L and Sylvester C. (2011). Assessment and treatment of anxiety disorders in children and adolescents. *Current Psychiatry Reports* **13**: 99–110.

43. American Academy of Child and Adolescent Psychiatry. (2007). Practice parameter for the assessment and treatment of children and adolescents with anxiety disorders. *Journal of the American Academy of Child and Adolescent Psychiatry* **46**: 267–283.

44. Kennedy SJ, Rapee RM and Edwards SE. (2009). A selective intervention program for inhibited preschool-aged children of parents with anxiety disorder: effects on current anxiety disorders and temperament. *Journal of The American Academy of Child and Adolescent Psychiatry* **48**: 602–609.

45. Neil AL and Christensen H. (2007). Australian school-based prevention and early intervention programs for anxiety and depression: a systematic review. *Medical Journal of Australia* **186**: 305–308.

46. Rapee RM, Kennedy SJ, Ingram M, et al. (2010). Altering the trajectory of anxiety in at-risk young children. *American Journal of Psychiatry* **167**: 1518–1525.

47. Bayer JK, Hiscock H, Scalzo K, et al. (2009). Systematic review of preventive interventions for children's mental health: what would work in Australian contexts? *Australian and New Zealand Journal of Psychiatry* **43**: 695–710.

48. Bayer JK, Rapee RM and Hiscock H. (2011). The Cool Little Kids randomised controlled trial: population-level early prevention for anxiety disorders. *BMC Public Health* **5**: 11:11 [Epub ahead of print]

49. Gosch EA, Flannery-Schroeder E, Mauro CF, et al. (2006). Principles of cognitive-behavioral therapy for anxiety disorders in children. *Journal of Cognitive Psychotherapy* **20**: 247–262.

50. Park RJ and Goodyer IM. (2000). Clinical guidelines for depressive disorders in childhood and adolescence. *European Child and Adolescent Psychiatry* **9**: 147–161.

51. American Academy of Child and Adolescent Psychiatry. (2007). Practice parameter for the assessment and treatment of children and adolescents with depressive disorders. *Journal of The American Academy of Child and Adolescent Psychiatry* **46**: 1503–1526.

52. Horowitz J and Garber J. (2006). The prevention of depressive symptoms in children and adolescents: a meta-analytic review. *Journal of Consulting and Clinical Psychology* **74**: 401–415.

53. Garber J, Clarke GN, Weersing VR, et al. (2009). Prevention of depression in at-risk adolescents – a randomized control trial. *The Journal of The American Medical Association* **301**: 2215–2224.

54. Maloney D, Jones J, Walter G and Davenport R. (2008). Addressing mental health concerns in schools: does "School-Link" achieve its aims? *Australasian Psychiatry* **16**: 48–53.

55. Sawyer MG, Pfeiffer S, Spence SH, et al. (2009). School-based prevention of depression: a randomised controlled study of the beyondblue schools research initiative. *Journal of Child Psychology and Psychiatry* **51**: 199–209.

56. Lenze SN, Pautsch J and Luby J. (2011). Parent-child interaction therapy emotion development: a novel treatment for depression in preschool children. *Depression And Anxiety* **28**: 153–159.

57. Dudley M, Goldney R and Hadzi-Pavlovic D. (2010). Are adolescents dying by suicide taking SSRI antidepressants? A review of observational studies. *Australasian Psychiatry* **18**: 242–245.

58. Australian Bureau of Statistics. (2007). National Survey of Mental Health and Wellbeing: Summary of Results.

59. Walter G. (2009). "Nessun Dorma ("None Shall Sleep"). . . . at least not before we digest TASA. *Journal of the American Academy of Child and Adolescent Psychiatry* **48**: 977–978.

60. Anthony J and Scott P. (1960). Manic-depressive psychosis in childhood. *Journal of Child Psychology and Psychiatry* **1**: 17–25.

61. Geller B and Luby J. (1997). Child and adolescent bipolar disorder- A review of the past ten years. *Journal of the American Academy of Child And Adolescent Psychiatry* **36**(9): 1168–1176.

62. Weller EB, Weller RA and Fristad MA. (1995). Bipolar disorders in children: misdiagnosis, under-diagnosis and future directions. *Journal of the American Academy of Child and Adolescent Psychiatry* **34**(6): 709–714.

63. Jairam R, Andreson R and Redwin R. (2006). Paediatric Bipolar Disorder; Perspectives on Course and Outcome for the book. *New Developments in Mania Research*. New York: Nova Science Publishers.

64. Kowatch RA, Fristad M, Birmaher B, et al. (2005). Treatment guidelines for children and adolescents with bipolar disorder. *Journal of the American Academy of Child and Adolescent Psychiatry* **44**(3): 213–235.

65. Jairam R, Hanstock T, Cahill C, et al. (2008). The changing face of bipolar disorder: adolescence to adulthood. *Minerva Pediatrica* **60**: 59–68.

66. Reddy YCJ, Srinath S and Jairam R. (2007). "Paediatric bipolar disorder – from the perspective of India". In: RS Diler (ed.), *Paediatric Bipolar Disorder – A global perspective,* pp. 91–107. New York: Nova science publishers.

67. Biederman J, Mick E, Bostic JQ, et al. (1998). The naturalistic course of pharmacologic treatment of children with manic-like symptoms: a systematic chart review. *Journal of Clinical Psychiatry* **59**: 628–637.

68. Jairam R, Srinath S, Girimaji SC and Seshadri SP. (2004). A prospective 4–5 year follow-up of juvenile onset bipolar disorder. *Bipolar Disorders* **6**(5): 386–394.

69. Strober M, Morrell W, Lampert C and Burroughs J. (1990). Relapse following discontinuation of lithium maintenance therapy in adolescents with bipolar I illness: a naturalistic study. *American Journal of Psychiatry* **147**: 457–461.

70. Birmaher B, Axelson D, Strober M, et al. (2006). Clinical course of children and adolescents with bipolar spectrum disorders. *Archives of General Psychiatry* **63**: 175–183.

71. DelBello MP, Hanseman D, Adler CM, et al. (2007). Twelve-month outcome of adolescents with bipolar disorder following first hospitalisation for a manic or mixed episode. *American Journal of Psychiatry* **164**: 582–590.

72. Mattai AK, Hill JL and Lenroot RK. (2010). Treatment of early-onset schizophrenia. *Current Opinion in Psychiatry* **23**: 304–310.

73. Walker E. (2002). Risk factors and the neurodevelopmental course of schizophrenia. *European Psychiatry: The Journal of The Association of European Psychiatrists* **17**: 363–369.

74. Schultze-Lutter F, Ruhrmann S, Berning J, et al. (2010). Basic symptoms and ultrahigh risk criteria: symptom development in the initial prodromal state. *Schizophrenia Bulletin* **36**: 182–191.

75. Kulhara P, Banerjee A and Dutt A. (2008). Early intervention in schizophrenia. *Indian Journal of Psychiatry* **50**: 128–134.

76. McGorry PD, Nelson B, Amminger GP, et al. (2009). Intervention in individuals at ultra high risk for psychosis: a review and future directions. *Journal of Clinical Psychiatry* **70**: 1206–1212.

77. Francey SM, Nelson B, Thompson A, et al. (2010). Who needs antipsychotic medication in the earliest stages of psychosis? A reconsideration of benefits, risks, neurobiology and ethics in the era of early intervention. *Schizophrenia Research* **119**: 1–10.

78. Bachmann CJ, Lehr D, Theisen FM, et al. (2009). Aripiprazole as an adjunct to clozapine therapy in adolescents with early-onset schizophrenia: a retrospective chart review. *Pharmacopsychiatry* **42**: 153–157.

79. Vitiello B, Correll C, Van Zwieten-Boot B, et al. (2009). Antipsychotics in children and adolescents: increasing use, evidence for efficacy and safety concerns. *European Neuropsychopharmacology* **19**: 629–635.

80. IHDP. (1990). Enhancing the outcomes of low-birth-weight, premature infants. *The Journal of the American Medical Association* **263**: 3035–3042.

19
Early Intervention for Delirium

David Meagher[1] and Walter Cullen[2]

[1]*Department of Psychiatry, University of Limerick Medical School, Limerick, Ireland*
[2]*Department of General Practice, University of Limerick Medical School, Limerick, Ireland*

Key points

1. Delirium is common across all health care settings and has a major adverse impact upon outcomes that is predicted by the occurrence and severity of delirium.

2. Patients at high risk can be readily identified and a variety of interventions can reduce delirium incidence and severity of emergent cases.

3. Problems with delayed or nondetection occur in approximately 50% of cases of delirium.

4. Improved identification can be achieved through routine and systematic screening for cognitive impairment and neuropsychiatric symptoms of delirium.

5. Evidence to support pharmacological management of delirium is gathering with the increasing emergence of randomised studies, including some placebo-controlled designs.

6. Improved delirium care requires fundamental changes to the organisation of health care environments that require the combined efforts of clinicians and health care management.

Delirium – a key target for early intervention

Delirium is an acute neuropsychiatric syndrome that is characterised by a complex constellation of cognitive impairments and neuropsychiatric disturbances that reflect generalised

Early Intervention in Psychiatry: EI of nearly everything for better mental health, First Edition.
Edited by Peter Byrne and Alan Rosen.
© 2014 John Wiley & Sons, Ltd. Published 2014 by John Wiley & Sons, Ltd.

impairment of brain function. It is common in many clinical settings, occurring in approximately one in five hospitalised patients, with rates of up to 90% reported among patients in palliative and intensive care settings [1]. No other psychiatric disorder has such penetration across health care settings – this frequency, along with the complexity of clinical presentation where typically one half of the cases are not detected [2], makes more timely intervention a key health care priority.

Delirium is especially common in patients with diminished cognitive function and/or multiple chronic illnesses, so that these predisposing factors interact with acute precipitants to result in acute brain failure. Many of these factors are highly preventable (and many have a significant iatrogenic component) such that better service organisation can allow for preventative measures to produce better patient outcomes and reduced health care costs. Early intervention includes strategies that embrace primary prevention as well as more optimal management of emergent cases so as to reduce the serious consequences of delirium and its complications.

The impact of delirium on health care outcomes

Optimising delirium care is an important health care priority for several reasons. In addition to its frequency, delirium has a considerable impact on patient outcomes and health care costs. Patients with delirium experience more prolonged hospitalisations, more complications, greater costs of care, reduced subsequent functional independence, and increased in-hospital and subsequent mortality [3]. Importantly, these adverse health and social outcomes are predicted by the presence of delirium and are relatively independent of confounding factors such as morbidity level, baseline cognition, age and frailty. In addition, delirium may be an accelerating and possibly causal factor in the development of dementia [4, 5].

Primary prevention of delirium
Delirium risk factors

Efforts at early intervention are assisted by studies that have identified a range of patients, illness and treatment factors predict the likelihood of developing delirium. The vulnerability of certain individuals to delirium, or "delirium readiness" emphasizes how a variety of predisposing factors interact with acute precipitating insults to produce the acute brain failure of delirium.

Inouye and Charpentier [6] developed a model comprising four predisposing factors (cognitive impairment, severe illness, visual impairment, and dehydration) and five precipitating factors (polypharmacy, catheterization, use of restraints, malnutrition, any iatrogenic event) that predicted a 17-fold variation in the relative risk of developing delirium. Baseline risk is especially important such that patients with high baseline vulnerability can develop delirium even in response to minor precipitants.

Table 19.1 shows a detailed list of factors. Certain factors are more relevant in particular settings and patient groups, but age extremes, pre-existing cognitive problems, severe comorbid illness, and psychotropic medication exposure are robust predictors of delirium risk across populations. Many risk factors are modifiable while others can help assess

Table 19.1   Risk factors for delirium

A. Patient
Age
Pre-existing cognitive impairment
Previous delirium episode
CNS disorder
Increased blood–brain barrier permeability
Poor nutritional status

B. Illness
Severity of comorbidity
Burns
HIV/AIDS
Organ insufficiency
Infection (e.g.UTI)
Hypoxemia
Fracture
Hypothermia/fever
Metabolic disturbances
Dehydration
Low serum albumin
Nicotine withdrawal
Uncontrolled pain

C. Intervention
Perioperative
Type of surgery (e.g. hip)
Emergency procedure
Duration of operation
Catheterization

D. Medications
Polypharmacy
Drug/alcohol dependence
Psychoactive drug use
Specific drugs (e.g. anticholinergics)

E. Environment
Social isolation
Sensory extremes
Visual deficit
Hearing deficits
Immobility
Novel environment
Stress
Use of restraints

risk–benefit balance of surgical and other interventions in deciding upon optimal care, especially in frail elderly patients with cognitive impairments. Minimising exposure to modifiable factors has been the focus of intervention studies (see below) that demonstrate that delirium is highly preventable. Many interventions involve elements of good medical and nursing care (e.g. avoiding unnecessary polypharmacy, correcting sensory deficits). That these practices need to be protocolised within complex interventions reflects the standard of routine care provided in real-world settings, such that delirium may be a marker of the dysfunctionality of health care systems.

Nonpharmacological interventions

Primary prevention of delirium through nonpharmacological risk-reduction strategies has been demonstrated in elderly medical [7, 8] and surgical [9–11] populations. Moreover, these studies also indicate that incident delirium is less severe and of shorter duration when it occurs in the setting of active management of delirium proneness. Simple interventions (e.g. consensus guidelines, educational interventions) have limited impact [12, 13] which is unsurprising given the complex range of factors involved in delirium causation, which are more amenable to multifaceted interventions.

Multifaceted interventions include many common elements that focus upon assisting orientation, enhancing efficacy (e.g sensory), sleep, pain relief, optimising physiological parameters (electrolytes, hydration), physical therapy/mobilisation and active review by specialist nurses [7, 9] or geriatricians/geriatric psychiatrists [14]. A widely adopted intervention, the Hospital Elder Life Program (HELP), targeting six risk factors using standardized protocols can reduce the incidence and duration of delirium episodes relative to controls [7]. Other randomized works comparing perioperative geriatric consultation with usual care in elderly hip fracture patients found reduced delirium incidence and severity in the intervention group [15–17].

Overall, the evidence indicates that improving awareness of the importance of delirium through proactive education of staff involved in the care of patients at high risk of delirium combined with risk factor reduction, systematic screening for delirium, and patient-tailored treatment of emergent delirium can reduce incidence, severity and duration of incident delirium and delirium-related mortality [9, 10, 17]. The impact of interventions depends on degree of implementation [15]. However, these measures appear more effective in preventing delirium in patients at high risk for reasons other than dementia [10, 16, 17, 18]. Moreover, the impact upon longer-term outcomes such as independence and mortality at 1 year follow-up is less impressive, especially in populations with high rates of comorbid dementia [19].

The timing of preventative interventions may also be a key factor. 'Prehabilitation' involves risk factor reduction to optimise preparedness for nonemergency procedures or other interventions that represent key periods of risk for delirium. Bjorkelund et al. [11] described an intervention that commenced during the pre-hospital period and focused on optimising preparedness for surgery in patients with hip fracture (addressing hydration, oxygenation, analgesia, polypharmacy and optimising care environment routines) that significantly reduced delirium incidence.

The success with which these programmes can be applied to other settings where risk factors for delirium may differ (e.g. palliative care, community-based settings) is less clear. Siddiqi et al. [20] described a delirium prevention programme for care homes based upon elements with demonstrated effectiveness in hospitalised patients. Marcantonio et al. [21] conducted a randomized trial of a delirium abatement program for post-acute nursing facilities involving nurse-led detection and treatment which increased delirium detection (12–41%) but did not reduce delirium persistence at 1 month follow-up. Of note, the implementation rates for the intervention were modest reflecting the challenges of providing for delirious patients in such settings. Gagnon et al. [13] used a simple intervention targeting clinician awareness of delirium risk and monitoring of medication changes that was aligned to involving families in delirium recognition but did not significantly reduce delirium incidence, perhaps reflecting the different risk factor profile in palliative care (e.g. opioid exposure, vital organ failure). Moreover, the intervention was minimal, emphasised education and monitoring rather than implementation of specific protocolised interventions and as such highlights the knowledge–practice divide. These studies highlight the need to tailor interventions to the particular needs of different settings and patient groups.

The success of complex delirium prevention programmes is linked to system factors [22, 23] that include: (a) involvement of clinical leaders, (b) support from senior management, (c) linking the implementation of programmes to periods of system change (e.g. realignment of care pathways), (d) educational elements that are sustained and engaging, (e) mechanisms to support decision-making that are integrated to everyday routines (e.g. electronic care pathways), (f) monitoring procedures to promote continued adherence. In general, improving delirium care through formalised interventions is best achieved where it is supported by activities that promote enthusiasm, support implementation, remove barriers and allow for progress monitoring.

The workload and cost implications of interventions are key considerations. The 'HELP' programme, for example requires skilled interdisciplinary staff and trained volunteers to implement standardised protocols and the use of copyrighted protocols involves a fee. However, preliminary studies suggest that proactively dealing with delirium risk can be cost neutral [24] and reduces nursing workload caused by disturbed behaviours [25]. Given the evidence that the impact of delirium reflects more prolonged hospitalisations and need for interventions to address complications [26], better management of delirium and its complications should reduce health care costs.

Pharmacological prophylaxis

The prevailing neurochemical theory of delirium emphasises dopaminergic and cholinergic systems in the pathophysiology of delirium. As a consequence, interest has focused upon the impact of agents that diminish dopaminergic or enhance cholinergic function. Studies have explored the impact of neuroleptic and procholinergic agents in prevention of delirium in high-risk populations.

Neuroleptic agents

Studies have explored the impact of prophylactic use of typical antipsychotic agents upon delirium incidence. Kalisvaart et al. [27] in a randomized, double-blind, prophylaxis study using either low-dose haloperidol or placebo given up to 3 days prior to and 3 days following hip surgery found significantly shorter and less severe delirium associated with shorter length of stay in the active treatment group but without a significant impact upon delirium incidence.

Other studies have focused on atypical antipsychotic agents; Prakanrattana and Prapaitrakool [28] reported a significantly reduced delirium incidence in patients receiving a single 1 mg dose of risperidone versus placebo when emerging from cardiac surgery. Similarly, Larsen et al. [29] reported a double-blind placebo-controlled trial of olanzapine

5 mg given the day before and after orthopaedic surgery for elderly patients where the active treatment group experienced significantly reduced delirium incidence and a greater likelihood of being discharged to home rather than to a rehabilitation facility.

Procholinergic strategies

The use of procholinergic strategies is also supported by neurochemical theories of delirium. Although some work with rivastigmine suggests that sustained use may protect against delirium in patients with dementia [30], studies with donepezil [31, 32] have not identified a prophylactic effect, perhaps due to the limited duration of use prior to delirium risk exposure.

Other strategies

Careful management of agitation and pain in severely ill patients can reduce delirium incidence. The use of the α-2 agonist dexmedetomidine for post-operative sedation is associated with reduced incidence of delirium and reduced ventilator time compared with midazolam in patients undergoing mechanical ventilation [33] or sedation after cardiac surgery versus propofol or fentanyl/midazolam [34]. Pandharipande et al. [35] linked lorazepam use with increased risk of delirium in ICU patients. A placebo-controlled study of melatonin (0.5 mg nocte for up to 14 days) in elderly medical admissions found significantly reduced delirium incidence [36].

Careful titration of analgesia can reduce delirium incidence; Tokita et al. [37] found lower delirium incidence and superior pain control in elderly using patient-controlled epidural anaesthesia with bupivacaine and fentanyl compared to continuous epidural mepivacaine. An open-label study found that opioid rotation from morphine to fentanyl was associated with better pain control and reduced delirium severity [38]. Protocolised care to optimise use of medications in ICU for pain and agitation can reduce duration of mechanical ventilation, improve pain management and reduce delirium symptoms [39].

Overall, the evidence in respect of antipsychotic agents is encouraging, but there are uncertainties as to their role across settings, with limited work in high-risk elderly medical inpatients and in patients with comorbid dementia. In addition, the interaction between pharmacological and nonpharmacological interventions needs to be clarified. Moreover, optimal doses and timing of treatment is uncertain since studies have focused on low dose brief exposure.

Improving the identification of patients at risk of delirium

In addition to factors shown in Table 19.1, a variety of neuropsychological, biological and pathophysiological measures may allow for better identification of delirium risk and/or may be markers of the process by which delirium emerges.

Neuropsychological markers of delirium proneness

Pre-existing cognitive impairment is a well-recognised risk factor for delirium, with comorbid dementia evident in more than 50% of delirium occurring in hospitalised elderly. In addition, more subtle impairments of neuropsychological functioning are associated with increased delirium risk in nondemented patients. These include tests of attention, vigilance, memory, visuospatial function graphomotor speed and executive function [40–45].

Cognitive performance in the immediate post-operative period also predicts delirium likelihood [28]. Lowery et al. [46] found that impaired cognitive performance is common during the post-operative period in patients who do not develop delirium, although impairments differed with nondelirious patients experiencing a decrease in vigilance whereas delirious patients were impaired in the accuracy of attention. This work emphasises the need to qualify the character and extent of the acute deterioration of cognition that equates with delirium since impairment of cognitive performance is common during periods of high morbidity or exposure to interventions that confer elevated delirium risk, including many who do not develop syndromal delirium. These studies also highlight how formal neuropsychological testing can identify patients at risk of delirium for whom preventative actions are especially recommended.

Biological markers of delirium

Biological markers may assist in recognition and monitoring of delirium. The EEG shows generalised slowing in delirium and can distinguish delirium from dementia [47], but generalised slowing lacks specificity and the practicalities of performing EEG on delirious patients limits widespread use. Other works have linked peripheral measures of anticholinergic activity to delirium proneness [48] but findings are inconsistent. Post-operative delirium characterised by reduced serum levels of amino acids with tryptophan levels below 40 µg/mL is suggested as a measure for delirium detection [49]. However, this pattern may reflect the physiological response to surgery rather than a specific pathophysiological mechanism for delirium.

Delirium symptoms overlap with features of sickness behaviour that occurs in inflammatory responses. C-reactive protein is a marker of the acute phase of the inflammatory response that predicts delirium incidence in elderly medical admissions but lacks specificity for delirium and may be of greater use in monitoring progress [50]. Delirium often occurs in infectious states that involve cytokine activation and therapeutic use of cytokines can induce delirium. Studies of cytokine levels and delirium incidence have been inconsistent, with some indicating elevated proinflammatory cytokines in elderly medical admissions [51, 52] while a study in surgical patients found elevated chemokine levels in the immediate post-operative period without a significant rise in cytokine levels [53]. Cytokine and chemokines are associated with cognitive function and cholinergic activity such that their role as predisposing or precipitating factors or merely epiphenomena needs to be further explored.

Delirium detection

Delirium is poorly recognised in real-world practice where 50% or more of cases are diagnosed late or missed completely [54–56]. Early detection of delirium can allow for more timely and effective intervention while poor detection is associated with poorer outcomes that include elevated mortality [57, 58]. Low detection rates have been reported among cases that involve hypoactive clinical presentation [58], comorbid dementia [59], a history of previous psychiatric problems [54], prominent pain [54] and occur in the perioperative period [60].

The accurate detection of delirium is obfuscated by the continued use of a range of synonyms which reflect delirium occurring in different patient groups and treatment settings (e.g. acute confusion, ICU psychosis, toxic encephalopathy) rather than discrete scientific entities. Lakatos et al. [61] highlighted that delirium is not accurately diagnosed even where patients experience serious complications typical of delirium.

Screening

Delirium recognition in everyday practice is best achieved with routine screening. However, such practices are atypical and the reality is of *ad hoc* practices that lack a systematic approach with validated tools. In part, this reflects uncertainty regarding the optimal screening method – because delirium is primarily a cognitive disorder, bedside assessment of cognition is a critical element of diagnosis but limiting screening to cognitive assessment lacks specificity for delirium [62]. Screening may be best achieved by assessing for a combination of cognitive and noncognitive delirium features but including noncognitive features adds greater subjectivity to ratings. However, the problem of false negatives means that tools need to prioritise sensitivity over specificity.

Wong [63] reviewed bedside instruments for delirium detection with regard to sensitivity and specificity for DSM-IV delirium as well as suitability for use by various health care professionals. The Confusion Assessment Method (CAM) [64] was identified as the optimal instrument but with a number of caveats which are discussed below. Key considerations include the availability of time for testing and skill set of the tester; although the CAM is estimated to take approximately 5 minutes to complete, even this may have implications on clinical workload.

Cognitive tests

Bedside cognitive screening tests are sensitive to cognitive disorder but lack specificity to differentiate delirium from dementia. Other works have focused upon cognitive functions that are disproportionately affected in delirium but relatively preserved in normal ageing and early dementia [65], including tests of visual attention [66], visual perception and memory [67]. However, these tests require tester expertise and patient cooperation which is often lacking due to agitation and uncooperativeness in hyperactive patients, or lethargy and hypersomnolence in hypoactive patients. Leonard et al. [68] studied symptoms of depression and delirium in palliative care admissions and identified that any measure that required patient cooperation was sensitive to the presence of delirium, including self-report measures of mood. The extent to which inability to cooperate with testing is an indicator of delirium in different populations is a key consideration in determining approaches that allow assessment of uncooperative patients.

Delirium-specific screening tools

Other instruments incorporate neuropsychiatric and contextual features for delirium detection. Of these, the CAM is the most widely used delirium screening tool in general hospitals [64]. It is a brief (5 minute) four-item algorithm based on DSM-III-R criteria that has been adapted for use in the ICU [69] and nursing homes [70] where structured testing of each feature allows for more reliable rating. Wei et al. [71] reviewed the CAM scale attributes across studies and reported a sensitivity of 94%, specificity of 89% and inter-rater reliability typically over 70%. However, CAM accuracy is impacted upon by the background and training exposure of raters [72, 73] and the frequency of comorbid dementia in the population under study [59, 71]. CAM sensitivity can be increased by using structured cognitive tests but involves more prolonged administration time. Its accuracy in identifying more difficult cases such as those with hypoactive presentations requires greater study.

Other instruments emphasise observed patient behaviour. The Delirium Rating Scale (DRS) [74], Revised Delirium Rating Scale (DRS-R98) [75] and Memorial Delirium Assessment Schedule (MDAS) [76] are well-recognised delirium symptom assessment and diagnostic scales but are too detailed for the purposes of screening. The NEECHAM [77] takes less than 5 minutes and includes cognitive, behavioural and physiological items. It has high sensitivity with moderate specificity in medical and intensive care settings [78, 79]. The Nu-DESC is even briefer (1 minute), and assesses five delirium features including hypoactive symptoms [80]. It has high sensitivity and specificity in palliative care and internal medicine settings but requires that the rater account for the patient's medical condition. Interestingly, it does not include ratings of either inattention or context of disturbances but compares favourably with the CAM in recovery room patients [81] and surgical wards [82].

Improving delirium detection

Despite these tools, delirium detection remains a major obstacle to improved delirium care in everyday practice. In general, nurses are less adept at cognitive assessment whilst doctors struggle with the challenge of accurately identifying the context of delirium-possible presentations within time-pressurised settings where information regarding acuity of onset, symptom pattern over time, and baseline cognitive, functional and characterological attributes may be difficult to obtain. Moreover, presentations of delirium that involve hypoactivity and/or comorbid dementia are common and pose particular challenges in accurate identification. Heightened awareness of delirium along with systematic assessment for core features of delirium such as inattention and altered consciousness can allow for more consistent recognition.

Approaches to delirium detection need to be tailored to the characteristics of the setting where they are to be applied with particular consideration of the time available, the expertise of health care staff responsible for screening and the availability of expert clinicians to clarify diagnosis. In general, delirium detection is a two-stage process involving initial screening with a brief, simple and sensitive instrument followed by formal diagnosis using DSM-IV criteria and/or assisted by an instrument with high specificity for delirium. Instrument selection should be guided by the particular skills of the assessor as well as the ease with which the patient population can be assessed. An observational scale is preferable if initial screening involves staff who are not skilled in cognitive assessment. More recently, Sands et al. [83] described a single probe "do you think X has been more confused lately" in screening for delirium in a palliative care setting and found greater sensitivity (80%) compared to the CAM (40%). The CAM was administered by medical students with minimal training, but this level of training is typical of many of the staff who screen for delirium in highly pressurised modern health care environments with high staff and patient turnover. Further studies of this approach are awaited.

Computer-assisted technologies can allow for more consistent application of cognitive assessment in routine practice by a range of health care staff. Lowery et al. [46] incorporated an attention-testing battery into a wristwatch while many other cognitive tests that are sensitive to delirium can be readily incorporated into computerised devices that allow for greater consistency and ease of interpretation. Osse et al. [84] developed a wrist actigraphic device to detect alterations in motion that indicate delirium post-operatively.

Educational interventions can improve delirium diagnostic and management skills [21, 85–88]. Typical approaches involve interactive techniques that are based on identified needs of the learner. The longer-term impact of such interventions is less clear, but some work has demonstrated that improvements in knowledge are maintained over periods as long as 18 months and improved practice can be sustained by reminder strategies that are incorporated into daily ward routines and regular follow-up training [89]. Moreover, adherence to formalized delirium screening improves where it is supported by random accuracy spot checks but diminishes when monitoring is discontinued [89].

The increasing recognition of the frequency of delirium in post-acute and community-based settings is an important but understudied target for improving delirium detection and management. Siddiqi et al. [20] identified a delirium point prevalence of 14% among patients in residential care, although other work in similar settings has highlighted variable recognition [21]. Educational interventions and specific management programmes tailored to these settings may enhance detection [21].

Systematic screening of at-risk patients using instruments that are simple, brief, sensitive, and not prone to language or educational effects can improve detection of cognitive disorder. This has been demonstrated with the use of 'Mini-Cog', but such detection must be linked to appropriate investigation and treatment practices [90].

The prodromal phase of delirium

The onset of delirium is typically acute, with symptoms occurring over hours or days. The extent to which a recognizable prodromal phase occurs is less certain with studies suggesting that full syndromal illness is preceded by noncognitive symptoms, deterioration in cognition function [91], both cognitive and noncognitive symptoms [92] and/or a variety of nonspecific complaints including reduced pain tolerance, anxiety, general malaise, and being 'not themselves' [93]. Matsushima et al. [94] found prodromal changes of background slowing on EEG (θ/α ratio) and sleep disturbance associated with changing consciousness in a small study of CCU patients developing delirium. Osse et al. [84] identified early changes in activity levels (measured on an actigraphic device) that are associated with subsequent delirium. The identification of symptoms of emerging delirium represents an important mechanism by which earlier intervention can be facilitated.

Optimising delirium treatment: secondary prevention

The evidence for primary prevention of delirium is complemented by studies indicating that when delirium occurs, earlier and more optimal management can improve outcomes.

Nonpharmacological therapeutic interventions

In contrast to studies of delirium prevention, studies investigating the impact of nonpharmacological interventions upon reducing the burden of incident delirium have been less impressive [2]. Removing underlying causes, general support and symptom-focused interventions make good clinical sense in the management of every patient with delirium, but more formalised approaches using specialist assessment aligned to reduction of factors that can aggravate delirium progression have not demonstrated a major impact. Most studies have focused on frail elderly medical populations, including high rates of comorbid dementia, where the course of delirium may be less modifiable. Existing research indicates that nonpharmacological treatments impact modestly upon the duration of delirium and possibly length of inpatient stay [9, 19] but longer-term outcomes such as discharge to independent living and mortality appear unaltered [14, 16, 19].

The link between the poor outcomes of delirium and complications that can be prevented by good nursing suggests that focusing upon such practices may improve outcomes. However, systematic detection combined with optimising nursing care, family support and patient sensory efficacy while minimising medication exposure was not associated with significant benefits [16]. The reality is that even for patients with recognised delirium, the care environment differs considerably from that described in research studies and care in real-world settings combines these approaches with pharmacological interventions.

Pharmacological treatment

Delirium pharmacotherapies have evolved from their use to alleviate symptoms such as agitation and psychosis in other psychiatric disorders. There is limited appreciation of any specific effect in correcting neurochemical derangements that underpin delirium and clinicians typically associate positive effects to sedative and antipsychotic effects [87]. The lack of placebo-controlled studies of delirium treatment, along with concerns regarding risk of adverse effects in highly morbid populations with high rates of comorbid dementia, has resulted in many treatment guidelines recommending that psychotropic agents should be reserved for patients with symptoms that pose risk issues or interfere with their capacity to receive other treatments. However, the increasing bulk of prospective studies, including placebo-controlled designs, supports the judicious use of pharmacological interventions in the management of incident delirium.

Neuroleptic agents

Neuroleptic agents have long been the clinical standard for pharmacotherapy of delirium. Systematic reviews of prospective studies using antipsychotic agents have concluded that more than two-thirds of delirious patients experienced clinical improvement, typically after 2–6 days of treatment [95]. Hua et al. [96] found comparable response rates in elderly hospitalised patients receiving haloperidol (87.5%) and olanzapine (82%) that were significantly greater (31%) than a 'no drug treatment' group. Two placebo-controlled studies have demonstrated more rapid recovery in elderly medical [97] and ICU [98] patients treated with low-dose quetiapine. The use of antipsychotic agents is limited by concerns regarding possible increased mortality when used in agitated elderly dementia patients.

However, the extent to which this risk applies to the short duration of use in delirium (typically less than 1 week) [95] is unclear. One retrospective analysis linked increased mortality to medical comorbidity rather than antipsychotic exposure [99].

Benzodiazepines

Benzodiazepines are generally reserved for delirium due to seizure-related or withdrawal delirium. However, benzodiazepine use should be limited because they can be deliriogenic [48] and aggravate existing delirium [100].

Procholinergic strategies

The cholinergic deficiency hypothesis of delirium suggests that treatment with agents that enhance cholinergic function could be therapeutic but evidence remains lacking. A placebo-controlled trial of rivastigmine in intensive care patients with delirium was halted due to absence of a clinical effect and concerns regarding elevated mortality in the rivastigmine group [101].

Overall, these studies question the extent to which delirious patients receive optimal care and suggest that careful use of nonpharmacological and pharmacological treatments can improve outcomes. Clearly, further delirium treatment research is needed, including adequately powered randomized, placebo-controlled clinical trials addressing efficacy and safety. However, mounting evidence from prospective trials is supportive of current clinical practice and consistent with neurochemical hypotheses for delirium.

Optimising treatment

Delirium is highly heterogeneous in clinical presentation which limits the extent to which consistent approaches to management occur in clinical practice. These inconsistencies are underpinned by a lack of consensus in therapeutic guidelines and variable awareness of the evidence to support interventions, including beliefs regarding their mechanism of action [87]. More consistent management of delirium can be facilitated by educational interventions that improve detection skills [102], protocols that tailor treatment to specific delirium symptoms [39], use of rating scales to guide choice of agent and dose [33] and computerised decision support mechanisms [23, 103].

Improving outcomes in delirium
How does delirium contribute to poor outcomes?

The poor outcomes associated with delirium may be a consequence of: (a) the underlying causes of delirium, (b) complications of active delirium, (c) poor cooperation with medical care during hospitalization, (d) direct neurotoxicity of the delirious state, (e) toxicity of treatments used to manage delirium.

Delirious patients are prone to serious complications that include feeding problems, dehydration, pneumonia, urinary incontinence, falls, intravenous line removal, pressure sores, uncooperative behaviour and problems with consent [61, 104, 105]. These are closely related to particular symptoms of delirium (e.g. pressure sores and hypoactivity, falls and agitation) with poor outcomes predicted by the severity and duration of delirium symptoms [106, 107]. One-quarter of elderly medical patients with delirium die within 1 month of its onset [108] with a recent study estimating that the risk of mortality increases by 11% for every additional 48 hours of delirium [109].

Nondetection is associated with especially poor outcomes; Kakuma et al. [57] prospectively studied prevalent delirium in emergency department attenders followed for 18 months. After adjusting for age, sex, functional level, cognitive status, comorbidity and number of medications, delirium was significantly associated with increased mortality, especially where it was not detected by the ER staff.

Delirium has traditionally been conceptualised as a transient neurobiological state with high reversibility potential. However, many delirious patients develop persistent difficulties including so-called *long-term cognitive impairment*. Importantly, these difficulties occur in patients deemed 'cognitively intact' prior to experiencing delirium. Delirium can thus be the beginning of a journey of cognitive decline resulting in dementia, with increasing recognition that delirium is more than a mere harbinger for dementia and may be an aggravating or even causal factor in more sustained cognitive disorder. Progression from acute to chronic cognitive disorder is a well-recognised complication of alcohol-related neuropsychiatric disturbance where the acute cognitive disturbances of Wernicke's encephalopathy can progress to a more persistent state of cognitive impairment termed Korsakoff's dementia. Such relationships may also apply between delirium and dementia. Fong et al. [5] found that the occurrence of delirium was associated with more rapid subsequent decline in cognition in Alzheimer's patients independent of factors such as age and previous cognitive function.

Persistent cognitive deficits may be related to a previously undiagnosed dementia that progresses during and after delirium resolution. Undetected dementia is frequent in both community-dwelling and hospitalised older people (20%) [110]. Moreover, delirium proneness is related to baseline cognitive function, including subtle disturbances of attention and related domains that are not necessarily recognised or perceived as clinically significant. Studies that include detailed pre-delirium neuropsychological testing and explore pathophysiological mechanisms can clarify the relationship between pre-existing impairments and cognitive impairments that follow delirium.

Improving delirium management post-hospitalisation

The occurrence of delirium has not only important implications for the immediate treatment of underlying causes and delirium symptoms, but also for subsequent care where ongoing risk factors can be minimised while addressing any residual functional deficits or psychological sequelae. Treatment of delirium should continue until symptoms have fully resolved but the role of continued treatment thereafter is uncertain, with on one hand concerns regarding the safety of sustained exposure to psychoactive agents in elderly patients while other evidence points to a protective effect of antipsychotic agents for patients at high risk. Alexopoulos et al. [111] found consensus among elderly care experts that treatment for delirium should be continued for at least a week after response. However, in reality many delirious patients are discharged before full resolution of symptoms and continued monitoring and treatment is often overlooked in post-discharge planning.

Kiely et al. [112] found that 16% of patients in skilled nursing facilities met the criteria for delirium while Marcantonio et al. [105] found that 15% of elderly admissions had delirium immediately after admission to post-acute care. These studies emphasize that transfer of patients with active delirium to therapeutic settings that are less equipped to cater to the many challenges of delirium is common even though delirium is frequently a marker of severe and urgent physical morbidity.

Delirium is a distressing experience for patients and their caregivers. Delirium-recovered patients may be uncomfortable discussing their delirium episodes because they equate it with being "senile" or "mad" [113]. The psychological aftermath of delirium is understudied, but recent work suggests that around 50% of patients can recall the episode [114, 115]. Breitbart et al. [114] explored perceptions of the delirium experience among patients with a resolved delirium episode and found that distress correlated with severity of perceptual disturbances for patients and functional loss for their spouses. Similarly, Fann et al. [92] found that level of distress was closely linked to delirium severity and in particular to psychosis and level of psychomotor disturbance. In nondemented elderly patients with delirium, O'Keeffe [115] found that more than half could recall psychotic symptoms and many were still distressed by their recollections 6 months later.

Persistent psychological disturbances are a particular target for interventions that can impact upon subsequent help-seeking behaviour. Formal follow- up visits can facilitate post-delirium adjustment by allowing for discussion of the meaning of delirium and planning of how to minimize future risk (e.g. by addressing risk factors such as medication exposure and sensory impairments).

Early intervention in delirium: penetrating the health care agenda

Delirium is a key target in our increasingly aged delirium-prone society because of its unrivalled penetration of health care settings and demonstrated preventability. Delirium is a multifactorial condition with a highly heterogeneous course that provides multiple opportunities for more timely intervention. Historically, delirium has been relatively overlooked – involving patients with complex multimorbidity, trivialised as a symptom of other morbidity, lacking clear guidance on management and not within the remit of any particular medical specialty.

The past decade has witnessed increased recognition of the significance of delirium as evidenced by increased research output but with inconsistent application in everyday practice. The quality of delirium care could be considered a sensitive marker of (dys)functionality in our health systems, highlighting the need for greater cohesion in everyday clinical management, more emphasis on educational programming and research funding, as well as administrative structures to ensure that this extremely common and prognostically significant condition is addressed across health care services. Optimum delirium care requires better appreciation of its importance both at the bedside interface with individual patients and by policy makers at national and international levels. In short, meaningful change needs to occur from bench to bedside to boardroom.

Delirium is a predictable and preventable occurrence. Patients at high risk are readily identified by factors such as age, medical problems and pre-existing cognitive problems, but quality of care is a key factor and delirium has a significant iatrogenic component to causation. Systematic cognitive screening can improve detection. Moreover, evidence exists for preventative and treatment interventions that are underutilised in real-world practice. Improving delirium care is thus a systems issue where a considerable gap between knowledge and practice must be bridged. Studies must focus on identifying barriers to change and how knowledge transfer can be improved. Factors which motivate health care managers, such as costs and patient safety, can drive a new agenda with more active participation by health care funding agencies. The support of senior managers is an important determinant of the success in implementing complex interventions [28] but this must be linked to thoughtful practices that incorporate good clinical care with systems management.

The challenges of dealing with delirium are increasingly rooted between the sometimes conflicting needs of improved risk management within organisations versus the provision of individualised, patient-focused care that promotes autonomy and dignity. Complications are often documented more thoroughly than actual clinical causes such as delirium [61]. Concerns regarding the safety of delirious patients at risk of falls and wandering can drive restrictive care practices that inhibit reorientation, mobility and self-efficacy, all of which are recognised elements of delirium management that maximise the likelihood of optimal recovery. Less restrictive care can be facilitated by electronic alarms and pressure mats to monitor patient behaviour and alert staff when vulnerable patients are at risk of wandering or falls [116]. Increased emphasis on 'capacity targets' drives a system of rapid turnover that is poorly conducive to addressing the detailed assessment and care planning that delirious patients need. This philosophy has extended to proposals to withhold payments for costs generated by preventable complications like delirium [117]. However, such developments risk further complicating accurate documentation of delirium and have the potential of excluding high-risk patients from care. Managers and clinicians must work towards a balanced approach which considers all these elements. One obvious target is to develop systems that allow for better coordination of interdisciplinary efforts and monitoring of delirium-relevant outcomes.

A plan for improved delirium care

The challenge of improving delirium care requires a range of measures that include the following.

(a) Promoting awareness of delirium by including its detection and management as a key educational component of medical and nursing programmes at undergraduate and postgraduate levels.

(b) Ensuring that delirium risk status monitoring becomes embedded into daily routines across all health care settings, including hospitalised and community-based settings.

(c) Greater application of preventative measures, particularly in high-risk patients.

(d) Well-designed studies that explore the respective roles of nonpharmacological and pharmacological interventions in delirium management across populations.

(e) Earlier and more consistent detection of delirium through formal systematic screening in everyday practice across health care settings. Computer-assisted and other technologies can facilitate more accurate assessment.

(f) Linkage of delirium identification to evidence-based action through protocolised management based upon a more coherent understanding of role of interventions in managing specific clinical presentations of delirium.

(g) Research that addresses key uncertainties regarding management, including the duration of treatment, risk–benefit ratio in highly morbid patients, the relevance of different clinical presentations and impact of comorbidities upon treatment choices.

(h) Strategies to promote the active management of the post-delirium phase, including the risk for subsequent episodes and prevention of secondary psychological sequelae.

(i) More robust monitoring of the frequency of delirium and its impact upon outcomes.

References

1. Siddiqi N, House AO and Holmes JD. (2006). Occurrence and outcome of delirium in medical inpatients: a systematic literature review. *Age and Ageing* **35**: 350–364.
2. National Institute for Health and Clinical Excellence. (2010). Delirium: diagnosis, prevention and management. Clinical guideline 103. www.nice.org.uk/CG103 (accessed 10 April 2013).
3. Trzepacz PT, Meagher D and Leonard M. (2010). Delirium. In: J Levenson (ed.), *Textbook of Psychosomatic Medicine*, Washington, DC: American Psychiatric Press, Inc.
4. MacLullich AMJ, Beaglehole A, Hall RJ and Meagher DJ. (2009). Delirium and long-term cognitive impairment. *International Review of Psychiatry* **21**(1): 30–42.
5. Fong TG, Jones RN, Shi P, et al. (2009). Delirium accelerates cognitive decline in Alzheimer disease. *Neurology* **72**: 1570–1575.
6. Inouye SK and Charpentier PA. (1996). Precipitating factors for delirium in hospitalized elderly patients: predictive model and interrelationships with baseline vulnerability. *The Journal of the American Medical Association* **275**: 852–857.
7. Inouye SK, Bogardus ST, Charpentier PA, et al. (1999). A multicomponent intervention to prevent delirium in hospitalized older patients. The *New England Journal of Medicine* **340**: 669–676.
8. Vidán MT, Sánchez E, Alonso M, et al. (2009). An intervention integrated into daily clinical practice reduces the incidence of delirium during hospitalization in elderly patients. *Journal of the American Geriatrics Society* **57**: 2029–2036.
9. Milisen K, Foreman MD, Abraham IL, et al. (2001). A nurse-led interdisciplinary intervention program for delirium in elderly hip-fracture patients. *Journal of the American Geriatrics Society* **49**: 523–532.
10. Lundström M, Olofsson B, Stenvall M, et al. (2007). Postoperative delirium in old patients with femoral neck fracture: a randomized intervention study. *Aging Clinical and Experimental Research* **19**: 178–186.
11. Bjorkeland KB, Hommel A, Thorngren KG, et al. (2010). Reducing delirium in elderly patients with hip fracture: a multi-factorial intervention study. *Acta Anaesthesiologica Scandinavica* **54**: 678–688.
12. Young LJ and George J. (2003). Do guidelines improve the process and outcomes of care in delirium? *Age and Ageing* **32**: 525–528.
13. Gagnon P, Allard P, Gagnon B, et al. (2012). Delirium prevention in terminal cancer: assessment of a multicomponent intervention. *Psychooncology* **21**:187–194.

14. Cole MG, Primean FJ, Bailey RF, et al. (1994). Systematic intervention for elderly inpatients with delirium: a randomized trial. *Canadian Medical Association Journal* **151**: 965–970.

15. Inouye SK, Bogardus ST Jr, Williams CS, et al. (2003). The role of adherence on the effectiveness of nonpharmacologic interventions: evidence from the delirium prevention trial. *Archives of Internal Medicine* **163**: 958–964.

16. Cole MG, McCusker J, Bellavance F, et al. (2002). Systematic detection and multidisciplinary care of delirium in older medical inpatients: a randomized trial. *Canadian Medical Association Journal* **167**: 753–759.

17. Marcantonio ER, Flacker JM, Wright RJ and Resnick NM. (2001). Reducing delirium after hip fracture: a randomized trial. *Journal of the American Geriatrics Society* **49**: 516–522.

18. Bogardus ST Jr, Desai MM, Williams CS, et al. (2003). The effects of a targeted multicomponent delirium intervention on postdischarge outcomes for hospitalized older adults. *American Journal of Medicine* **114**: 383–390.

19. Pitkala KH, Laurila JV, Strandberg TE, et al. (2008). A multicomponent geriatric intervention for elderly inpatients with delirium: effects on costs and health-related quality of life. *Journals of Gerontology. Series A, Biological Sciences and Medical Sciences* **63**: 56–61.

20. Siddiqi N, Young J, House AO, et al. (2011). Stop Delirium! A complex intervention to prevent delirium in care homes: a mixed-methods feasibility study. *Age and Ageing* **40**: 90–98.

21. Marcantonio ER, Bergmann MA, Kiely DK, et al. (2010). Randomized trial of a delirium abatement program for postacute skilled facilities. *Journal of the American Geriatrics Society* **58**: 1019–1026.

22. Bradley EH, Webster TR, Schlesinger M, et al. (2006). Patterns of diffusion of evidence-based clinical programmes: a case study of the Hospital Elder Life Program. *Quality and Safety Health Care* **15**: 334–338.

23. Holroyd-Leduc JM, Abelseth GA, Khandwala F, et al. (2010). A pragmatic study exploring the prevention of delirium among hospitalized older hip fracture patients: Applying evidence to routine clinical practice using clinical decision support. *Implement Science* **5**: 81.

24. Leslie DL, Marcantonio ER, Zhang Y, et al. (2008). One-year health costs associated with delirium in the elderly population. *Archives of Internal Medicine* **168**: 27–32.

25. Pretto M, Spirig R, Milisen K, et al. (2009). Effects of an interdisciplinary nurse-led Delirium Prevention and Management Program (DPMP) on nursing workload: a pilot study. *International Journal of Nursing Studies* **46**: 804–812.

26. Milbrandt EB, Deppen S, Harrison PL, et al. (2004). Costs associated with delirium in mechanically ventilated patients. *Critical Care Medicine* **32**: 955–962.

27. Kalisvaart KJ, de Jonghe JFM, Bogaards MJ, et al. (2005). Haloperidol prophylaxis for elderly hip surgery patients at risk for delirium: a randomized, placebo-controlled study. *Journal of the American Geriatrics Society* **53**: 1658–1666.

28. Prakanrattana U and Prapaitrakool S. (2007). Efficacy of risperidone for prevention of postoperative delirium in cardiac surgery. *Anaesthesia and Intensive Care* **35**: 714–719.

29. Larsen KA, Kelly SE, Stern TA, et al. (2010). Administration of olanzapine to prevent postoperative delirium in elderly joint-replacement patients: a randomized, controlled trial. *Psychosomatics* **51**: 409–418.

30. Dautzenberg PL, Mulder LJ, Olde Rikkert MG, et al. (2004). Delirium in elderly hospitalized patients: protective effects of chronic rivastigmine usage. *International Journal of Geriatric Psychiatry* **19**: 641–644.

31. Liptzin B, Laki A, Garb JL, et al. (2005). Donepezil in the prevention and treatment of postsurgical delirium. *American Journal of Geriatric Psychiatry* **13**: 1100–1106.

32. Sampson EL, Raven PR, Ndhlovu PN, et al. (2007). A randomized, double-blind, placebo-controlled trial of donepezil hydrochloride (Aricept) for reducing the incidence of postoperative delirium after elective total hip replacement. *International Journal of Geriatric Psychiatry* **22**, 343–349.

33. Riker RR, Shehabi Y, Bokesch PM, et al. (2009). Dexmedetomidine vs midazolam for sedation of critically ill patients: a randomized trial. *The Journal of the American Medical Association* **301**: 489–499.

34. Maldonado JR, van der Starre P, Wysong A and Block T. (2004). Dexmedetomidine: can it reduce the incidence of ICU delirium in postcardiotomy patients? Proceedings of 50th Annual Meeting of the Academy of Psychosomatic Medicine. *Psychosomatics* **45**: 145–175.

35. Pandharipande P, Shintani A, Peterson J, et al. (2006). Lorazepam is an independent risk factor for transitioning to delirium in intensive care unit patients. *Anesthesiology* **104**: 21–26.

36. Al-Aama T, Brymer C, Gutmanis I, et al. (2010). Melatonin decreases delirium in elderly patients: a randomized, placebo-controlled trial. *International Journal of Geriatric Psychiatry* **26**: 687–694.

37. Tokita K, Tanaka H, Kawamoto M and Yuge O. (2001). Patient-controlled epidural analgesia with bupivacaine and fentanyl suppresses postoperative delirium following hepatectomy. *Masui. Japanese Journal of Anesthesiology* **50**: 742–746.

38. Morita T, Takigawa C, Onishi H, et al. (2005). Opioid rotation from morphine to fentanyl in delirious cancer patients: an open-label trial. *Journal of Pain and Symptom Management* **30**: 96–103.

39. Skrobik Y, Ahern S, Leblanc M, et al. (2010). Protocolized intensive care unit management of analgesia, sedation, and delirium improves analgesia and subsyndromal delirium rates. *Anesthesia and Analgesia* **111**: 451–463.

40. Trzepacz PT, Brenner R, Coffman G and Van Thiel DH. (1988). Delirium in liver transplantation candidates: discriminant analysis of multiple test variables. *Biological Psychiatry* **24**: 3–14.

41. Fann JR, Roth-Roemer S, Burington BE, et al. (2002). Delirium in patients undergoing hematopoietic stem cell transplantation. *Cancer* **95**: 1971–1981.

42. Greene NH, Attix DK, Weldon BC, et al. (2009). Measures of executive function and depression identify patients at risk for postoperative delirium. *Anesthesiology* **110**: 788–795.

43. Lowery DP, Wesnes K and Ballard CG. (2007). Subtle attentional deficits in the absence of dementia are associated with an increased risk of post-operative delirium. *Dementia and Geriatric Cognitive Disorders* **23**: 390–394.

44. Wallbridge HR, Benoit AG, Staley D, et al. (2010). Risk factors for postoperative cognitive and functional difficulties in abdominal aortic aneurysm patients: a three month follow-up. *International Journal of Geriatric Psychiatry* **26**: 818–824.

45. Smith PJ, Attix DK, Weldon BC, et al. (2009). Executive function and depression as independent risk factors for postoperative delirium. *Anesthesiology* **110**: 781–787.

46. Lowery DP, Wesnes K, Brewster N and Ballard C. (2008). Quantifying the association between computerised measures of attention and confusion assessment method defined delirium: a prospective study of older orthopaedic surgical patients, free of dementia. *International Journal of Geriatric Psychiatry* **23**: 1253–1260.

47. Thomas C, Hestermann U, Kopitz J, et al. (2008). Serum anticholinergic activity and cerebral cholinergic dysfunction: an EEG study in frail elderly with and without delirium. *BMC Neuroscience* **15**: 86.

48. Mussi C, Ferrari R, Ascari S and Salvioli G. (1999). Importance of serum anticholinergic activity in the assessment of elderly patients with delirium. *Journal of Geriatric Psychiatry and Neurology* **12**: 82–86.

49. Robinson TN, Raeburn CD, Angles EM and Moss M. (2008). Low tryptophan levels are associated with postoperative delirium in the elderly. *American Journal of Surgery* **196**: 670–674.

50. Macdonald A, Adamis D, Treloar A and Martin F. (2007). C-reactive protein levels predict the incidence of delirium and recovery from it. *Age and Ageing* **36**: 222–225.

51. de Rooij SE, van Munster BC, Korevaar JC and Levi M. (2007). Cytokines and acute phase response in delirium. *Journal of Psychosomatic Research* **62**: 521–525.

52. Adamis D, Treloar A, Martin FC, et al. (2007). APOE and cytokines as biological markers for recovery of prevalent delirium in elderly medical inpatients. *International Journal of Geriatric Psychiatry* **22**: 688–694.

53. Rudolph JL, Ramlawi B, Kuchel GA, et al. (2008). Chemokines are associated with delirium after cardiac surgery. *Journals of Gerontology. Series A, Biological Sciences and Medical Sciences* **63**: 184–189.

54. Kishi Y, Kato M, Okuyama T, et al. (2007). Delirium: patient characteristics that predict a missed diagnosis at psychiatric consultation. *General Hospital Psychiatry* **29**: 442–445.

55. Collins N, Blanchard MR, Tookman A and Sampson EL. (2010). Detection of delirium in the acute hospital. *Age and Ageing* **39**: 131–135.

56. Han JH, Zimmerman EE, Cutler N, et al. (2009). Delirium in older emergency department patients: recognition, risk factors, and psychomotor subtypes. *Academic Emergency Medicine* **16**: 193–200.

57. Kakuma R, du Fort GG, Arsenault L, et al. (2003). Delirium in older emergency department patients discharged home: effect on survival. *Journal of the American Geriatrics Society* **51**: 443–450.

58. Fang CK, Chen HW, Liu SI, et al. (2008). Prevalence, detection and treatment of delirium in terminal cancer inpatients: a prospective survey. *Japanese Journal of Clinical Oncology* **38**: 56–63.

59. Inouye SK, Foreman MD, Mion LC, et al. (2001). Nurses' recognition of delirium and its symptoms: comparison of nurse and researcher ratings. *Archives of Internal Medicine* **161**: 2467–2473.

60. Gupta N, Sharma P and Meagher D. (2010). Predictors of delayed identification of delirium in a general hospital liaison psychiatry service: a study from North India. *Asian Journal of Psychiatry* **3**: 31–32.

61. Lakatos BE, Capasso V, Mitchell MT, et al. (2009). Falls in the general hospital: association with delirium, advanced age, and specific surgical procedures. *Psychosomatics* **50**: 218–226.

62. Eissa A, Andrew MJ and Baker RA. (2003). Postoperative confusion assessed with the Short Portable Mental Status Questionnaire. *ANZ Journal of Surgery* **73**: 697–700.

63. Wong CL, Holyrod-Leduc J, Simel DL and Straus SE. (2010). Does this patients have delirium? Value of bedside instruments. *The Journal of the American Medical Association* **304**: 779–786.

64. Inouye SK, van Dyke CH, Alessi CA, et al. (1990). Clarifying confusion: the confusion assessment method. *Annals of Internal Medicine* **113**: 941–948.

65. Wiechmann A, Hall JR and Bryant SE. (2011). The utility of the spatial span in a clinical geriatric population. *Aging, Neuropsychology and Cognition* **18**: 56–63.

66. Meagher D, Leonard M, Donnelly S, et al. (2010). A comparison of neuropsychiatric and cognitive profiles in delirium, dementia, comorbid delirium-dementia and cognitively intact controls. *Journal of Neurology, Neurosurgery and Psychiatry* **81**: 876–881.

67. Brown LJE, McGrory S, McLaren L, et al. (2009). Cognitive visual perceptual deficits in patients with delirium. *Journal of Neurology, Neurosurgery and Psychiatry* **80**: 594–599.

68. Leonard M, Spiller J, Keen J, et al. (2009). Symptoms of depression and delirium assessed serially in palliative care inpatients. *Psychosomatics* **50**: 506–514.

69. Ely EW, Gordan S, Francis J, et al. (2001). Evaluation of delirium in critically ill patients: validation of the Confusion Assessment Method for the Intensive Care Unit (CAM-ICU). *Critical Care Medicine* **29**: 1370–1379.

70. Dosa D, Intrator O, McNicoll L, et al. (2007). Preliminary derivation of a Nursing Home Confusion Assessment Method based on data from the Minimum Data Set. *Journal of the American Geriatrics Society* **55**: 1099–1105.

71. Wei LA, Fearing MA, Sternberg EJ and Inouye SK. (2008). The confusion assessment method: a systematic review of current usage. *Journal of the American Geriatrics Society* **56**: 823–830.

72. Ryan K, Leonard M, Guerin S, et al. (2009). Validation of the confusion assessment method in the palliative care setting. *Palliative Medicine* **23**: 40–45.

73. Barnes J, Kite S and Kumar M. (2010). The recognition and documentation of delirium in hospital palliative care inpatients. *Palliative Support Care* **8**: 133–136.

74. Trzepacz PT, Baker RW and Greenhouse J (1988). A symptom rating scale for delirium. *Psychiatry Research* **23**: 89–97.

75. Trzepacz PT, Mittal D, Torres R, et al. (2001). Validation of the Delirium Rating Scale–revised-98: comparison with the delirium rating scale and cognitive test for delirium. *Journal of Neuropsychiatry and Clinical Neurosciences* **13**: 229–242.

76. Breitbart W, Rosenfeld B, Roth A, et al. (1997). The Memorial Delirium Assessment Scale. *Journal of Pain and Symptom Management* **13**: 128–137.

77. Neelon VJ, Champagne MT, Carlson JR and Funk SG. (1986). The NEECHAM scale: construction, validation, and clinical testing. *Nursing Research* **45**: 324–330.

78. Immers HE, Schuurmans MJ and van de Bijl JJ. (2005). Recognition of delirium in ICU patients: a diagnostic study of the NEECHAM confusion scale in ICU patients. *BMC Nursing* **4**: 7.

79. Hattori H, Kamiya J, Shimada H, et al. (2009). Assessment of the risk of postoperative delirium in elderly patients using E-PASS and the NEECHAM Confusion Scale. *International Journal of Geriatric Psychiatry* **24**: 1304–1310.

80. Gaudreau JD, Gagnon P, Harel F, Tremblay A and Roy MA. (2005). Fast, systematic, and continuous delirium assessment in hospitalized patients: the nursing delirium screening scale. *Journal of Pain and Symptom Management* **29**: 368–375.

81. Radtke FM, Frannck M, Schneider M, et al. (2008). Comparison of three scores to screen for delirium in the recovery room. *British Journal of Anaesthesia* **101**: 338–343.

82. Radtke FM, Franck M, Schust S, et al. (2010). A comparison of three scores to screen for delirium on the surgical ward. *World Journal of Surgery* **34**: 487–494.

83. Sands MB, Dantoc BP, Hartshorn A, et al. (2010). Single Question in Delirium (SqiD): testing its efficacy against psychiatrist interview, the Confusion Assessment Method and the Memorial Delirium Assessment Scale. *Palliative Medicine* **24**: 561–565.

84. Osse RJ, Tulen JH, Hengeveld MW and Bogers AJ (2009). Screening methods for delirium: early diagnosis by means of objective quantification of motor activity patterns using wrist-actigraphy. *Interactive Cardiovascular and Thoracic Surgery* **8**: 344–348.

85. Devlin JW, Marquis F, Riker RR, et al. (2008). Combined didactic and scenario-based education improves the ability of intensive care unit staff to recognize delirium at the bedside. *Critical Care* **12**: R19.

86. Ramaswamy R, Dix EF, Drew JE, et al. (2011). Beyond grand rounds: a comprehensive and sequential intervention to improve identification of delirium. *Gerontologist* **51**: 122–131.

87. Meagher DJ. (2010). Impact of an educational workshop upon attitudes towards pharmacotherapy for delirium. *International Psychogeriatrics* **22**: 938–946.

88. van den Boogaard M, Pickkers P, van der Hoeven H, et al. (2009). Implementation of a delirium assessment tool in the ICU can influence haloperidol use. *Critical Care* **13**: R131.

89. Pun BT, Gordon SM, Peterson JF, et al. (2005). Large-scale implementation of sedation and delirium monitoring in the intensive care unit: a report from two medical centers. *Critical Care Medicine* **33**: 1199–1205.

90. Borson S, Scanlan J, Hummel J, et al. (2007). Implementing routine cognitive screening of older adults in primary care: process and impact on physician behavior. *Journal of General Internal Medicine* **22**; 811–817.

91. de Jonghe JF, Kalisvaart KJ, Dijkstra M, et al. (2007). Early symptoms in the prodromal phase of delirium: a prospective cohort study in elderly patients undergoing hip surgery. *American Journal of Geriatric Psychiatry* **15**: 112–121.

92. Fann JR, Alfano CM, Burington BE, et al. (2005). Clinical presentation of delirium in patients undergoing hematopoietic stem cell transplantation. *Cancer* **103**: 810–820.

93. Duppils GS and Wikblad K (2004). Delirium: behavioural changes before and during the prodromal phase. *Journal of Clinical Nursing* **13**: 609–616.

94. Matsushima E, Nakajima K, Moriya H, et al. (1997). A psychophysiological study of the development of delirium in coronary care units. *Biological Psychiatry* **41**: 1211–1217.

95. Meagher D and Leonard M. (2008). The active management of delirium: improving detection and treatment. *Advances in Psychiatric Treatments* **14**: 292–301.

96. Hua H, Wei D and Hui Y. (2006). Olanzapine and haloperidol for senile delirium: a randomised controlled observation. *Chinese Journal of Clinical Rehabilitation* **10**: 188–190.

97. Tahir TA, Eeles E, Karapareddy V, et al. (2010). A randomised controlled trial of quetiapine versus placebo in the treatment of delirium. *Journal of Psychosomatic Research* **69**: 485–490.

98. Devlin JW, Roberts RJ, Fong JJ, et al (2010). efficacy and safety of quetiapine in critically ill patients with delirium: a prospective, multicenter, randomized, double-blind, placebo-controlled pilot study. *Critical Care Medicine* **38**: 419–427.

99. Elie M, Boss K, Cole MG, et al. (2009). A retrospective, exploratory, secondary analysis of the association between antipsychotic use and mortality in elderly patients with delirium. *International Psychogeriatrics* **21**: 588–592.

100. Breitbart W, Marotta R, Platt MM, et al (1996). A double-blind trial of haloperidol, chlorpromazine, and lorazepam in the treatment of delirium in hospitalized AIDS patients. *American Journal of Psychiatry* **153**: 231–237.

101. van Eijk MM, Roes KC, Honing ML, et al. (2010). Effect of rivastigmine as an adjunct to usual care with haloperidol on duration of delirium and mortality in critically ill patients: a multicentre, double-blind, placebo-controlled randomised trial. *Lancet* **376**: 1829–1837.

102. Van den Boogard M, Pickkers P, van der Hoeven H, et al (2009). Implementation of a delirium assessment tool in the ICU can influence haloperidol use. *Critical Care* **13**: R131.

103. Fick DM, Steis MR, Mion LC and Walls JL (2011). Computerized decision support for delirium superimposed on dementia in older adults. *Journal of Gerontological Nursing* **37**: 39–47.

104. Saravay SM, Kaplowitz M, Kurek J, et al. (2004). How do delirium and dementia increase length of stay of elderly general medical inpatients. *Psychosomatics* **45**: 235–242.

105. Marcantonio ER, Kiely DK, Simon SE, et al. (2005). Outcomes of older people admitted to postacute facilities with delirium. *Journal of the American Geriatrics Society*. **53**: 963–969.

106. Leslie DL, Zhang Y, Holford TR, et al. (2005). Premature death associated with delirium at 1-year follow-up. *Archives of Internal Medicine* **165**: 1657 1662.

107. Kiely DK, Marcantonio ER, Inouye SK, et al. (2009). Persistent delirium predicts greater mortality. *Journal of the American Geriatrics Society* **57**: 55–61.

108. McCusker J, Cole M, Abrahamowicz M, et al. (2002). Delirium predicts 12-month mortality. *Archives of Internal Medicine* **162**: 457–463.

109. González M, Martínez G, Calderón J, et al. (2009). Impact of delirium on short-term mortality in elderly inpatients: a prospective cohort study. *Psychosomatics* **50**: 234–238.

110. Sampson EL, Blanchard MR, Jones L, et al. (2009). Dementia in the acute hospital: prospective cohort study of prevalence and mortality. *The British Journal of Psychiatry* **195**: 61–66.

111. Alexopoulos GS, Streim J, Carpenter D, et al. (2004). Using antipsychotic agents in older patients. *The Journal Of Clinical Psychiatry* **65**(Suppl 2) 5–99.

112. Kiely DK, Bergmann MA, Jones RN, et al. (2004). Characteristics associated with delirium persistence among newly admitted post-acute facility patients. *Journals of Gerontology. Series A, Biological Sciences and Medical Sciences* **59**: 344–349.

113. Schofield I. (1997). A small exploratory study of the reaction of older people to an episode of delirium. *Journal of Advanced Nursing* **25**: 942–952.

114. Breitbart W, Gibson C and Tremblay A (2002). The delirium experience: delirium recall and delirium-related distress in hospitalized patients with cancer, their spouses/caregivers, and their nurses. *Psychosomatics* **43**: 183–194.

115. O'Keeffe S. (2005). The experience of delirium in older people. *International Psychogeriatrics* **17**: S2: 120.

116. Schofield I. (2008). Delirium: challenges for clinical governance. *Journal of Nursing Management* **16**: 127–133.

117. Pronovost PJ, Goeschel CA and Wachter RM. (2008). The wisdom and justice of not paying for "preventable complications". *The Journal of the American Medical Association* **299**: 2197–2199.

20
Early Intervention for Self-Harm and Suicidality

Sarah Steeg, Jayne Cooper and Nav Kapur
Centre for Suicide Prevention, Centre for Mental Health and Risk, University of Manchester, Manchester, UK

Introduction

Self-harm itself is not a medical diagnosis but is a term used to describe an act, for which there are many different meanings and functions for individuals. There is a range of disorders associated with self-harm and interventions should address underlying conditions that may perpetuate the behaviour. For some individuals, motivations behind self-harm may be multiple and can change over time. Treatment options should be considered in view of the individual's specific needs, their vulnerability and protective characteristics and with clinicians seeking a full picture of the reasons behind the self-harm act. These may include social circumstances, the immediate environment the individual will be returning to, physical health, interpersonal relationships and coping styles and underlying psychiatric conditions, including alcohol and drug misuse. Interventions may aim to deal with one or more of these contributing factors but should take into account the complexity behind self-harm behaviour. Throughout this chapter we use the term 'self-harm' to describe intentional acts of self-poisoning or self-injury irrespective of motivation [1], that is, the acts may or may not involve suicidal intent. We will consider the importance of acting early to support people who self-harm, summarise the current recommendations for treatment and review the evidence that the guidance is based on.

Epidemiology of self-harm

It is estimated that there are around 220,000 presentations to Accident and Emergency (A&E) departments in England (equivalent to emergency rooms or departments

Early Intervention in Psychiatry: EI of nearly everything for better mental health, First Edition.
Edited by Peter Byrne and Alan Rosen.
© 2014 John Wiley & Sons, Ltd. Published 2014 by John Wiley & Sons, Ltd.

elsewhere) each year [2] and recent estimates of annual rates indicate 300–500 individuals per 100,000 in England will attend hospital having self-harmed [3], rising to 1400 per 100,000 amongst adolescent females [4]. People who present to hospital with self-harm may represent the visible 'tip of the iceberg' of the problem of self-harm in the general population. Many people will not present to services following self-harm and figures based on self-reporting suggest that around 1 in 40 adults have self-harmed in their lifetime [5]. Self-harm attendances to general hospitals are not routinely audited but both short- and long-term monitoring has been set up in a number of hospitals [3, 6] allowing the investigation of trends and providing an overview of how self-harm is managed in hospitals in England. The majority – up to 80% – of hospital presentations are acts of self-poisoning, around 15% self-cutting and the remainder involve other methods, predominantly more violent methods such as attempted hanging and jumping from a height or a combination of these methods [3, 7]. People who present to hospital having self-harmed are not always offered a psychosocial assessment by a mental health specialist [6], yet hospital attendance is an opportunity for services to intervene [8], with general hospitals existing as an important base for secondary prevention of self-harm. Services for self-harm patients attending hospital vary, with some providing mental health liaison teams situated within the A&E departments available 24 hours a day, and others with more limited access to mental health specialists [6]. Hospitals have an important role not only in treating the self-harm episode itself but also in identifying the need for follow-up care to address existing problems that may not have otherwise reached the attention of services, such as depression and alcohol misuse.

Why intervene early for self-harm?

All acts of self-harm serve as a warning sign for an increased risk of suicide, but those who repeat self-harm are at further elevated risk [9]. When we compare the outcomes of people who repeat to those who do not, we see that those who have attended hospital more than once tend to have poorer outcomes. They have more than twice the risk of suicide than people with a single episode, with this increase more pronounced amongst females where the risk is threefold [9]. In terms of the possible psychological process, repeat self-harm may operate on a trajectory with multiple episodes increasing individuals' tolerance to the negative elements of the experience whilst also resulting in cognitive sensitisation [10, 11].

By analysing attendance patterns of people who present to hospital more than once, it is clear that repetition tends to happen quickly and is common. Between one in seven and one in five people were found to re-attend within a year [3, 12, 13], though repetition is likely to happen sooner. For those that do repeat within a year, it is estimated that one in three will happen within a month and one in ten within 5 days [12]. The timing of repeat attendances, based on individuals presenting to hospitals in Manchester, UK between 2005 and 2009, is illustrated below (Figure 20.1). With respect to the risk of suicide, studies have found that suicide rates were highest in the 6-month period following a self-harm episode [14]. These findings suggest that it would be advantageous for interventions to begin soon after a self-harm episode and that there is the potential for early intervention to have a significant impact on preventing non-fatal self-harm repetition and suicide. A study of suicidal ideation and self-harm across 17 countries found that the time period between onset of suicidal ideation and self-harm was consistently short; 6 in 10 acts occurred within

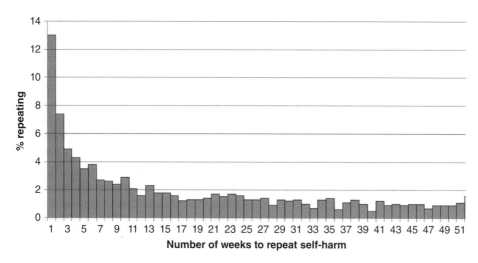

Figure 20.1 Number of weeks to repeat self-harm amongst individuals who repeated within a year (*N* = 1643). Between 2005 and 2009, 1643/10459 individuals presenting to hospitals in Manchester had at least one repeat self-harm episode within a year (all individuals were followed up to the end of 2010)

a year of initial ideation [5]. Service users state a need for aftercare to begin immediately or very soon after discharge from the hospital [15] and where interventions have achieved this, both staff and service users viewed the immediacy of the intervention positively [16].

Evaluating efficacy of interventions

There are various ways in which interventions for self-harm have been evaluated for effectiveness. Randomised controlled trials (RCTs) have been conducted on a range of interventions, including, brief psychological and behavioural therapies, postal and telephone 'contact-based' interventions and pharmacological therapy [17, 18]. These tend to be conducted in groups of patients with particular characteristics that make them suitable for the specific treatment. It is possible, however, to pool results from trials with similar characteristics to attempt to estimate efficacy of similar treatments, so-called meta-analysis. We can also use information collected from self-harm attendances to hospitals to detect patterns in attendances and clinical management. Repetition of self-harm points to ongoing distress and unresolved problems. Incidence of repeat self-harm, therefore, is often used as an outcome to measure efficacy of interventions. However, reasons behind self-harm can be numerous and complex, and information gleaned from qualitative discussions with service users and clinicians provides valuable insight into the mechanisms through which interventions have an effect and can uncover more subtle changes in behaviour following interventions.

The importance of specialist psychosocial assessment

Current national guidance in England [19] recommends that a full psychosocial needs assessment and mental state examination should follow each hospital presentation involving self-harm and highlights the importance of emergency department and local mental health services to jointly plan liaison psychiatric services available 24 hours a day. The assessment should be carried out by professionals, who may include psychiatric nurses, social workers and psychiatrists, who are trained to carry out assessments specifically for people who have self-harmed and where adequate supervision is provided. People who self-harm repeatedly may not experience the same motivation behind each act. An assessment at each episode, therefore, increases the likelihood that appropriate help will be offered. Research using observational data from hospitals where self-harm attendances are monitored has demonstrated that receiving psychosocial assessment upon presentation to hospital can improve outcomes for certain groups of patients [20–22]. Whilst these findings are not generated from controlled conditions, as is the case in RCTs, they are informative because they report real-world, population-level scenarios. Patients who discharged themselves from hospital before any assessment could be carried out had three times the rate of repetition compared to those who were assessed [22]. Recent estimates are that around six in ten patients who attend hospital with self-harm receive a psychosocial assessment by a mental health specialist [6, 20], although this proportion varies widely by hospital [6]. Studies have found that specialist psychosocial assessment is associated with reduced risk of repetition in centres where higher proportions of patients are assessed [21]. This suggests that when mental health specialists in general hospitals assess more people, presumably by including more people deemed lower risk, the benefits in terms of the reduced number of repeat attendances are greater.

Of course data from observational studies cannot prove causation but these findings indicate that for some individuals the assessment itself may be beneficial. This effect may operate through a number of mechanisms, and has been explored by interviewing service users about their experiences. Service users placed value on psychosocial assessments conducted in a manner that promoted hope and acceptance. Positive experiences of assessment had the potential to promote future therapeutic engagement with services. However, assessments where service users felt staff were judgemental or did not instil hope for change, or where arrangements for follow-up care did not materialise, could disengage service users and counteract feelings of hope [23]. Interestingly, a recent RCT of 'therapeutic assessment', consisting of a 30-minute intervention based on cognitive analytic therapy alongside standard psychosocial assessment, found that adolescents receiving the intervention had higher levels of attendance at follow-up appointments than those receiving standard assessment alone [24].

Guidance: general principles

The current evidence for what might be effective in treating people who self-harm has recently been systematically reviewed and incorporated into guidance published in the United Kingdom by the National Institute for Health and Clinical Excellence (NICE) [17]. There is no single treatment that is known to be especially effective at treating self-harm, though recommendations have emerged nonetheless. Most interventions aim to identify and address the underlying problems that lead an individual to self-harm. Whilst there is no single treatment, there are overarching principles of care that have been set out to guide health care professionals on the best approach to take when working with people who self-harm. Central to working effectively with people who self-harm is building a trusting, supportive and engaging therapeutic relationship and aiming to maintain continuity of relationships. Interventions should involve working collaboratively with service users, involving them fully in decisions relating to their care and encouraging the development of autonomy and independence. Because of the stigma associated with self-harm [25] and the negative experiences of services reported by some service users [17, 23], health care professionals should ensure services are delivered in a nonjudgemental and sensitive manner. When service users were given more responsibility for their own care alongside a genuinely compassionate relationship with professionals [26], they were more likely to view services positively. Service users' accounts of recovery from self-harm and its associated conditions can offer valuable insight into what works. Common threads running through people's accounts of stopping self-harm include accessing services that fit with their needs, establishing therapeutic relationships (either with individual health professionals, statutory or non-statutory services, local community groups or online support networks), gaining an understanding of the reasons they self-harmed, addressing psychological symptoms, building autonomy and being able to use alternative coping strategies [17, 27, 28]. Recovery often correlated with increased levels of engagement with life pursuits and increased quality of interpersonal ties and use of social support [2].

Interventions: psychological

There are indications that psychological therapies may be effective in improving outcomes. Findings from a number of RCTs were pooled to evaluate the relationship between brief psychological therapy following self-harm and outcomes for service users [17]. The types and lengths of therapies varied between studies but included brief problem-solving therapy, cognitive behavioural therapy and psychodynamic interpersonal therapy, ranging from 3 to 12 sessions. These studies measured outcomes in terms of repeat self-harm with some also reporting changes in psychological measures such as depression, hopelessness and suicidal ideation. An intervention involving four sessions of brief psychodynamic interpersonal therapy, which involves identifying and working to resolve interpersonal difficulties that may be associated with psychological distress, was tailored for people who have self-harmed, and delivered following an episode of self-poisoning. The intervention was found to reduce both suicidal ideation and further self-harm in a sample of people who had self-poisoned and presented to hospital [29]. Another trial involving individuals who had attempted suicide reported improvement in a number of variables including measures of hopelessness, suicidal ideation and problem-solving following brief cognitive-behavioural and problem-solving–based therapies [30]. Problem-solving therapy focuses on individuals' existing approaches to dealing with problems and aims to develop structured solutions and more effective techniques with which to deal with problems. A recent study investigated changes in peoples' problem-solving appraisal over the 6-month period following a suicide attempt [31]. Both groups – those receiving cognitive behavioural therapy for suicide prevention and controls – experienced improvements in problem-solving, but the treatment group experienced significantly faster rates of improvement. This demonstrates that these skills are likely to be impaired at the time of a self-harm act and during the sensitive period immediately after but that early intervention may speed up the process of recovering these skills. Other brief, structured therapies have shown promise, such as cognitive-behavioural therapy designed especially for preventing suicide attempts. By working with clients to develop adaptive ways of responding to specific thoughts and beliefs that were associated with previous acts of self-harm [32, 33], incidence of repeat self-harm in the treatment group was reduced. However, not all studies have reported such clear benefits and studies such as these involve selected samples which mean their findings cannot be generalised to all people who self-harm; RCTs, by their nature, involve predefined sets of patients with differing degrees of psychiatric disorder and self-harm history. Whist individual studies have reported improvements following intervention for those with a history of self-harm [34, 35], the pooled evidence suggests that psychological interventions may be more effective for those who do not have a history of self-harm [17], possibly indicating that early intervention modifies the effect of treatment. It is also possible that these individuals would still have had poorer outcomes if they had received intervention at the first self-harm episode, due to higher prevalence of mental disorder in this group, and is an area that needs further investigation.

Treatment options are often considered in terms of their cost-effectiveness meaning that longer-term and more intensive psychological therapies are likely to be reserved for people with more enduring and severe mental disorder and highest risk of repeat self-harm. Dialectical behaviour therapy has become an established longer-term psychological intervention for those with recurrent self-harm [36], particularly for those with borderline personality traits. Treatment for people with borderline personality disorder is discussed in another chapter within this book. Considerably briefer psychological treatments have also been designed with cost effectiveness in mind, including a cognitive analytical-derived, one to three session intervention for repeated self-harm, designed to be deliverable by non-therapists as well as trained psychotherapists [37].

In summary, whilst pooled evidence in support of psychological therapy to reduce self-harm is limited, it is appreciated that therapies may be beneficial when tailored specifically to patients' needs. NICE guidance suggests practitioners should consider offering 3 to 12 sessions of psychological therapy to those who have self-harmed. The treatment could involve features of cognitive-behavioural, psychodynamic or problem-solving therapies and should be designed specifically for people who self-harm and carried out by trained and supervised therapists working collaboratively with clients.

Interventions: pharmacological

In consideration of the available clinical evidence, it is not recommended that pharmacological treatment is offered as an intervention specifically for self-harm. There are a number of mental health conditions associated with self-harm, including depression, borderline personality disorder and alcohol and drug misuse. These may be identified upon assessment of a person's mental state, and, where this is the case, an appropriate pharmacological, psychological or social intervention should be considered. Separate guidance exists for treating people with these associated conditions (www.nice.org.uk), many of whom self-harm. Given the high prevalence of repeat self-harm, clinicians prescribing psychotropic medication should consider the toxicity of drugs when used in overdose [38]. Certain antidepressants have been associated with higher rates of case-fatality when used in self-poisoning [39].

Interventions: 'contact-based'

Psychological therapies – even those that are delivered short term – are costly and are not available to all patients who self-harm [17]. There are also varying levels of uptake and completion of therapy with reported levels of compliance with aftercare arrangements of around half [40, 41], though may increase with 'assertive' follow-up by specialist self-harm teams [42, 43]. Interventions of a less-intensive nature have focused on the provision of information via postcards [44], short letters and telephone calls [45], usually timed so that they are received shortly after a self-harm episode and at regular intervals over a set time period. These interventions often operate in conjunction with usual care and can contain information 'signposting' to statutory/voluntary services and crisis telephone numbers. Reviews of these studies [17, 18], found some modest indications that these interventions may have reduced the number of repeated self-harm episodes in the treatment group. However, no recommendations have been made based on these interventions because of lack of firm evidence. The extent to which such minimal intervention could potentially be harmful in a group of patients who are likely to have complex needs has not been fully explored [46] and warrants further investigation. Regarding the content of the correspondence, service users have expressed concern over interventions that are generic in nature and it is generally accepted that there should be some degree of personalisation to contact-based interventions [16, 47]. Interventions involving non face-to-face contact, such as information leaflets, a follow-up telephone call soon after discharge and appropriately timed letters with a carefully composed personal element to them were perceived by service users to be an important element of care [16]. The timing of the intervention – beginning upon presentation to hospital and tapering off over the following months – was identified by service users as appropriate to their needs, corresponding to their feelings of increased need in the short-term period following the self-harm. The effectiveness of these 'light touch' interventions may be related to the quality and availability of existing (routine) care and the extent to which service users' positive experiences are mirrored by their subsequent encounters with mental health services. In summary, it would seem premature to introduce contact-based interventions into routine clinical practice.

Mechanisms of efficacy: evidence from service users

Whilst the evidence from RCTs is moderate, by considering the findings alongside qualitative evidence from service users who have experienced treatment, we can build a picture of what might be most likely to be helpful for people who self-harm. Benefits may exist, beyond measures of repeat self-harm, to initiating and maintaining contact with individuals following self-harm. Some service users report feeling encouraged and supported by such contact, though these benefits are not so easily measurable in RCTs [48]. The more subtle shifts in people's behaviour that would not be detected by measuring repeat hospital attendances or self-report repeat self-harm measures can be explored in qualitative interviews with service users which often show that people view these interventions positively [48]. Interventions may increase the level of engagement with services, which could be particularly advantageous for those who have traditionally been difficult to engage, such as young people. A trial of an intervention involving a 'therapeutic assessment' following self-harm [24], referred to the above, found no evidence that the intervention improved psychopathology and functioning for adolescents; however, levels of attendance at follow-up appointments and engagement with treatment were higher. This initial positive engagement could potentially be useful as a basis for further therapeutic intervention. Service users are likely to engage with interventions when they are delivered in context of their specific needs [28] and when they view them as acceptable and appropriate to their needs [15].

Early intervention in patients with high suicide risk

Shifting the focus of this chapter more explicitly towards suicide, interventions that address non-fatal self-harm are likely to target a portion of people at risk of suicide. Though suicide is rare in the general population, it is relatively common in people who present to hospital having self-harmed [13]. Key to reducing the risk of suicide is addressing the risk of further self-harm. It is estimated that for people who have died by suicide, between one-fifth and two-thirds will have attended hospital with a non-fatal self-harm act in the preceding year [13].

Some other broad strategies to reduce suicide which have some evidence base include:

- Training to gatekeepers (schools, health professionals inter alia as well as to professionals in high-risk settings such as prison or military service)

- Reduction in access to means of suicide (at national and local level), and

- Effective mental health care [49].

The first and last of these are the essence of early intervention, and the greatest challenge is to engage people with mental health problems into mental health services. There are national guidelines for suicide prevention and an international perspective (www.who.int/mental_health/prevention/suicide/suicideprevent/en/).

The second area, access to methods [50], should not be something health professionals leave to national or local government, although legislation (eg. to reduce pack sizes of analgesics) may play a very important role [51]. The choice of medication prescribed to individual patients at risk of suicide should take account of potential toxicity in overdose [51, 52]. Access to methods also includes vigilance of the media reporting of suicide, where detailed information about the methods used or simplistic representations of individuals' motives are known to provoke 'copycat' suicides (http://www.samaritans.org/media-centre/media-guidelines-reporting-suicide).

As well as the impact that individually delivered interventions may have on a person's risk of future suicide, actions taken at a wider level may act to protect against potentially harmful societal changes associated with increased suicide rates.

Local mental services can implement changes that may reduce suicide rates, for example:

- The provision of 24-hour crisis care

- Clear local policies for dual diagnosis patients (co-morbidity of severe mental illness and alcohol/substances misuse), and

- Routinely undertaking multidisciplinary reviews to discuss lessons learned after a completed suicide [53].

The evidence for these activities comes from a large, national study carried out over 10 years in England where areas that made these changes saw a reduction in suicides (with larger falls in highly deprived areas despite larger caseloads), but those areas that did not implement saw no changes [53]. As recommended with assessment and careful follow-up of safe-harm presentations, this is the key activity at an individual level to prevent suicide [54]. Often this is simply about the comprehensive treatment and assessment of people with mental health diagnoses, and frequently we now see the evidence concurs with conventional clinical wisdom, for example, that long-term lithium use reduces suicide rates [55].

It is widely accepted that during periods of economic recession, rates of suicide increase [56], reflecting higher prevalence of mental distress in the general population. In 2009, an excess 4900 suicides in 54 American and European countries followed the economic downturn beginning in 2008 [56]. These severe consequences appeared to be most pronounced in countries with the sharpest drops in employment [56]. The short time between onset of economic downturn and rise in suicide rate suggests the damaging effects of economic recession are felt quickly. There is some evidence that the way governments deal with economic crises can determine the extent to which the population suffers; initiatives which invest public money in efforts to increase rates of employment have been shown to moderate the effect of unemployment on suicide [57]. These programmes are in contrast to 'austerity measures' which fail to address high unemployment whilst imposing restrictions on social protection. In England, around 1000 excess suicides were estimated to occur between 2008 and 2010 [58], a period during which the rise of unemployment rose each year. The rises were found to be most pronounced in regions with the greatest job losses [58]. There is also likely to be a relationship, exacerbated by 'austerity measures', between reduced expenditure on statutory and voluntary mental health services and a deterioration of the population's mental health [51].

Conclusion

People who self-harm do not consistently receive adequate treatment [6, 59] and may face negative attitudes from clinical staff [25], yet appropriate management and intervention can improve individual outcomes and reduce the burden on services. Early intervention for self-harm and suicidality also requires systematic attention to those who repeat self-harm, given their increased risk. Whilst robust evidence is limited, delivering interventions with service users' individual needs in mind and ensuring they are designed to fit within the person's existing care, is likely to enhance their efficacy. A clear and consistent set of arrangements, which foster good therapeutic relationships, may be as important as the specific modality of treatment.

National and local structures should be in place to sustain early intervention efforts and reduce suicide rates, including 24-hour crisis care, clear local policies for dual diagnosis patients, and a multidisciplinary review to discuss lessons learned after a suicide death.

References

1. Hawton K, Harriss L, Hall S, et al. (2003). Deliberate self-harm in Oxford, 1990–2000: a time of change in patient characteristics. *Psychological Medicine* **33**(6): 987–995.
2. Hawton K, Bergen H, Casey D, et al. (2007). Self-harm in England: a tale of three cities. Multicentre study of self-harm. *Social Psychiatry and Psychiatric Epidemiology* **42**: 513–521.
3. Bergen H, Hawton K, Waters K, et al. (2010). Epidemiology and trends in non-fatal self-harm in three centres in England: 2000–2007. *British Journal of Psychiatry* **197**: 493–498.
4. Hawton K, Bergen H, Waters K, et al. (2012). Epidemiology and nature of self-harm in children and adolescents: findings from the multicentre study of self-harm in England. *European Child and Adolescent Psychiatry* **21**(7): 369–377.
5. Nock MK, Borges G, Bromet EJ, et al. (2008). Cross-national prevalence and risk factors for suicidal ideation, plans and attempts. *British Journal of Psychiatry* **192**: 98–105.
6. Cooper J, Steeg S, Bennewith O, et al. (2013). Are hospital services for self-harm getting better? An observational study examining management, service provision and temporal trends in England. *BMJ: British Medical Association* **3**(11): e003444.
7. Gunnell DJ, Bennewith O, Peters TJ, et al. (2004). The epidemiology and management of self-harm amongst adults in England. *Journal Of Public Health* **27**(1): 67–73.
8. Larkin GL and Beautrais AL. (2010). Emergency departments are underutilized sites for suicide prevention. *Crisis* **31**(1): 1–6.
9. Zahl DL and Hawton K. (2004). Repetition of deliberate self-harm and subsequent suicide risk: long-term follow-up study of 11 583 patients. *British Journal of Psychiatry* **181**: 70–75.
10. Joiner T. (2002). The trajectory of suicidal behaviour over time. *Suicide and Life-Threatening Behavior* **32**(1): 33–41.
11. Joiner T. (2008). *Why People Die by Suicide*. Cambridge, MA: Harvard University Press.
12. Kapur N, Cooper J, King-Hele S, et al. (2006). The repetition of suicidal behavior: a multicenter cohort study. *Journal of Clinical Psychiatry* **67**: 1599–1609.
13. Owens D, Horrocks J and House A. (2002). Fatal and non-fatal repetition of self-harm. *British Journal of Psychiatry* **181**: 193–199.
14. Cooper J, Kapur N, Webb R, et al. (2005). Suicide after deliberate self-harm: a 4-year cohort study. *American Journal Of Psychiatry* **162**: 297–303.
15. Hume M and Platt S. (2007). Appropriate interventions for the prevention and management of self-harm: a qualitative exploration of service-users' views. *BMC Public Health* **7**: 9.
16. Cooper J, Hunter C, Owen-Smith A, et al. (2011). "Well it's like someone at the other end cares about you." A qualitative study exploring the views of users and providers of care of contact-based interventions following self-harm. *General Hospital Psychiatry* **33**(2): 166–176.
17. National Institute for Health and Clinical Excellence. (2011). The long term care and treatment of self-harm. Clinical Guideline 133. http://guidance.nice.org.uk/CG133.
18. Hawton K, Arensman E, Townsend E, et al. (1998). Deliberate self harm: systematic review of efficacy of psychosocial and pharmacological treatments in preventing repetition. *BMJ: British Medical Association* **317**(7156): 441–447.
19. National Institute for Health and Clinical Excellence. (2004). The short-term physical and psychological management and secondary prevention of self-harm in primary and secondary care. Clinical Guideline 16. http://guidance.nice.org.uk/CG16.
20. Bergen H, Hawton K, Waters K, et al. (2010). Psychosocial assessment and repetition of self-harm: the significance of single and multiple repeat episode analyses. *Journal of Affective Disorders* **127**: 257–265.
21. Kapur N, Murphy E, Cooper J, et al. (2008). Psychosocial assessment following self-harm: results from the multi-centre monitoring of self-harm project. *Journal of Affective Disorders* **103**: 285–293.
22. Crawford MJ and Wessely S. (1999). Does initial management affect the rate of repetition of deliberate self-harm? Cohort study. *BMJ: British Medical Association* **317**: 985.

23. Hunter C, Chantler K, Kapur N, et al. (2013). Service user perspectives on psychosocial assessment following self-harm and its impact on further help-seeking: A qualitative study. *Journal of Affective Disorders* **145**: 315–323.

24. Ougrin D, Zundel T, Ng A, et al. (2011). Trial of therapeutic assessment in London: randomised controlled trial of therapeutic assessment versus standard psychosocial assessment in adolescents presenting with self-harm. *Archives of Disease in Childhood* **96**: 148–153.

25. Saunders KEA, Hawton K, Fortune S, et al(2012). Attitudes and knowledge of clinical staff regarding people who self-harm: A systematic review. *Journal of Affective Disorders* **139**(3): 205–216.

26. Bywaters P and Rolfe A. (2002). *Look Beyond the Scars: Understanding and Responding to Self-Injury and Self-Harm*. London: NCH.

27. Kool N, van Meijel B and Bosman M. (2009). Behavioral change in patients with severe self-injurious behavior: a patient's perspective. *Archives of Psychiatric Nursing* **23**: 25–31.

28. Sinclair J and Green J. (2005). Understanding resolution of deliberate self-harm: qualitative interview study of patients' experiences. *BMJ: British Medical Association* **330**: 1112.

29. Guthrie E, Kapur N, Mackway-Jones K, et al. (2001). Randomised controlled trial of brief psychological intervention after deliberate self-poisoning. *BMJ: British Medical Association* **323**: 1–5.

30. Stewart CD, Quinn A, Plever S, et al. (2009). Comparing cognitive behavior therapy, problem solving therapy, and treatment as usual in a high risk population. *Suicide and Life-Threatening Behavior* **39**: 538–547.

31. Ghahramanlou-Holloway M, Bhar SS, Brown GK, et al. (2012). Changes in problem-solving appraisal after cognitive therapy for the prevention of suicide. *Psychological Medicine* **42**(6): 1185–1193.

32. Brown GK, Ten Have T, Henriques GR, et al. (2005). Cognitive therapy for the prevention of suicide attempts: a randomized controlled trial. *JAMA: The Journal of the American Medical Association* **294**: 563–570.

33. Slee N, Garnefski N, van der Leeden R, et al. (2008). Cognitive-behavioural intervention for self-harm: randomised controlled trial. *British Journal of Psychiatry* **192**: 202–211.

34. Hatcher S, Sharon C, Parag V, et al. (2011). Problem-solving therapy for people who presentto hospital with self-harm: Zelen randomised controlled trial. *British Journal of Psychiatry* **199**: 310–316.

35. McAuliffe C, Corcoran P, Keeley H, et al. (2006). Problem-solving ability and repetition of deliberate self-harm: a multicentre study. *Psychological Medicine* **36**: 45–55.

36. Linehan MM, Comtois KA, Murray AM, et al. (2006). Two-year randomized controlled trial and follow-up of dialectical behavior therapy vs therapy by experts for suicidal behaviors and borderline personality disorder. *Archives of General Psychiatry* **63**: 757–766.

37. Sheard T, Evans J, Cash D, et al. (2000). A CAT-derived one to three session intervention for repeated deliberate self-harm: A description of the model and initial experience of trainee psychiatrists in using it. *The British Journal of Medical Psychology* **73**: 179–196.

38. Kendall T, Taylor C, Bhatti H, et al. (2011). Longer term management of self harm: summary ofNICE guidance. *BMJ: British Medical Association* **343**: d7073.

39. Bergen H, Murphy E, Cooper J, et al. (2009). A comparative study of non-fatal self-poisoning with antidepressants relative to prescribing in three centres in England. *Journal of Affective Disorders* **123**: 95–101.

40. Nordentoft M and Sogaard M. (2005). Registration, psychiatric evaluation and adherence to psychiatric treatment after suicide attempt. *Nordic Journal of Psychiatry* **59**(3): 213–216.

41. Van Heeringen C. (1992). The management of noncompliance with outpatient after-care in suicideattempters: A review. *Italian Journal of Suicidology* **2**: 79–83.

42. Van Heeringen C, Jannes S, Buylaert W, et al. (1995). The management of non-compliance with referral to out-patient after-care among attempted suicide patients: A controlled intervention study. *Psychological Medicine* **25**: 963–970.

43. Murphy E, Steeg S, Cooper J, et al. (2010). Assessment rates and compliance with assertive follow-up after self-harm: cohort study. *Archives of Suicide Research* **14**(2): 120–134.
44. Carter GL, Clover K, Whyte IM, et al. (2005). Postcards from the EDge project: randomised controlled trial of an intervention using postcards to reduce repetition of hospital treated deliberate self poisoning. *BMJ: British Medical Association* **331**(7520): 805.
45. Kapur N, Cooper J, Bennewith O, et al. (2010). Postcards, green cards and telephone calls: therapeutic contact with individuals following self-harm. *British Journal of Psychiatry* **197**(1): 5–7.
46. Evans MO, Morgan HG, Hayward A, et al. (1999). Crisis telephone consultation for deliberate self-harm patients: effects on repetition. *British Journal of Psychiatry* **175**: 23–27.
47. Owens C, Farrand P, Darvill R, et al. (2010). Involving service users in intervention design: a participatory approach to developing a text-messaging intervention to reduce repetition of self-harm. *Health Expectations* **14**: 285–295.
48. Owens C. (2010). Interventions for self-harm: are we measuring outcomes in the most appropriate way? *British Journal of Psychiatry* **197**: 502–503.
49. Mann JJ, Apter A, Bertolote J, et al. (2005). Suicide prevention strategies: a systematic review. *JAMA: The Journal of the American Medical Association* **294**: 2064–2074.
50. Yip P, Caine E, Yousuf S, et al. (2012). Means restriction for suicide prevention. *Lancet* **9834**: 2393–2399.
51. Hawton K and Haw C. (2013). Economic recession and suicide. *BMJ: British Medical Association* **347**: f5612.
52. Hawton K, Bergen H, Simkin S, et al. (2010). Toxicity of antidepressants: rates of suicide relative to prescribing and non-fatal overdose. *The British Journal of Psychiatry* **196**(5): 354–358. doi: 10.1192/bjp.bp.109.070219
53. While D, Bickley H, Roscoe A, et al. (2012). Implementation of mental health service recommendations in England and Wales and suicide rates, 1997–2006: a cross-sectional and before-and-after observational study. *Lancet* **379**: 1005–1012.
54. De Leo D, Dello Buono M, Dwyer J. (2002). Suicide among the elderly: the long-term impact of a telephone support and assessment intervention in northern Italy. *British Journal of Psychiatry* **181**: 226–229.
55. Cipriani A, Hawton K, Stockton S, et al. (2013). Lithium in the prevention of suicide in mood disorders: updated systematic review and meta-analysis. *British Medical Journal* **346**: f3646.
56. Chang S-S, Stuckler D, Yip P, et al. (2013). Impact of 2008 global economic crisis on suicide: time trend study in 54 countries. *BMJ: British Medical Association* **347**: f5239.
57. Stuckler D, Basu S, Suhrcke M, et al. (2009). The public health effect of economic crises and alternative policy responses in Europe: an empirical analysis. *Lancet* **374**: 315–323.
58. Barr B, Taylor-Robinson D, Scott-Samuel A, et al. (2012). Suicides associated with the 2008-10 economic recession in England: time trend analysis. *BMJ: British Medical Association* **345**: e5142.
59. Taylor T, Hawton K, Fortune S, et al. (2009). Attitudes towards clinical services among people who self-harm: systematic review. *British Journal of Psychiatry* **194**: 104–110.

21
Early Intervention in Bipolar Disorder

Paddy Power[1], Philippe Conus[1], Craig Macneil[1] and Jan Scott[2]
[1]*Treatment and early Intervention in Psychosis Program (TIPP), Service of General Psychiatry, Department of Psychiatry CHUV, Lausanne University, Switzerland*
[2]*Newcastle University & Centre for Affective Disorders, Institute of Psychiatry, UK*

Introduction
The status of EI in bipolar affective disorder

Early intervention (EI) for patients with bipolar affective disorders (BPAD) is in its infancy. This is despite the fact that they constitute the second largest group of patients attending EI in psychosis (EIP) services [1]. There is a remarkable absence of research directed towards EI in BPAD and there are very few specific EI services for affective disorders. It is only when affective disorders are severe enough to be complicated by psychotic features that they fall into the remit of most EIP services. In some EIP services they are actually excluded, while in others they are simply subsumed within the larger non-affective group with no specific guidelines for managing their different needs. It is only very recently that a body of literature is emerging about the wider BPAD population attending Youth Mental Health services [2]. EI in affective disorders is very much the poor cousin. This is very surprising, given its high prevalence, morbidity, mortality, burden, social cost [3] and good potential for prevention [4].

Part of the reason for this emphasis on schizophrenia-spectrum disorders in EI is that schizophrenia has traditionally been viewed as the more serious and enduring condition, with long delays in accessing treatment, and a prognosis that is largely dependent on the initial course of the illness. BPAD is a rather more complicated condition, not least because it commonly presents with depressive episodes indistinguishable from unipolar depression, has divergent phases of illness, and may not be complicated by psychosis.

Manic episodes are more acute in onset and shorter in duration, giving less opportunity for EI.

However, despite these shortcomings, interest in EI in BPAD is beginning to emerge and early evidence indicates that the rationale for EI in BPAD is just as compelling as that for psychotic disorders [4, 5].

The aim of EI in BPAD

The rationale for EI is that by investing resources into this early phase of illness, one not only can ameliorate and prevent unnecessary suffering but one can also maximize the chances of a full recovery and minimize the risk of relapse, thereby reducing the overall burden and costs for individuals, families and society [3]. In some individuals it may even be possible to prevent the onset of the illness altogether.

However, it is also clear that concepts that are central to EIP such as 'at risk mental state', duration of untreated psychosis (DUP) and the 'critical period' need re-evaluation when applied to BPAD. For example, estimates of the duration of untreated BPAD will vary widely depending on whether it is calculated from the onset of any mood change or is just limited to onset of mania [5]. Likewise interventions that might be quite appropriate in treating emerging schizophrenia may be very inappropriate in BPAD. However, the general EI principles of early detection, prevention and phase-specific interventions being maintained through a 'critical period' are very likely to hold true for BPAD as long as they are modified accordingly [4].

Does EI in BPAD matter?

BPAD is a serious and potentially chronic condition that places a huge burden on society. BPAD is ranked sixth in a World Bank study of the global burden of diseases (ahead of Schizophrenia which was ranked eighth) [4] and ranked fourth among 10–24-year olds [7]. It is the disorder associated with the greatest loss of 'human capital' (i.e. the gap between individuals' pre-morbid potential and their post onset functioning) [5]. McCrone et al. [3] estimated that compared to schizophrenia, BPAD affects 3 times as many individuals (1.4 vs. 0.5%), costs services in England nearly as much annually (£1.6 billion vs. £2.2 billion) and is a greater cost of lost employment (£5.2 vs. £4 billion) to the nation annually.

Similar to the field of psychosis, there is good evidence that a large proportion of patients presenting to services with BPAD for the first time have already had untreated episodes for several years. Several large studies have indicated that it is not unusual for people with bipolar disorder to experience a delay of over 10 years between the initial onset of symptoms, obtaining the correct diagnosis and receiving treatment [8]. Initial mood episodes typically develop in adolescence and have the potential to seriously disrupt the individuals' capacity to establish their own independence and consolidate their emotional, social, educational and vocational trajectories. Delays in accessing treatment increase the risk of progression to severe stages of the illness with accompanying risk of hospitalisations, co-morbidity, poorer clinical outcomes and suicide [9]. Though symptomatic remission with treatment in the first episode is the norm (70–95%), functional recovery from the first episode is much poorer (35–56%) [5] and relapse rates (80%) are very high [10]. There is therefore a clear rationale for intervening earlier during this initial phase of the disorder.

Clinical and demographic features of BPAD
What actually is first-episode BPAD?

Traditionally, BPAD is separated into two types: Bipolar Type I and II. Type I requires at least one manic episode while Type II requires only a hypomanic episode. Type II not uncommonly progresses later to Type I. The stability of the diagnosis is high (between 70 and 90%) and individuals commonly fall into one of two further categories of BPAD, the depressive polarity (60%) and the manic polarity (40%) [11]. Bipolar spectrum disorders encompass a broader category of mood states that include Cyclothymia.

Such a broad categorisation makes defining the first episode of BPAD a challenge. It is also complicated by the multidimensional nature of episodes, which are the presence of depression, mania, psychosis and their cyclical nature. Strictly speaking, BPAD should not be diagnosed until an individual has experienced two distinct episodes of mood disorder, one of which needs to be a manic, hypomanic or mixed manic episode (International Statistical Classification of Diseases and Related Health Problems, Tenth Revision—ICD-10, World Health Organisation). If an individual has already been diagnosed with 'unipolar' depressive episodes prior to developing a manic, hypomanic or mixed episode, then technically the first depressive episode would in hindsight constitute the initial episode of BPAD. If an individual experiences their first acute mania/hypo/mixed mania with no history of depression, then according to ICD-10 one should reserve judgement until the person develops a second episode of mania/hypomania/depression and classify the first episode as a manic/hypomanic episode (not BPAD). However, this seems an academic distinction that fails to take into account the longitudinal course of BPAD.

This is further complicated by the rather arbitrary boundaries defining the different mood states and episodes (see Figure 21.1). If it was possible to identify these initial

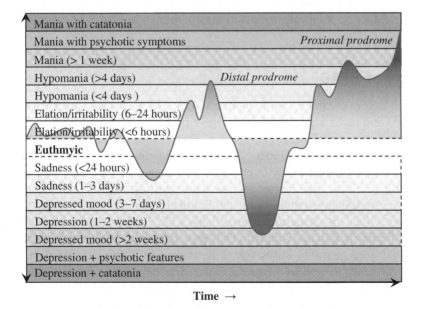

Time →

Figure 21.1 Course of mood swings and clinical thresholds

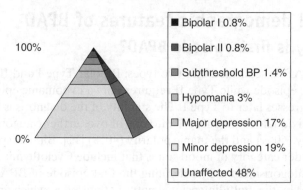

100%

0%

- Bipolar I 0.8%
- Bipolar II 0.8%
- Subthreshold BP 1.4%
- Hypomania 3%
- Major depression 17%
- Minor depression 19%
- Unaffected 48%

Figure 21.2   Distribution of mood disorders in the general population

mood episodes more accurately as episodes of BPAD, then one might be able to prevent the onset of potentially more damaging manic episodes. It also might avoid the risk of unwittingly triggering the onset of mania by the use of antidepressants during depressive phases in those at high risk of BPAD. In those presenting with just one episode of mania/hypo/mixed mania, defining this as the first episode of BPAD would ensure more appropriate advice and treatment in the long term.

How common is bipolar disorder and who is affected?

BPAD (Type I and II) affects 0.8–1.6% of the population [4]. Type I has an annual inception rate of 4 per 100,000 [12, 13] and is relatively evenly distributed across urban and rural populations. It is twice as likely to affect those living in socially deprived areas [13] possibly because of a higher incidence among immigrant populations. The male:female ratio is equal. These figures refer only to people meeting full diagnostic criteria. If one includes the broader category of bipolar spectrum disorders then 2.8–6.5% of the population are affected [4] (see Figure 21.2).

Aetiology of BPAD

Aetiological factors are important to mention as they identify those most at risk of developing BPAD and reveal opportunities for prevention. In reality, there are many different pathways that ultimately lead to the onset of BPAD and the factors along the way are complex, varied and dynamic. Genetics has been estimated to account for 59% of BPAD [14]. So far a myriad of genes have been implicated but as yet none has proven specific for BPAD. Early developmental factors such as Winter/Spring birth, obstetric complications, early brain injuries, delayed milestones, childhood adjustment and behavioural problems carry a higher risk [15]. Structural brain changes have been a relatively consistent but nonspecific finding in patients with BPAD. Neurochemical findings suggest abnormalities in the Opioid neuropeptide, Purinergic, Glutamatergic, Tachykinin Neuropeptide and Cholinergic systems, as well as the intracellular signalling pathways and oxidative stress [16]. Drugs and medications that act on the Serotonergic and Dopaminergic systems such as ecstasy, amphetamines, cocaine, methylphenidate, antidepressants and L-Dopa can trigger a first episode or aggravate further episodes in those susceptible to BPAD. Similarly, medications such as steroids that act on the Adrenocortical Axis can trigger episodes of BPAD. ACTH is more likely to induce mania while Prednisolone is more likely to induce depression. Other triggers particularly in the elderly are operative procedures under GA and physical illnesses such as stokes in the non-dominant cerebral hemisphere. Organic brain conditions are rare in younger patients and I present the most common, including HIV, SLE, and MS. Psychological factors such as perfectionism [17], negative self-esteem [18], need for approval [19] and coping styles that avoid negative emotion [20] are more prevalent in people with a diagnosis of BPAD. Social factors such as childhood adversity, stressful life events, sexual abuse and migration are also more common in people who develop BPAD [4]. Finally, sleep deprivation has been reported as an immediate precipitant in the onset of many cases of mania [21], and seasonal factors also affect mood with mania more likely to occur in Spring while depression in the autumn [22].

While each of these above factors carry risks across the general population, at the individual level each person carries his or her own unique constellation of risks (and protective factors) for developing BPAD. Like most other common illnesses, it is likely that a sizeable proportion of the general population carries a relatively high risk for BPAD but is fortunate to never actually develop the condition as they are not exposed to the lifestyle/environmental factors that trigger the onset or progression of the condition.

Natural history of BPAD

Onset of BPAD is rare before puberty [23, 24] (see Figure 21.3) though there is controversy about the high rates of childhood BPAD reported in the United States [25]. In those with adolescent onset, the first episode is typically depression developing around the age of 15 with the first manic episode occurring 1 year later. The depressive features are similar to adult episodes and are often associated with psychomotor retardation. However, manic

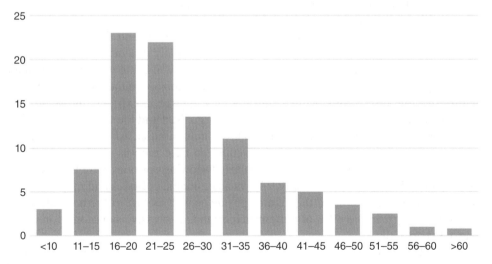

Figure 21.3 Age of onset of bipolar affective disorder. Baldessarini et al. (2012). Reproduced with permission of John Wiley & Sons

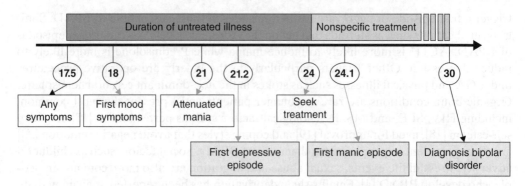

Figure 21.4   Average age at different stages of emergence of BPAD

episodes show more variable features with controversies over the nature of the core symptoms in younger patients, for example childhood BPAD can be diagnosed by the presence of irritability [26]. Overall, the age of onset of the first manic episode peaks in 15–24-year olds [24]. In some study samples a second peak is seen again in the middle age (45–54-year olds), while the first hypomanic episode is seen to have only one peak age of onset in middle age adults [13].

Between 63 and 90% of BPAD patients experience their first episode as depression [13, 27]. The vast majority then experience their first manic episode by their mid-20s [28]. Even though most will have experienced some manic symptoms by age 21 [6, 25] they are not diagnosed with BPAD until age 30 (Figure 21.4).

Untreated, a person with BPAD will typically experience 10 episodes in a lifetime with around 4 episodes per decade. These episodes tend to occur with gradually increasingly frequency up to the fifth episode and then the frequency stabilises for the remainder. Episodes usually last between 4 and 13 months and full symptomatic remission is the norm. Manic episodes tend to last 3–4 months if untreated while depressive episodes typically last 6–9 months untreated and remit spontaneously. Rapid cycling bipolar disorder is reserved for those with more than 4 episodes per year.

Psychotic features complicate the more severe acute manic and depressive episodes. They are very common (70–88%) in mania [29] but relatively rare in depressive episodes. Mood incongruent psychotic features and psychosis between acute episodes of mania or depression would suggest schizoaffective disorder or schizophrenia. Confusion may be a feature of rapid onset cases, while catatonia may emerge in extreme end-stage cases. Behaviours can be highly risky, unpredictable, disorganised and life threatening.

Remission from acute episodes usually takes a few months. About 80–90% of first episode manic patients will have achieved remission by 6 months [4]. However, residual cognitive deficits are common [4], particularly following episodes complicated by psychotic features. Depression commonly follows acute manic episodes and may be seen as partly reactive to the trauma of the manic episode as well as part of the natural cycle of the condition. As many as 40% of patients experience depressive symptoms for 40% of the next 3 years [30].

Co-morbidity with other Axis I conditions (anxiety disorders, addictions, etc.) is common, particularly in younger onset cases while organic co-morbidity is common in elderly presentations. Substance use (e.g. cannabis) and alcohol abuse is a common trigger for BPAD occurring in up to 69% of young patients with first onset BPAD [31]. Co-morbidities are associated with longer delays in accessing treatment and poorer prognosis [32, 33]. There is considerable debate about the overlap of some Axis II conditions and their association with BPAD in children and adolescents, for example attention deficit hyperactivity disorder (ADHD) and emotional unstable personality disorder (EUPD). It is possible that a small proportion of patients diagnosed with ADHD and EUPD are actually experiencing early onset BPAD. It is also possible that these disorders increase the risk of other disorders such as substance use which themselves increase the risk of BPAD. BPAD itself is likely to be a primary cause of co-morbid complications through its psychological impact and disruption to education, employment, relationships and self-esteem.

Long-term disability is a major concern. Repeated relapses may result in progressive cognitive decline, neuroanatomical changes and increasing poor response to treatment [4]. Between 30 and 60% of BP patients failing to regain full occupational and social functioning [4] and a quarter of patients failing to achieve employment even 30 years after their first manic episode [34]. These lifestyle factors and the iatrogenic effects of medication no doubt contribute to the high rates of complicating physical health problems (and reduced life expectancy) seen in up to a third of BPAD patients [4].

Between 10 and 15% of BP patients commit suicide [35, 36] and 25 and 50% attempt suicide [4]. Suicide is twice as common in males and tends to occur in the earlier years of the illness while later in females. Phase of illness is particularly relevant as those in the depressive phase are 18 times more likely while those in mixed affective phases are 37 times more likely [37]. Those with psychotic features are 5 times more at risk. Rates are higher among those treated in hospital versus those never hospitalised. Co-morbidity increases the risk of suicide substantially. Pharmacotherapy has been shown to reduce suicide risk in the long term [38].

The clinical staging model of BPAD

The Clinical Staging Model used in medical conditions such as cancer (e.g. Stages I–IV) can be equally applicable to psychiatric disorders [2, 39]. The model assumes that earlier stages of illness may respond effectively to more benign interventions, and that a certain percentage of individuals will naturally progress from early stages to more advanced stages if untreated. This model provides a clinical rationale for EI. The effectiveness of earlier interventions can be measured by their capacity to prevent progression to more advanced stages of illness. The challenge is to identify who is most at risk of progression and targeting stage-specific treatments more effectively so that the risk of unnecessary treatment is minimised. This model has already been applied to schizophrenia [39], BPAD [40] and eating disorders. The following below outlines this model in BPAD Type I.

Stage 0: Asymptomatic at-risk group

Genetic vulnerability is one of the most important predisposing factors for BPAD [14]. First degree relatives of affected cases carry a 10–15% risk of developing BPAD and this risk increases with the degree of familial loading, for example, having two affected parent carries a 25% risk while a monozygotic twin carries a 45% risk. In reality, only 20% of bipolar patients have an affected relative. Complicating this is that relatives of patients with other disorders also carry a high risk of BPAD, for example offspring of patients with schizophrenia carry 5 times the average population risk of BPAD.

It is likely that only a small fraction of those carrying a high genetic risk actually ever develop the condition and do so only in response to the interaction of developmental and environmental factors mentioned above [41]. Identifying who is most at risk and under what circumstances is a challenge. Falsely attributing risk would be common. This is an important consideration as more genetic/biomarkers become available [42] as their detection may produce unwanted iatrogenic effects stigmatising individuals, particularly if preventative measures are not readily available. A number of centres are already developing biobanks for genomic medical research, for example the Bipolar Biobank set up in 2008 at the Mayo Clinic with the aim of early identification and medical intervention for individuals at risk.

Stage 1: The bipolar prodrome

Most BPAD patients experience a prodrome before their first manic episode [43]. This phase of illness is best conceptualised as comprising the *distal* and *proximal* prodrome or 'at risk' syndrome phases (see Figure 21.5) [15].

The *distal* prodrome of the first manic episode is characterised by a distinct shift from pre-morbid states to one in which the earliest manifestations of mood disorder emerge (e.g. anxiety, depression, sleep disturbance and emotional instability). Spontaneous remission may be the norm and only a small proportion might progress to the next stage of the disorder (typically in response to extra triggers or additional risk factors). In clinical practice it is often quite difficult to differentiate what is developmental, situational and what represents a distinct pathological shift towards a prodrome, for example a sleepless exam stressed teenager using drugs. This period includes episodes of clinical depression and hypomania. These depressive episodes are more likely to be associated with an abrupt onset, psychomotor retardation, agitation, pathological guilt, irritability and hypersomnia [44, 45]. Attenuated self-limiting episodes of elation (lasting less than 4 days) often emerge about 2 years prior to the transition to BPAD [46]. The features include increased energy, activity, sociability, libido, self-esteem, risk taking, emotional spontaneity, irritability and decreased need for sleep. It may be associated with improved functioning but be a distinctly uncharacteristic shift in personality functioning towards greater risk taking. A

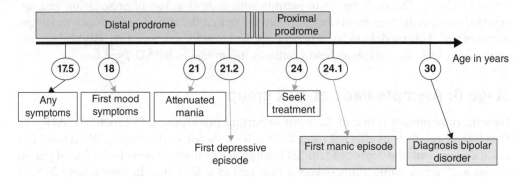

Figure 21.5   The distal and proximal prodrome of the first manic episode

proportion will progress on to hypomania with elation, irritability, disorganisation, insomnia, attentional deficits, grandiosity, paranoia, aggression and more detrimental risk taking. It is likely than only a minority of these episodes is likely to progress on to the proximal prodrome and Stage 2.

The *proximal* prodrome is the phase when attenuated manic/mixed affective features emerge in the immediate lead up to the first manic episode (Stage 2). It is typically short lasting, a few days to a few weeks [46]. For the majority, these features may progress incrementally into a manic episode while for a minority they may wax and wane erratically from day to day (see Figure 21.1) before the transition.

Unlike in schizophrenia, there are as yet no well-established Ultra high risk (UHR) criteria for BPAD. However, Bechdolf et al. [47] have developed the Bipolar At-Risk (BAR) criteria, which comprise the peak age of onset (15–25), genetic loading, sub-threshold mania, cyclothymia or depressive symptoms. A pilot follow-up study of 22 individuals meeting the BAR criteria found that 23% developed a proxy to first episode mania within an average of 265 days (compared with 0.7% of the control group who did not meet these criteria). Their results suggested the BAR criteria had high specificity and sensitivity.

Similarly, Conus et al. [48] have developed the First Episode Mania Prodrome Inventory that combines pre-morbid risk factors, recent markers of vulnerability and attenuated symptoms of mood disorder. Though highly specific in BPAD patients when tested retrospectively its sensitivity in truly identifying UHR patients has yet to be tested.

Stage 2: First acute manic episode of BPAD and its recovery

Only a third of BPAD patients' first presentation to services is with a manic episode (the rest will have already presented with a depressive episode). About 70–88% of those presenting first with manic episodes have complicating psychotic features [29]. Most individuals with manic psychosis do not seek help on their own initiative, usually come to the attention of services via police, family or community agencies, and require hospitalisation [49]. Initial presentations may not be easy to distinguish from non-affective psychotic illnesses and substance use disorders. Though standard acute inpatient treatment will produce full remission from mania in 6 weeks for 50% of first episode patients, this may take longer in younger patients, males, those with longer duration of untreated mania and co-morbid psychotic features [29]. By 1 year, over 90% of adult onset patients will have achieved remission from their first episode of mania. In adolescent first episode mania the remission rates are 85% [50]. Follow-up treatment however is difficult to maintain and drop-out rates are high. In the adolescent group only a third maintain good treatment adherence [50]. Prophylactic use of mood stabilisers is often reserved for those with more established histories. Relapse is unfortunately common and the majority of patients progress onto Stage 3 (below).

Stage 3: Relapsing episodes followed by remissions

In the short term, nearly 40% of first episode manic patients will experience a relapse within 2 years (24% mania, 13% depression) and another 20% will switch to another phase of illness without remission. The vast majority of these relapses occur within a year of remission from the first manic episode [29]. Manic relapses are more likely after manic psychosis, while depression is much more likely after mixed manic first episodes [29].

In the long term, it is likely that most first episode manic patients will experience further episodes of BPAD. However, as yet there are no lifelong prospective studies to provide details. Relapses tend to be triggered in the same manner as the initial episode, or follow cessation of medication. Psychosocial sequelae are common and the risks of post manic depression and suicide are high. With each relapse there is greater risk of incomplete remission (Stage 4) and failure to respond to medication such as Lithium and Olanzapine [4]. About 20% develop chronic persistent affective symptoms (usually depression complicated by degrees of cognitive impairment). Women with later onset of illness are more likely to fall into this group.

Stage 4: No remission or partial remission with relapses

There is no agreed definition of treatment resistance in BPAD disorder [51]. It is complicated by the diversity of mood states and the varied speeds with which these mood states respond to treatment. However, it includes treatment refractory and persistent mania, depression, rapid cycling and the 20% of BPAD patients who develop chronic features of mood disturbance complicated by cognitive deficits and enduring disability. Treatment resistance is more likely in those with earlier age of onset, co-morbidity, psychotic features, longer duration of untreated illness (DUI), poor treatment adherence and rapid cycling BPAD [51]. About 8% of treated first episode manic patients will not have achieved remission from mania by 12 months [29].

Evidence that EI at different stages in BPAD works

There is now substantial evidence that EI is effective in first episode psychosis. Many of these trials include individuals with first episode manic, depressive and schizoaffective psychoses. However, there are very few trials specifically designed for EI in BPAD and a systematic review by Gonzalez et al. [52] revealed that none of psychological therapies in BPAD met their criteria for EI. There is one published study of outcomes of a small sample ($n = 16$) of first episode BPAD patients attending an EI service [53] but no comparison was made with BPAD patients attending generic services. There is one study in Denmark, of relapse rates in a sample of 158 patients discharged from hospital after their first, second or third episodes BPAD to either a specialised service for BPAD or a generic standard service [54]. This randomised controlled trial demonstrated that treatment within a specialised mood disorder clinic early in the course of bipolar disorder substantially reduced readmissions and increased patient satisfaction with care.

Existing EI services specifically for BPAD

Apart from the Copenhagen Affective Disorder Clinic above [54], one other such service has been described recently in the literature. The Jano Programme was set up in 2005 in Valdecilla Hospital, Santander, Spain [52] and provides psychiatric management, psychoeducation, psychotherapy and family therapy for patients in the early stage of bipolar disorder as well as undertaking a number of research trials. It caters for patients present-ing between the ages of 16 and 55 with BPAD developing as either a manic episode within the previous 5 years or a depressive episode within the previous 10 years. It has yet to be formally evaluated.

What an ideal model for EI in BPAD would look like

Given the diversity of services and health systems internationally, no one model could possibly fit all circumstances. However, there are essential components that should be common to all and then specific components reserved for particular settings. Some compo-nents (e.g. early detection strategies) have significant implications and their introduction should wait until other basic elements (e.g. acute care) are operating effectively to receive them. Some bring with them cost savings (e.g. reduced hospital usage due to relapse pre-vention strategies) and if set up in a timely manner can then allow for self-generating fund-ing for additional components (e.g. using savings from acute hospital funds to run recovery day-programmes).

There is a vigorous debate about whether it is better to start reforming from the front end or the back end of services when establishing EI models. There is also a tension between EI services that are rigidly disorder specific (e.g. psychosis) and youth mental health services that are deliberately disorder nonspecific, for example Headspace. Each model has its pros and cons. They all risk excluding or failing to meet the needs of a pro-portion of patients with or at risk of BPAD.

For BPAD, the added difficulty is that the diagnosis is often retrospective, that is with patients very likely to be already engaged with a service for depression long before they develop their manic episode. Therefore, any EI programme attempting to address BPAD should ideally start by screening young people with depression to identify those with greater risk of BPAD [5] as well as those with unrecognized manic symptoms (current or past). Such services would therefore specifically should be embedded within a wider generic mental health service preferably spanning across the adolescent/adult divide and with well-integrated programmes across diagnostic streams. Given the sheer number of cases of mood disorders in adolescence, the model will also need to work across the primary–secondary care interface [2]. The worst outcome would be for patients who are forced to move from one specialised team to another if their illness progresses through pro-drome to depression to mania and to psychosis as well as having to transfer from CAMHS to AMHS as they turn 18.

It is clearly preferable to structure services in such a way that they have very accessi-ble generic 'catch all' front end capacity (e.g. Youth Mental Health model) with back-end specialist clinical/diagnostic streams (Figure 21.6). These specialist clinical streams could then be phase specific, for example early detection, acute inpatient or recovery teams com-bining relevant interventions, for example medication clinics, cognitive behaviour therapy (CBT) intervention teams, group programmes or family interventions.

Careful consideration should be given to the 'care pathway' and to ensure the model is 'client centred'. Ideally, all patients should have one keyworker/case manager/primary clinician/psychiatrist who follows them through from beginning to the end of the service.

An ideal EI programme for BPAD should incorporate the following components. Each focuses on particular steps in the care pathway and clinical staging.

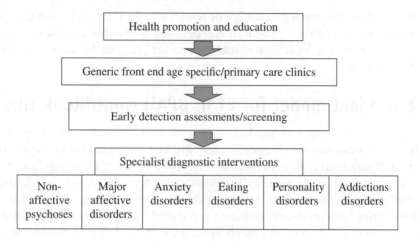

Figure 21.6   Ideal model

Health education programmes and raising awareness

There is a prima facia case for providing health education and preventative programmes for high-risk groups such as the offspring of affected parents or first degree relatives. There is also a good case for early detection training for professionals who are more likely to come in contact with those in the early stages of the illness, such as teachers, tutors, emergency services, police, and primary care staff. This also should include parents and carers of offspring with affected first degree relatives.

Genetic counselling, provided in a sensitive and timely manner highlighting the benefits of early detection and prevention, should be offered to parents and prospective parents, if one or both has bipolar disorder, given that the risk of one of their children developing BPAD is 10% and major depression 25%.

Improving the accessibility and appeal of 'front end' mental health

Given that most first episode BPAD patients will present in late teens and early adulthood during an acute phase of depression or mania 'soft' 'primary care' front end access into mental health services needs to be particularly receptive to their developmental issues and the needs of parents and carers. But these front end services also need to be particularly robust and responsive in facilitating rapid access to emergency psychiatric care for acutely unwell patients as young manic patients are particularly difficult to engage and challenging.

Specialist early detection services/teams that include BPAD in their remit

As access improves and patients are identified much earlier, it becomes more of a challenge to accurately categorise their earlier subtle presentations into traditional diagnostic groupings. Rapid access to assessments by specialists in early detection of BPAD is essential. Otherwise patients presenting with other disorders (e.g. EUPD, ADHD or substance use disorders) will be mistakenly diagnosed and started on treatment for BPAD. Given the relatively low incidence rate, it would be inappropriate to set up diagnostic-specific early detection teams and it would be far more cost-effective to embed these specialist clinicians within generic assessment teams, so they can provide backup for the more complex minority of early cases which are not so obvious to the average clinician.

These specialists would undertake a more careful timeline of mood changes over the lifespan accessing sources of information from family, primary care, student support services etc. This might help identify previously unrecognised episodes of mania in patients presenting with depression. It will also help exclude other conditions such as emotionally unstable personality disorder, substance use disorders etc. The goal is then to identify whether the patient is either at high risk or already experiencing BPAD and if so then what stage (see stages above) are they at in the condition. In the future it might be possible to accurately predict each individual's risk of progression to the next stage of illness and which treatment is likely to provide the most effective response and protection.

Specialist interventions for the BPAD ultra high risk population (Stage 1 interventions)

Specialist interventions for the BPAD UHR group would include general counselling and psychoeducation for patients and carers about BPAD with a focus on prevention through the recognition of early symptoms, triggers, stress management, sleep hygiene, dangers of substance use and risks of antidepressants. Self-monitoring and management of mood through mindfulness interventions and use of smartphone apps may provide some benefits. Judicial use of medication may also be helpful with even consideration for prophylactic mood stabilisers [43], particularly if antidepressants are being prescribed in those who are more acutely depressed and have either a history of untreated mania or a strong family history of BPAD.

Interventions in episodes of BPAD (Stage 2–4 interventions)

Once acute episodes of BPAD have developed, then care should be provided by a mental health service for at least 3 years after symptom remission has been achieved. If presenting with an acute first episode, antidepressant or anti-manic medication should be introduced as soon as organic factors have been ruled out. The type, combination and duration of these medications depend on phase and stage of illness (see below) and medical management is central to the treatment plan. However, psychosocial interventions are crucial to functional recovery and the prevention of secondary morbidity. Long-term self-monitoring and management (akin to physical illness such as diabetes) is a realistic goal for many patients.

Service setting   Home-based treatment is a challenge during the acute first episode of mania or of major depression with a history of previous untreated mania. If psychotic symptoms are present, then hospitalisation is advisable unless carers can provide 24/7 supervision and the patient is genuinely engaged in the process otherwise the risks are too high. Only 20% of patients with manic psychosis can be managed at home by EI services during the acute phase of first episode manic psychosis [49] considerably less than first episode non-affective psychosis (45%). Involuntary hospitalisation rates are very high and the use of emergency services such as police intervention is common. Steps may have to be taken to safeguard assets and protect others from patients' temporary lack of mental capacity, for example driving, financial affairs, work responsibilities and child care. Advance directives should be considered after the first episode as a way of putting in place contingencies in case of future episodes.

Pharmacotherapy   About 80% of people with BPAD receive some form of treatment during their lifetime [49] but at any given time, 60% are untreated or inappropriately treated.

First manic episode: Pure mania/hypomania without psychotic features may respond to monotherapy alone with either a mood stabiliser or antipsychotic. However, anti-manic doses are needed (e.g. for Lithium blood levels of 0.8–1.0 are required). Olanzapine is possibly one of the more efficacious anti-manic antipsychotic in mania [55] and one would question the rationale for prescribing 'antidepressant' atypicals such as Quetiapine during acute manic episodes though they may minimise the risk of subsequent depressive features and side effects. Benzodiazepines are usually required for sedation and insomnia. Sleep is a good barometer of response to treatment.

Failure to respond within 7 days of starting a mood stabiliser, or the presence of psychotic features will generally require the addition of antipsychotic medication. Initial doses of antipsychotic medication should be low but may need to be increased every few days during the acute phase until manic symptoms start to settle. Doses of antipsychotic medication can usually then be gradually reduced and ceased during the first 3 months of recovery, but the mood stabiliser should continue as a prophylactic measure.

Treatment of Depression in BP Disorder: Two thirds of BPAD patients experience a major depressive episode before their first manic episode, that is during Stage I of their illness. Certain criteria (see Stage 1 above) can better identify their potential for mania, particularly if antidepressants are being considered. If antidepressants are required then they should be used for brief periods only [56], for example 3 months or until remission from depression is achieved (whichever is sooner). Mood stabilisers should be considered as a combination treatment in these patients, particularly if the depression fails to improve, or higher doses or longer-term use of antidepressants is required or there are high-risk indicators of mania.

Depression commonly follows first episode of mania. If psychosocial interventions fail to address the post manic adjustment and self-esteem issues then the next step is to carefully reduce the dose of antipsychotic medication. Failing this then adding an antidepressant is advisable but only if the patient is already on mood stabilisers as the risk of antidepressants triggering a manic episode is high. Antidepressants should be ceased shortly after the depression has lifted and SNRIs or TCA should be avoided as they are more likely than SSRIs to trigger mania [56].

If psychotic features complicate depression, then combination therapy (antidepressant plus antipsychotic medication) or even antidepressants alone are better than monotherapy with an antipsychotic [57]. Quetiapine is recommended because of its antidepressant effects [58] but it can be quite sedating. Aripiprazole may be more activating but it can aggravate agitation and irritability. Antipsychotics should be withdrawn gradually within several months of remission of symptoms and longer-term use of mood stabilisers should be considered in order to prevent relapse. ECT, though very effective in this group, is rarely required in practice except in the elderly or those with catatonia.

Prophylactic treatments to prevent progression to stage 3 and 4: Long-term (18 months minimum) prophylaxis with mood stabilisers should be the norm after first episode mania. In practice, only half of the first episode manic patients are prescribed a mood stabiliser and this is often for only a few months [59]. Adherence is particularly poor at this stage of the illness. Prophylaxis with antipsychotics either alone or in combination with mood stabilisers should be reserved often for those with more severe or intractable forms of BPAD. Prophylactic doses are generally lower than acute phase doses. Patients should be actively engaged in monitoring blood levels, side effects and medication complications such as hypothyroidism, metabolic syndrome and renal impairment. Specially designed medication 'pocket books' for patients are particularly helpful in keeping a record.

Typical practice might be to continue prophylactic medication for at least 18 months after remission from the first episode of mania, 3 years after the first relapse and 5 years after remission from repeated relapses. We would recommend further tailoring the duration of an individual's prophylactic treatment to take into account the extent of additional risk factors. For example, someone with a younger age of onset and strong family history might merit longer prophylaxis, particularly if there were very significant risk behaviours during the acute episode. As yet there is unfortunately no reliable prognostic indicator to guide such individualised regimens. Ceasing prophylactic medication should be gradual, stepwise and cautious as relapses during this period are common.

Treatment refractory BPAD (stage 4 treatment)

If the condition is at risk of becoming treatment resistant (see above) then a thorough diagnostic review should be undertaken that includes a review of organic factors, Axis II considerations, medication regimens and blood levels. Inadequate treatment and medication non-adherence are possibly the most common causes.

Combined medication regimens are recommended if mania or depression persist. Switching mood stabilisers or even in severe cases adding a second mood stabiliser may be required. ECT should be considered if all else fails.

Psychological interventions Three forms of psychological intervention have been reported to be effective in BPAD. They are psychoeducation, CBT (including family-based CBT interventions), interpersonal and social rhythm therapy (ISRP) [52, 60]. ISRP was found to be the least effective [61]. Large RCTs by Scott et al. [62] and Colom [63] found that both psychoeducational interventions and cognitive behavioural therapy were more effective when undertaken early in the course of the disorder. Smaller studies by Jones and Burrell Hodgson [64] and Macneil et al. [65] found that modified cognitive behavioural therapy for EI in bipolar disorder was efficacious and well tolerated. In a RCT of CBT plus medication versus medication alone, Lam et al. [66] found that relapses were significantly less and delayed with the combined CBT intervention and produced cost savings of £1400 per patient compared to medication alone.

Psychological interventions early in the course of bipolar disorder focus on the challenge of engagement, identifying and addressing barriers to medication adherence, psychoeducation, early signs identification, self-monitoring using mood diaries, coping strategies with life events, sleep hygiene, relapse prevention, addressing the impact of the disorder on the person's sense of self, reducing potential for post manic depressive reactions and secondary morbidity, social rhythm stabilisation and reintegration and improving functional outcome and involving families [67]. Identifying and working with unhelpful core beliefs also offers considerable promise [19]. Sessions can be provided either in individual or group format, for example the *Bipolar Programme* in St Patrick's Hospital, Dublin operates a 5-day closed group programme during the last week in hospital and then a weekly afternoon group session for 12 weeks follow-up.

Most patients need a considerable amount of time and counselling to process the enormity of what has happened. Residual manic symptoms may hinder this process but a certain amount of denial is healthy and driving the message home too much can risk depressing patients, particularly if they already have very negative preconceptions about the illness.

Self-help resources   Aids such as mood timelines, 'mood diaries', 'lithium passports', relapse signatures, patients own clinical files, will help patients develop more confidence in self-management under the guided supervision of their treating clinician.

There is a rapidly expanding array of self-help books now available on BPAD (see www.mdf.org.uk and www.rcpsych.ac.uk\). In addition, there are several educational videos and documentaries, for example Stephen Fry's series. These go a long way to help demystify the condition and normalise the treatment, particularly for first episode patients and carers.

Family interventions   Family interventions are amongst the most promising psychosocial approaches and have been found to be at least as effective as individually based CBT [68]. Family-based interventions in BPAD tend to focus on 'debriefing' the often complex and frustrating pathway to care, addressing guilt and confusion, psychoeducation, understanding family members' explanatory models, addressing problematic communication styles and problems solving difficulties if these are present, assisting in mood monitoring and relapse planning [67, 69].

Vocational/educational/psychosocial interventions   Functional recovery (including psychosocial, educational and vocational recovery) is often poor in BPAD and is correlated with pre-morbid neuroticism, ongoing depressive symptoms and cognitive impairment [70, 71]. Recovery of educational and vocational functioning can be challenging, given the impact of manic or depressive symptoms on the developmental trajectory. Patients need practical advice about what to tell prospective employers, colleges, insurance companies, licensing authorities (driving, guns, etc.) and visa application authorities. This can be assisted by practical interventions within a case-management model including liaison by the health professional with schools, colleges, universities or workplaces, role-playing some of the challenges of commencing or returning to work or study, assisting the re-establishment of necessary sleep-wake cycles, and ongoing monitoring and support in the study/workplace [67, 72].

Discharge and long-term follow-up/recommendations Given the high risk of relapse and suicide in the first few years after the first episode, all patients should be assertively followed up if they drop out of treatment prematurely. Patients are most likely to drop out when they are about to relapse, or if they transfer from one service to another, or if their clinician changes. Careful proactive planning for these eventualities will reduce this risk.

For those who have made a good recovery, discharge planning and long-term recommendations are essential. Each patient's risk of relapse is different and until individualised prognostic indicators have been developed, the generally advice is to help the patients consider all the ramifications of stopping medication well in advance of any attempt to cease it. If a patient decides to take the risk, then they should be slowly weaned off prophylactic medication (preferably after 3 years if the risk is low). Relapse prevention counselling should be routinely provided and include the carers. If should include long-term recommendations about maintaining wellness and rehearse contingencies during high-risk periods or if early warning signs develop. The recommendations should include advice about the use of drugs, alcohol, certain medications such as steroids, as well as issues such as having children, child birth and post natal risk management, and ways of minimising risk to offspring.

Outcomes expected and how they would be evaluated
Prevention and early detection

With public health strategies focussing on prevention, one would expect the incidence to be reduced in the population served. However, early detection strategies are likely to temporarily increase the inception rate as previously undetected cases are discovered and new cases are detected earlier each year. Any evaluation would need to take into account the Duration of Untreated Illness (DUI) which one would expect to shorten as the EI strategies are rolled out. This effect on the incidence and DUI might take several years to wash out.

Pathways to care and access to evidence-based interventions

Attention to these areas should provide measureable improvements in engagement rates, reduced delays, acuity and secondary morbidity, reduced hospitalisations and lengths of stay, improved rates of remission and time to remission, reduced relapse rates and time to relapse, improved functional outcomes and quality of life, reduced suicides and suicide attempts and finally reduced burden on carers.

Costs

In a comprehensive analysis of health service costs in England, McCrone et al. [3] estimated that annual savings of over £25 million per year could be achieved if EI services were rolled out nationally in the England for BPAD with psychosis. This was based on economic evaluations of several EI services restricted to those with psychosis and below the age of 35 years. Even though this group (with psychosis) is possibly the most expensive to treat [3], they represent only a half of the total population of new patients presenting annually with first episode BPAD [12]. The savings above of £25 million/year represent only a very small percent (less than 2%) of the total service costs for BPAD (estimated in England to be £1.6 Billion/annum). There needs to be a broader economic evaluation of potential savings if the EI model was rolled out for all patients presenting with first episode BPAD. It also needs to include the elderly (over 65s) with BPAD as they are 4 times more expensive to manage than those under 45-year olds [3].

Conclusions

EI in BPAD remains in its infancy. It is about 20 years behind the advances being made in EIP. However, the research evidence is gathering momentum and there is already a very clear rationale for intervening early in BPAD. It carries just as much if not more burden to society than schizophrenia and is possibly even more preventable. There is an urgent need to develop better 'at risk' screening tools and interventions for those in the prodromal phases. Treatment protocols for those with established illnesses remain crude and lack consideration of each individual's unique prognostic indicators. Conventional practice still grossly underestimates the extent of long-term sequelae and there needs to be far more attention given to psychosocial recovery and relapse prevention. EI has an extremely promising role in BPAD. The challenge now is to realise this with innovative services and timely interventions at different stages of illness.

References

1. Conus P and McGorry PD. (2002). First episode mania: a neglected priority for early intervention. *The Australian and New Zealand Journal of Psychiatry* **36**: 158–172.
2. Scott J, Leboyer M, Hickie I, et al. (2013). Clinical staging in psychiatry: a cross-cutting model of diagnosis with heuristic and practical value. *British Journal of Psychiatry* **202**(4): 243–245.
3. McCrone P, Dhanasiri S, Patel A, et al. (2008). *Paying the Price: The Cost of Mental Health Care in England to 2026*. London: The King's Fund.
4. Conus P, Macneil C and McGorry PD. (2013). Public health significance of bipolar disorder: implications for early intervention and prevention. *Bipolar Disorder*. doi: 10.1111/bdi.12137, Printed online ahead of print on Oct 16th.
5. Scott J. (2012). Beyond psychosis: the challenge of early intervention in bipolar disorder. *Revista de Psiquiatría y Salud Mental* **5**(1):1–4.
6. Drancourt N, Etain B, Lajnef M, et al. (2013). Duration of untreated bipolar disorder: missed opportunities on the long road to optimal treatment. *Acta Psychiatrica Scandinavica* **127**(2):136–144.
7. Gore FM, Bloem GC, Ferguson J, et al. (2011). Global burden of disease in young people aged 10–24 years: a systematic analysis. *Lancet* **377**: 2093–2102.
8. Berk M, Dodd S, Callaly P, et al. (2007a). History of illness prior to a diagnosis of bipolar disorder or schizoaffective disorder. *Journal of Affective Disorders* **103**(1–3): 181–186.
9. Altamura AC, Buoli M, Albano A, et al. (2010). Age at onset and latency to treatment (duration of untreated illness) in patients with mood and anxiety disorders: a naturalistic study. *International Clinical Psychopharmacology* **25**(3): 172–179.
10. Keller MB, Lavori PW, Coryell W, et al. (1993). Bipolar I: a five-year prospective follow-up. *Journal of Nervous and Mental Disease* **181**(4): 238–245.
11. Vieta E and Phillips M. (2007). Deconstructing bipolar disorder: a critical review of its diagnostic validity and a proposal for DSM-V and ICD-11. *Schizophrenia Bulletin* **33**(4): 886–892.

12. Lloyd T, Kennedy N, Fearon P, et al. (2005). Incidence of bipolar affective disorder in three UK cities: Results from the AESOP study. *British Journal of Psychiatry* **186**: 126–131.

13. Kroon JS, Wohlfarth TD, Dieleman J, et al. (2013). Incidence rates and risk factors of bipolar disorder in the general population: a population-based cohort study. *Bipolar Disorders* **15**: 306–313.

14. Lichtenstein P, Yip B, Björk C, et al. (2009). Common genetic determinants of schizophrenia and bipolar disorder in Swedish families: a population based study. *Lancet* **373**: 234–239.

15. Conus P, Ward J, Hallam KT, et al. (2008). The proximal prodrome to first episode mania – a new target for early intervention. *Bipolar Disorder* **10**: 555–565.

16. Machado-Vieira R, Carlos A and Zarate Jr CA. (2011). Proof of concept trials in bipolar disorder and major depressive disorder: a translational perspective in the search for improved treatments. *Depress Anxiety* **28**(4): 267–281.

17. Power MJ. (2005). Psychological approaches to bipolar disorders: A theoretical critique. *Clinical Psychology Review* **25**: 1101–1122.

18. Schwannauer M. (2003). In: Power, M. (ed), *A Handbook of Science and Practice: Mood Disorders*. West Sussex: John Wiley & Sons, Ltd, Chichester.

19. Ball J, Mitchell P, Malhi G, et al. (2003). Schema-focused cognitive therapy for bipolar disorder: reducing vulnerability to relapse through attitudinal change. *Australian and New Zealand Journal of Psychiatry* **37**: 41–48.

20. Thomas J, Knowles R, Tai S, et al. (2007). Response styles to depressed mood in bipolar affective disorder. *Journal of Affective Disorders* **100**: 249–252.

21. Wehr TA, Sack DA and Rosenthal NE. (1987). Sleep reduction as the final common pathway in the genesis of mania. *American Journal of Psychiatry* **144**: 201–204.

22. Geoffroy P, Bellivier F, Scott J, et al. (2013). Bipolar disorders with seasonal pattern: clinical characteristics and gender influences. *Chronobiology International* **30**(9): 1101–1107.

23. Douglas J, Scott J. (in press). Bipolar disorders in prepubertal children: fact or artifact. *Bipolar Disorder*.

24. Baldessarini R, Tondo L and Tohen M. (2012). Age at onset versus family history and clinical outcomes in 1,665 international bipolar-I disorder patients. *World Psychiatry* **11**(1): 40–46.

25. Post R, Luckenbaugh D, Grunze H, et al. (2010). Bipolar disorder in U.S. versus Europe. *Neuropsychopharmacology* **35**: S166–S167.

26. Pavuluri MN, Graczyk PA, Henry DB, et al. (2004). Child and family-focused cognitive behavioural therapy for pediatric bipolar disorder: development and preliminary results. *Journal of the American Academy of Child and Adolescent Psychiatry* **43**: 528–537.

27. Duffy A, Alda M, Crawford L, et al. (2007). The early manifestations of bipolar disorder: a longitudinal study of the offspring of bipolar parents. *Bipolar Disorder* **9**: 828–838.

28. Merikangas KR, Akiskal HS, Angst J, et al. (2007). Lifetime and 12-month prevalence of bipolar spectrum disorder in the National Co-morbidity Survey Replication. *Archives of General Psychiatry* **64**: 543–552.

29. Tohen M, ZarateJr CA, Hennen J, et al. (2003). The McLean-Harvard First-Episode Mania Study: prediction of recovery and first recurrence. *American Journal of Psychiatry* **160**: 2099–2107.

30. Joffe RT, MacQueen GM, Marriott M, et al. (2004). A prospective, longitudinal study of percentage of time spent ill in patients with bipolar I or bipolar II disorders. *Bipolar Disorder* **6**: 62–66.

31. Hasty MK, Macneil CA, Kader LF, et al. (2006). The developmental considerations for psychological treatment of first episode bipolar disorder, 5th International Conference on Early Psychosis, October, Birmingham, England.

32. Leboyer M, Henry C, Paillere-Martinot ML, et al. (2005). Age at onset in bipolar affective disorders: A review. *Bipolar Disorders* **7**: 111–118.

33. Strakowski SM, Williams JR, Fleck DE, et al. (2000). Eight month functional outcome from mania following a first psychiatric hospitalization. *Journal of Psychiatric Research* **34**(3): 193–200.

34. Tsuang MT, Woolson RF and Fleming JA. (1979). Long-term outcome of major psychoses. I. Schizophrenia and affective disorders compared with psychiatrically symptom-free surgical controls. *Archives of General Psychiatry* **36**: 1295–1301.

35. Hawton K, Sutton L, Haw C, et al. (2005). Suicide and attempted suicide in bipolar disorder: A systematic review of risk factors. *Journal of Clinical Psychiatry* **66**: 693–704.

36. Cassidy F. (2011). Risk factors of attempted suicide in bipolar disorder. *Suicide and Life-Threatening Behavior* **41**(1): 6–11.

37. Valtonen HM, Suominen K, Haukka J, et al. (2008). Differences in incidence of suicide attempts during phases of bipolar I and II disorders. *Bipolar Disorders* **10**(5): 588–596.

38. Rihmer Z and Gonda X. (2012). The effect of pharmacotherapy on suicide rates in bipolar patients. *CNS Neuroscience and Therapeutics* **18**(3): 238–242.

39. McGorry PD, Hickie IB, Yung AR, et al. (2006). Clinical staging of psychiatric disorders: a heuristic framework for choosing earlier, safer and more effective interventions. *Australian and New Zealand Journal of Psychiatry* **40**: 616–22.

40. Culebra NC. (2010). Early intervention in bipolar disorder: First episodes' designs and staging utility. *Early Intervention in Psychiatry* **4**(20): 1751–1785.

41. Elanjithara TE, Frangou S and McGuire P. (2011). Treatment of the early stages of bipolar disorder. *Advances in Psychiatric Treatment* **17**(4): 283–291.

42. Luby JL and Navsaria N. (2010). Pediatric bipolar disorder: evidence for prodromal states and early markers. *Journal of Child Psychology and Psychiatry* **51**: 459–471.

43. Howes OD and Falkenberg I. (2011). Early detection and intervention in bipolar affective disorder: targeting the development of the disorder. *Current Psychiatry Reports* **13**(6): 493–499.

44. Forty L, Smith D, Jones L, et al. (2008). Clinical differences between bipolar and unipolar depression. *British Journal of Psychiatry* **192**: 388–389.

45. Mitchell PB, Goodwin GM, Johnson GF, et al. (2008). Diagnostic guidelines for bipolar depression: a probabilistic approach. *Bipolar Disorders* **10**: 144–152.

46. Correll CU, Penzner JB, Lencz T et al. (2007). Early identification and high-risk strategies for bipolar disorder. *Bipolar Disorder* **9**: 324–338.

47. Bechdolf A, Ratheesh A, Wood S, et al. (2012). Rationale and first results of developing at-risk (prodromal) criteria for bipolar disorder. *Current Pharmaceutical Design* **18**(4): 358–375.

48. Conus P, Ward J, Lucas N, et al. (2010). Characterisation of the prodrome to a first episode of psychotic mania: results of a retrospective study. *Journal of Affective Disorders* **124**: 341–345.

49. Power P, Elkins K, Adlard S, et al. (1998). Analysis of the initial treatment phase in first-episode psychosis. *British Journal of Psychiatry* **172**(Suppl 33): 71–76.

50. DelBello MP, Hanseman D, Adler CM, et al. (2007). Twelve-month outcome of adolescents with bipolar disorder following first hospitalization for a manic or mixed episode. *American Journal of Psychiatry* **164**: 582–590.

51. Berk M, Conus P, Lucas N, et al. (2007b). Setting the stage: from prodrome to treatment resistance in bipolar disorder. *Bipolar Disorder* **9**: 671–678.

52. Gonzalez S, Artal J, Gomez E, et al. (2012). Early intervention in bipolar disorder: The Jano program at Hospital Universitario Marques de Valdecilla. *Actas Espanolas de Psiquiatria* **40**(2): 51–56.

53. Macmillan I, Howells L, Kale K, et al. (2007). Social and symptomatic outcomes of first-episode bipolar psychoses in an early intervention service. *Early Intervention in Psychiatry* **1**: 79–87.

54. Kessing LV, Hansen HV, Hvenegaard A, et al. (2013). Treatment in a specialised out-patients mood disorder clinic v. standard out-patient treatment in the early course of bipolar disorder: randomised clinical trial. *British Journal of Psychiatry* **202**: 212–219.

55. Lambert M, Conus P, Lubmann DI et al. (2005). The impact of substance abuse disorder on clinical outcome in 643 patients with first episode psychosis. *Acta Psychiatrica Scandinavica* **112**: 141–148.

56. Goodwin GM. (2009). Evidence-based guidelines for treating bipolar disorder: revised second edition – recommendations from the British Association for Psychopharmacology. *Journal of Psychopharmacology* **23**: 346–388.

57. Wijkstra J, Lijmer J, Balk FJ, et al. (2006). Pharmacological treatment for unipolar psychotic depression: Systematic review and meta-analysis. *British Journal of Psychiatry* **188**: 410–415.

58. Calabrese JR, Keck Jr PE, Macfadden W, et al. (2005). A randomized, double-blind, placebo-controlled trial of quetiapine in the treatment of bipolar I or II depression. *American Journal of Psychiatry* **162**: 1351–1360.

59. Conus P, Berk M and McGorry PD. (2006). Pharmacological treatment in the early phase of bipolar disorders: what stage are we at? *Australian and New Zealand Journal of Psychiatry* **40**: 199–207.

60. Lam DH, Burbeck R, Wright K, et al. (2009). Psychological therapies in bipolar disorder: the effect of illness history on relapse prevention – a systematic review. *Bipolar Disorders* **11**: 474–482.

61. Miklowitz DJ. (2006). A review of evidence-based psychosocial interventions for bipolar disorder. *Journal of Clinical Psychiatry* **67**: 28–33.

62. Scott J, Paykel E, Morris R et al. (2006). Cognitive–behavioural therapy for severe and recurrent bipolar disorders: randomised controlled trial. *British Journal of Psychiatry* **188**: 313–320.

63. Colom F. (2008). Long-term follow-up of psychotherapies in bipolar disorder. *Bipolar Disorder* **10**(Suppl 1): 20.

64. Jones SJ and Burrell-Hodgson G. (2008). Cognitive–behavioural treatment of first diagnosis bipolar disorder. *Clinical Psychology and Psychotherapy* **15**: 367–377.

65. Macneil C, Hasty M, Cotton S, et al. (2012). Can a targeted psychological intervention be effective for young people following a first manic episode? Results from an 18-month pilot study. *Early Intervention in Psychiatry* **6**: 380–388.

66. Lam D, McCrone P, Wright K, et al. (2008). Cost-effectiveness of relapse prevention cognitive therapy for bipolar disease: 30-month study. *British Journal of Psychiatry* **186**: 500–506.

67. Macneil C, Hasty M, Conus P, et al. (2009). *Bipolar Disorder in Young People: A Psychological Intervention Manual*. Cambridge: Cambridge University Press.

68. Miklowitz, DJ, Otto MW, Frank E, et al. (2007a). Intensive psychosocial intervention enhances functioning in patients with bipolar depression: results from a 9-month randomized controlled trial. *American Journal of Psychiatry* **164**(9): 1340–1347.

69. Miklowitz DJ and Goldstein MJ. (1997). *Bipolar Disorder: A Family-Focused Treatment Approach*. New York: The Guilford Press.

70. Pope M, Dudley R and Scott J. (2007). Determinants of social functioning in bipolar disorder. *Bipolar Disorders* **9**: 38–44.

71. Martinez-Aran A, Vieta E, Colom F, et al. (2000). Cognitive dysfunction in bipolar disorder: evidence of neuropsychological disturbances. *Psychotherapy and Psychosomatics* **69**: 2–18.

72. Wallace CJ and Tauber R. (2004). Supplementing supported employment with workplace skills training. *Psychiatric Services* **55**(5): 513–515.

22
Early Intervention in Eating Disorders

Leora Pinhas[1,2], Jennifer Wong[1] and D. Blake Woodside[2,3]
[1] Eating Disorders Program, The Hospital for Sick Children, Toronto, Ontario
[2] Department of Psychiatry, University of Toronto, Toronto, Ontario
[3] University Health Network, Toronto, Ontario

Introduction

Advocates of early intervention have argued that increasing the focus on the earlier stages of psychiatric illness improves patient outcomes and reduces costs [1, 2]. Early intervention has been extensively studied in the psychosis population, where the bulk of the evidence suggests that early intervention has just these effects. Such research has significant implications for the design of treatment delivery systems [2]. However, despite the interest in this area, there is controversy about the definition of 'early intervention' [3–5], which includes difficulties in identifying onset and characterising the nature of interventions suitable for earlier stages of illness. Nonetheless, concepts such as duration of untreated illness (DUI) developed to measure the length of time before treatment as part of the understanding of early intervention has been frequently applied to various mental health disorders including psychotic disorders, mood disorders and anxiety disorders [6, 7]. This concept has been useful as a predictor of outcome for many early interventions and research does suggest that earlier interventions in mental health disorders contribute to better overall outcomes [5].

There has been limited research into early intervention in the eating disorder (ED) population. There is therefore no consensus or standard as to what constitutes 'early intervention' in the ED context. While there are no studies specifically investigating treatments designed as early interventions in EDs *per se*, some studies investigating efficacy of various treatment modalities do reveal that earlier age of onset and shorter length of illness are associated with an increased likelihood of recovery. The literature describing the

Early Intervention in Psychiatry: EI of nearly everything for better mental health, First Edition.
Edited by Peter Byrne and Alan Rosen.
© 2014 John Wiley & Sons, Ltd. Published 2014 by John Wiley & Sons, Ltd.

outcomes of ED consists of follow-up (cohort) studies of children, adolescents and adults drawn from a variety of patient populations, including clinical case series or representative population-based surveys or registries, and primarily focus on anorexia nervosa (AN) [8]. To date, there is little to no information on bulimia nervosa (BN) or ED not otherwise specified (EDNOS) and there are no population-based outcome studies in children specifically [8]. DUI has yet to be applied to EDs. As a result, the data presented in the literature are often unclear about whether patients are treatment naive at the time of the study being reported. This makes it difficult to interpret the results of early interventions in EDs.

This chapter will review the data on the effects of early intervention in the treatment of various EDs, including AN, BN, binge-eating disorder (BED) and EDNOS. The evidence-based treatments that are often, although not exclusively, provided as early interventions will be reviewed. The barriers to early intervention will also be discussed.

Anorexia nervosa

AN is a serious and often chronic disorder characterised by very low body weight, intense fear of gaining weight and distorted body image [9]. Estimates of incidence of AN range from 1.6 to 8.3/100,000 person-years [10–15]. Twin birth cohort studies report lifetime prevalences, in women, of 0.51–2.2% [16–18], and in a recent cross-sectional study conducted in the United States with 10,123 adolescents examining prevalence of EDs, it was found that the lifetime prevalence estimates of AN was 0.3% [19] with a median age of onset of 12.3 years. The disorder is approximately 10 times more prevalent in females than in males [9]. Starvation in AN often leads to numerous physical complications and damage to vital organs including the brain and heart [20–27]. AN has one of the highest mortality rates of all psychiatric conditions, with a standardised mortality rate of 6–10 [28–31]. According to the guidelines set out by the American Psychiatric Association (APA), goals to consider when treating AN include restoring healthy weight, enhancing patient motivation to comply with treatment, providing psychoeducation and helping to change core cognitions and attitudes related to the ED [32, 33].

Short duration of illness and early age of onset as predictor variables in anorexia nervosa outcome

There are a small group of studies that examine the outcomes in AN that also provide some information on the effects of early intervention. In a study conducted by Eisler et al. [34], it was found that patients with AN who were less than 18 years of age and had been ill for less than 3 years (mean was 1.2 years) had better outcomes following family therapy treatment [34]. However, AN patients who had the illness for more than 3 years (mean was 5.9 years) had poorer outcomes. There was a clear association between the length of the illness and outcome; patients who had a poor outcome at the end of treatment had been ill for a significantly longer period than those who had a good outcome both at 1- and 5-year follow-ups [35, 36].

In a review conducted by Kreipe et al. (1996) examining the outcomes of three studies where the mean duration of illness prior to the onset of treatment averaged less than 12 months, excellent outcomes were reported. The authors also report that the duration of illness identified in patients treated in the adolescent medicine paediatric programmes is one-half to one-third that of patients treated in the child and adolescent psychiatry programmes, and treatment location (with more complex or chronic patients being seen by psychiatry) may be a significant factor relating to prognosis [37]. Moreover, Hall et al. conducted a follow-up study of 50 patients that they had assessed who were completely healthy at a minimum of 4 years since onset and found that only 20% of the sample were free from any physical or mental health issue. Once again, length of illness was found to be a factor related to outcome, with shorter length of illness predicting a better outcome [38]. One of the problems with this literature is that it is difficult to parse out the DUI as opposed to the duration of illness prior to the treatment that is being described. For example, comparing patients treated by adolescent medicine as compared to psychiatry. The results seem to be confounded by the greater likelihood of patients treated by psychiatry having had a more complex course. So, although they may be new patients to the psychiatry programme, they may have had previous treatment. Borrowing from researchers in psychosis, reporting on duration untreated in AN (DUAN) may improve the analysis and interpretation of the data. This of course would require a definition for the treatment.

Steinhausen [39, 40] addressed age of onset in two review papers. In the first, he compared adolescent subjects with AN to adult subjects with AN. There was a somewhat better global outcome for the adolescent patients in terms of recovery, improvement and chronicity, but there was no consensus on the prognostic value of age at onset. Only in some studies was the age associated with a better outcome [39]. In a more recent study with an expanded literature review [40], outcome in adolescent onset AN more clearly had a lower mortality rate and more favourable outcome, as measured by rates in recovery, improvement and chronicity.

Most studies of adolescents suggest that there are better outcomes compared to adults. Comparing studies of adults and adolescents is confounded by the earlier age of onset of adolescents, along with a tendency towards shorter duration. As a result, some authors believe that the shorter duration of illness is more important than the early onset [41]. Le Grange and Loeb (2007) also propose that adolescents fare better than adults because of the reduced severity and chronicity of their illness. It remains unclear if it is the shorter duration of illness, or early age of onset, or both are the variable(s) of interest.

Treatment of adolescents with anorexia nervosa

In children and adolescents, there are three primary elements to treatment of AN: outpatient-based family therapy, inpatient treatment and psychopharmacotherapy. The National Institute for Health and Clinical Excellence (NICE) guidelines from the United Kingdom suggest that family interventions should be the treatment of choice for adolescents with AN [8, 32]. Family therapy is more effective than individual therapy in producing higher rates of remission and lower rates of relapse and hospital admissions [35, 36, 42, 43].

The best-studied family therapy intervention was originally referred to as the Maudsley method and more recently as family-based treatment or FBT [44]. This is a manualised treatment consisting of three distinct phases. The first phase focuses on helping parents take charge and manage AN-related behaviours; the second phase slowly transitions control of these behaviours back to the adolescent and the third phase focuses on the impact of AN on adolescence. Sessions last around an hour and involve the entire family. The treatment includes approximately 15 sessions delivered over 9 months, initially occurring weekly and less often as time goes on [44].

A number of other models of family therapy have been described in the literature and appear to be effective, however, the studies that exist are limited [45, 46]. One model that has spread throughout Europe and is beginning to make inroads in North America is multifamily therapy (MFT) [36]. This therapy is an intensive group based therapy where six families participate in 4 days of group therapy as families. There are 4–12 one-day follow-up days that are spread out over the course of the next 6–12 months and occur about every 1–2 months [36]. Intensive MFT in the treatment of patients with AN results in dropout rates that are extremely low, roughly 2–3%, and inpatient admission rates reduced by 30%. In addition, length of stay for inpatients has decreased by 25%, while readmissions have been cut in half [45]. In 2001, Scholz and Asen showed (in their preliminary results) that the use of MFT in adolescents with EDs was acceptable to families and produced significant positive changes in symptoms and recovery rates [45]. Currently, there is limited research examining the effectiveness of MFT in relation to symptomatic improvement.

Inpatient care may be required in the course of treatment and generally occurs when a patient is considered to be medically unstable or too ill to respond to outpatient treatment. This regularly does occur early in the course of illness or in the early stages of treatment. In some cases, this can be the first presentation to treatment and does not predict the preceding length of illness. Some adolescents become quite medically unstable very quickly and this can occur soon after onset of illness. Length of stay varies from a few days to weeks or months [47–49]. Treatment is comprised of medical stabilisation and refeeding with the aim of increasing the patient's body weight towards a healthy weight. Treatment also includes other therapeutic interventions, most commonly family, individual, and group therapy [47–49]. Outcomes vary by study, with some predicting a good outcome in the majority of patients at 1-year follow-up [48], while more recent studies suggest as many as 60% of patients have a poor outcome at 1-year follow-up [47] and 8–32% have a poor outcome after 8 years of follow-up [50]. Outcome appears to be predicted by discharge weight, with higher weights predicting a better outcome [47, 48, 50].

Data on the effectiveness of psychotropic medication remain limited. There are no adequate well-designed studies that examine the effect of antidepressants in this population. Case reports and case series suggest that atypical antipsychotics, particularly olanzapine, may be helpful in this population [51–54]. More recent retrospective cohorts [55] and blinded and controlled studies [56] cast doubt on this hypothesis. While there are no reports of unexpected side effects [57], there appears to be no added benefits. However, the sample sizes of these studies are quite small (on average 20 patients) and may not have the statistical power to detect differences [55, 56].

Treatment of adults with anorexia nervosa

In contrast to the progress made with adolescents in recent years, the treatment of AN in adults continues to present a significant challenge. To date, there are no effective evidence-based treatments for adults with AN. The relative rarity of this condition, and the very high dropout rates from treatment studies are the primary barriers to the study of treatment for AN in adults. Completed studies are rare; one recent study examining the utility of fluoxetine on relapse prevention [58] showed no benefit from fluoxetine, but also had a 50% dropout rate, thus making the results difficult to interpret. There is a limited literature examining the correlates of successful inpatient treatment in AN [59, 60], and one small double-blind study suggesting a modest effect of adding olanzapine to inpatient treatment [61]. However, beyond these few papers, a review of the literature documents no evidence of the effectiveness of any specific treatment, psychotherapeutic or pharmaco-logic, for AN. There is no significant data examining the effect of early intervention in AN in adults, and there remains controversy about how to establish and date onset of illness in adults.

There are three sets of treatment guidelines for AN in adults: the APA guidelines [33], the NICE guidelines from Great Britain [32] and RANZCP (Australasian) Clinical Prac-tice Guidelines (CPGs) [62]. These provide recommendations for clinical treatment based on the best available evidence, which is slim. Both sets of guidelines emphasise the need to make a careful treatment plan, with clear goals, and matching the site of treatment to those goals. Outpatient treatment, usually consisting of cognitive-behavioural treatment (CBT) and nutritional advice, is unlikely to provide a benefit except for those patients with milder forms of the illness, although the NICE guidelines recommend an initial course of outpa-tient management. It is expected that patients with more than mild illness will require more intensive treatment, either in a residential or a partial hospitalisation setting.

Most intensive programmes have similar combinations of elements—behavioural change elements, including weight gain and normalised eating, and various types of psy-chological treatments. There is no clear evidence as to the optimal 'basket' of such addi-tional treatments. Treatments that do not include weight gain and nutritional rehabilita-tion are not recommended. A rate of weight gain of 1.0 kg/week is typical for intensive treatment. There is no evidence that slower rates of weight gain are beneficial in intensive treatment settings.

Bulimia nervosa

BN is characterised by episodes of binge eating followed by purging. There is a sense of loss of control with the binge eating and episodes of bingeing and purging occur at least twice a week for at least 3 months [9]. Prevalence rates of BN have been found to be higher than that of AN. In a review of epidemiological studies conducted by Hsu [63], it was reported that the prevalence of AN in women was found to be about 0.2–0.5%, and BN to be about 2–3% and can be as high as 10% in vulnerable populations, such as college-aged women [63, 64]. In a cross-sectional study conducted in the United States with 10,123 adolescents examining prevalence of EDs, it was found that the lifetime prevalence estimates of BN was 0.9%, with a median age of onset of 12.4 years [19]. BN is more common than AN, but the mortality rate is lower and the recovery rate higher than that of AN [65]. In a review conducted by Steinhausen and Weber (2009) examining published outcome stud-ies of BN from 1981 to 2007, it was determined that mean rates for recovery, improvement and chronicity ranged from 42.4% to 59.9%, 27% to 41.3% and 22.6% to 50.8%, respec-tively. Keel and Mitchell [65] found that 50% of patients previously diagnosed with BN are recovered 5 years after treatment.

Epidemiologic studies have reported that the highest incidence rates for BN are among females aged 20–24 years [66]. Typical age of onset has been reported to occur during young adulthood, with few cases starting during adolescence, which is in contrast to AN, where the onset after 25 years is less common [66].

Short duration of treatment and early age of onset as predictor variables in bulimia nervosa

The literature examining outcomes in patients with BN is scarce and has significant methodological shortcomings. In a systematic review conducted by Reas et al. [67] examining the prognostic value of duration of illness in BN and early intervention in BN, only five studies met inclusion criteria. Of the five studies that met methodological criteria for inclusion in the systematic review, only one of the studies found a significant negative association between the duration of illness and outcome. The other four studies in this systematic review [67] revealed no differences in duration of illness between those who had recovered at follow-up and those who did not. Steinhausen and Weber's (2009) review of 79 studies examining outcomes in BN revealed that duration of illness had been assessed in most of the studies, but found no effect on the course of illness. Most of the studies failed to find a significant association between age at onset and outcome. There is no consistent evidence to support that illness duration and age of onset results in better outcomes in BN. Once again, the lack of evidence to support early intervention may be due to the paucity of adequate research or possibly, once again, the failure to differentiate between duration of untreated BN (DUBN) from duration of BN.

Treatment in adolescents with bulimia nervosa

The evidence-based literature in the treatment of adolescents with BN is limited to a handful of studies. This is not surprising, given the later mean age of onset for BN. As in AN, family therapy, specifically FBT, appears to be an effective form of treatment for this population, with better outcomes at 6-month follow-up [68]. Family therapy has a similar outcome at 1-year follow-up to CBT-guided self-care [69]. A case series examining CBT in adolescents with bulimia reported that while some changes need to be made to account for developmental differences, with good adherence to treatment, an abstinence rate of 56% for binge eating and purging could be achieved [70].

The psychopharmacologic literature in BN in adolescence is very limited, with only 1 open trial examining 10 adolescents treated with fluoxetine [71, 72]. A confound in this literature is that older adolescents are typically included in adult medication trials, and their response is not described separately from the adults in the studies. Kotler et al. [71] examined 8 weeks of acute therapy with fluoxetine in 10 adolescents (average age 16.2 ± 1.2 years) with BN. The primary outcome measures were frequencies of binge eating and purging. Average weekly binges decreased significantly from 4.1 ± 3.8 to 0 ($p < 0.01$) and average weekly purges decreased significantly from 6.4 ± 5.2 to 0.4 ± 0.9 ($p < 0.005$).

Treatment in adults with bulimia nervosa

In contrast to AN, there are effective evidence treatments for BN in adults. This is may be in part due to the higher incidence of BN, which allows for easier recruitment into studies. There is evidence for the efficacy of self-help and psychoeducational treatments as a first step in the course of outpatient treatment of BN [73] regardless of the length of illness. CBT for BN has been extensively studied and has excellent efficacy [74]. Other forms of psychotherapy, such as interpersonal therapy (IPT), or dialectical behaviour therapy (DBT) [75] have also been studied and found to be as efficacious as CBT. However, response to IPT may be slower than CBT [74]. There is no evidence for the efficacy of psychodynamic psychotherapy as a treatment for BN and there is limited evidence supporting the efficacy of nutritional therapy alone in the treatment of BN.

The majority of patients with BN will respond to evidence-based, manualised outpatient psychotherapeutic approaches and, as is the case with manualised treatments, the best outcomes are achieved when treatment delivered adheres to the manual and is not altered [74]. A subset of patients will require a more intensive intervention. Day or partial hospitalisation can be an effective treatment for more severe cases of BN with approximately 50% of patients successfully completing the programme and about 50–70% [76, 77] remaining in remission upon follow-up of 1.5–2 years [78] These programmes will typically include nutritional rehabilitative approaches to reduce the dieting behaviours that are associated with binge eating, and additional psychotherapeutic elements thought to be helpful in assisting with the process of change or in preventing relapse [78]. Again, as is the case with AN, there is no evidence to support the inclusion or exclusion of specific psychotherapeutic elements in more intensive settings, although most will include CBT in one form or another. Treatments that encourage or support dieting behaviours are contraindicated in the treatment of BN.

Pharmacologic treatments have a role in BN. There is a fairly extensive literature on the use of antidepressants. The evidence suggests that most antidepressants, including selective serotonin reuptake inhibitors (SSRI), tricyclic antidepressants and monoamine oxidase inhibitors can be useful in the treatment of BN and can result in clinical improvement and even remission in some cases [79–81]. Most commonly, SSRIs are used in BN because of their more favourable side-effect profile [79–81]. SSRIs reliably cause a reduction in the intensity of the urge to binge, which may than assist patients in feeling more comfortable in experimenting with more normal eating habits without the fear that a normal meal might turn into a binge [82]. The medication is not a panacea, and will work best in conjunction with other evidence-based treatments such as CBT. There is no evidence for an enhanced benefit of one SSRI versus another or one class of antidepressant over another [79–81]. There is no evidence for the use of anxiolytics or antipsychotics in this population.

Binge-eating disorder

BED is characterised by binge eating that occurs twice a week for a minimum of 6 months and is not accompanied by purging behaviour [9]. It has only recently appeared in the DSM-IV (1994) and is listed under the category of EDNOS. The lifetime prevalence of BED in adults has been estimated to be 2.8%, with a higher prevalence found amongst women [83]. Approximately 3.5% of women and 2% of men reported having BED at some point in their lives [83]. The mean age of onset is older in BED and occurs between the ages of 22 and 25 years [83]. The course and outcome of BED is similar to that of BN with a standarised mortality ratio of 2.29 with 67.2% of patients being free of an ED diagnosis and 37.1% having a good outcome at 12-years follow-up [84].

There is limited data about the prevalence of BED in adolescents. Recent community-based surveys suggest that BED occurs in 1–2% of children and adolescents between the ages of 10 and 19 [85]. In one cross-sectional study conducted in the United States among American adolescents aged 13–18 years, the lifetime prevalence of BED was reported as 1.6%, with an average age of onset at 12.6 years and a higher incidence in girls [19]. In this same study, there was also a trend towards higher rates of BED in ethnic minorities. This same study found that among those with BED, 72.6% sought some form of treatment for other emotional or behavioural problems, but a much smaller proportion, 11.4%, sought treatment for their BED. BED differs from AN and/or BN in that more males suffer from this disorder [23]. Approximately 36% of obese patients with BED are males [86].

There is no literature on early interventions in BED for adolescents or adults. In fact, the evidence-based literature on treatment in adolescents with BED *per se*, is virtually non-existent.

Treatment of adults with binge-eating disorder

While there are effective evidence-based treatments for BED, caution must be exercised in interpreting these studies as many of the symptoms of BED are highly variable in frequency within the same patients, and placebo response rates can be high. It is also important to point out that the nature of the treatments for BED is significantly different than for BN, despite both illnesses sharing the symptom of binge eating. While the bingeing of BN is most often thought to be a response to hunger and dieting, the binge eating of BED is more related to satiety and self-soothing. So, while patients with BN need to be taught to reduce the rigid dietary restraint that leads to binge eating, patients with BED need to be taught to restrain their eating to a greater degree. Programmes that combine these two patient groups may find it difficult to manage the conflicting messages about dietary restraint required to treat the two groups.

There is good evidence for the effectiveness of manualised, evidence-based self-help in BED [87]. A specific variant of CBT, called CBT-BED, has also been found to be effective in the treatment of BED, as has IPT [88]. It is important for clinicians to ensure that patients with BED are aware that evidence-based treatments for BED are unlikely to have a significant effect of weight, and specifically are unlikely to produce rapid weight loss.

There is some evidence for the efficacy of pharmacotherapy in BED in adults, but again the results need to be viewed with some caution as many such trials have been industry funded and the amount of weight lost during the trials seems to be emphasised. Once again as with BN, antidepressants in general seem to provide some clinical improvement with the most common antidepressants in use being the SSRIs [89]. Anticonvulsants [90] also seem to have reasonable efficacy, although side effects may be at issue. Many of these results need to be interpreted with some caution as there have been some ongoing debates about illness definition, and there is room for more data from newer trials.

Eating disorder not otherwise specified

EDNOS is a residual category for those patients who do not meet full criteria for AN or BN, but are thought clinically to have meaningful problems with their eating. Research suggests that a very large proportion of patients in treatment setting have EDNOS [91–93], and that the prevalence in the community is high as well, ranging from 1.84 to 12% depending on the study [94]. The heterogeneity of this patient population makes it virtually impossible to study, and within the field, the main effort is focused on revising the diagnostic criteria to 'drain the EDNOS swamp' [95].

Duration of illness and eating disorders

DUI has yet to be applied to EDs, but has the potential to inform how early intervention in EDs may affect outcome. The work done in other areas of mental health can be used to inform the development of this much needed concept in EDs. Duration of untreated psychosis (DUP), the most extensively used predictor of this type, often refers to the time between onset of psychotic symptoms and start of antipsychotic medication [6, 7, 96]. Other models have considered such ideas as delay in intensive psychosocial treatment (DIPT) in the psychotic population as an associated potential predictor of outcome recognising that more than psychotropic medication plays a role in outcome [97]. Finally, over time it has become clear that DUP itself is comprised of various components and each of these components may play a different role in outcome [98, 99].

To apply these concepts to EDs, requires some modifications. First line treatment is not medication, but, psychotherapy and when necessary the stabilisation of nutritional status, with medication being more of an adjunctive treatment (see Table 22.1). Again as in psychosis, duration of untreated eating disorder (DUED), either DUAN or DUBN, has a number of potential components, all of which represent potential times where patients may experience a lag time or a barrier to access to treatment (see Table 22.1 and Figure 22.1). These categories are only conceptual at this stage and will require rigorous study before they can be reliably used to plan for early interventions or predict outcomes.

Barriers to early intervention

A number of barriers also impact access to care. At most, only about 30–50% of the individuals who struggle with an ED receive treatment [100–102]. Financial barriers are common in countries without publicly funded health care [100]. Low patient motivation may also impede access to care, as many patients choose not to seek treatment, even when recommended through a screening programme [102] patients also endorse perceived stigma (or shame) and social stereotyping, both within social networks and among clinicians as impacting access to care [103].

A significant barrier to the study of early intervention is the difficulty with early detection. General practitioners are at the forefront of early detection in the primary care setting. They are more likely to encounter patients with early/developing ED symptoms. Patients presenting in specialist clinics with EDs have often had a long duration of illness and it has been reported that although patients concealed their eating problems for many years, they had frequently consulted their general practitioner for secondary complications of the disorder [104]. The challenges of diagnosing cases of EDs in the primary care setting has been illustrated in two surveys of GPs, which found that they were unaware of the ED diagnosis in up to 50% of patients discovered by the researcher [104, 105]. Cases of EDs unknown to the general practitioner are common in general practice and go undetected even when a specialist is accessed for secondary complications of the ED

Table 22.1 Suggested definitions for duration of untreated illness time periods in EDs

Time period	Abbreviation	Definition
Duration untreated eating disorder	DUED	Duration of illness from first symptom to start of psychological treatment (e.g. CBT or FT)
Duration untreated with anorexia nervosa	DUAN	Duration of illness from first symptom to start of psychological treatment (e.g. CBT or FT)
Duration untreated with bulimia nervosa	DUBN	Duration of illness from first symptom to start of psychological treatment (e.g. CBT or FT)
Duration of untreated restriction	DUR	Duration of restriction from the start of successful restriction to the beginning of refeeding treatment
Duration of untreated purging	DUP	Duration of untreated purging from the first episode of purging to the beginning of medical treatment, that includes the monitoring and correction of the medical consequences of purging
Duration untreated with psychotropic medication	DUPMed	Duration of time from first symptoms of eating disorder to first medication trial
Time components along mental health treatment pathway		
Duration untreated to primary care	DUPC	Duration of illness from first symptom to attending primary care physician
Delay in referral to mental health care	DIRMH	Duration of time from first contact at primary care practice until referral is made to mental health programme
Delay due to waitlist	DWL	Duration of time when referral is made until patient is assessed by mental health Programme
Delay to mental health treatment	DIMH	Duration of time from mental health assessment until the first session of mental health treatment (psychological)
Duration until mental health team prescribes adjunctive medication	DUAdjMed	Duration of time from start of mental health assessment until start of psychotropic medication
Time components along medical treatment pathway		
Delay in referral to medical care	DIRMC	Duration of time from first contact at primary care practice until referral is made to medical treatment programme
Delay due to medical waitlist	DMWL	Duration of time when referral is made until patient is assessed by medical programme
Delay to medical treatment	DIMT	Duration of time from medical assessment until the first medical intervention by specialist medical treatment (may include inpatient treatment or refeeding)
Duration until medical team prescribes adjunctive medication	DUAdjMT	Duration of time from start of medical assessment until start of psychotropic medication when prescribed by medical doctor/paediatrician.

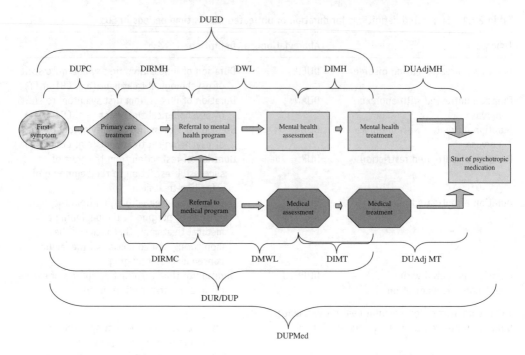

Figure 22.1   Components of untreated time periods along treatment path

[104, 106], regardless of the potential for early intervention and earlier age at diagnosis resulting in improved outcomes in patients with EDs [107].

It has been suggested that all high-risk patients presenting in primary care should be screened during routine office visits, and that the medical history is the most powerful tool for diagnosing EDs; physical examination and laboratory results might be normal [108]. The SCOFF questionnaire [109] has been suggested as a practical screening tool in the primary care setting, this tool consists of five yes/no questions. In countries where GPs are available and readily accessible, they have the potential to play a critical role in early detection, with the capability of initiating treatment before the illness becomes chronic; however, the literature suggests a need for better education and support.

Conclusion

The concept of early intervention in EDs is still in its infancy. While the literature suggests that early intervention predicts a better outcome for some disorders, it is still not clear what early intervention entails. Should there be specifically tailored treatments for early stage illness, or should patients receive the same treatment with the goal being better screening services that identify patients earlier? The data to answer this question simply does not exist. Even the definition for early or mild EDs has not been fully developed, with the criteria typically focused on medical or physiologic symptoms rather than psychological severity [110]. Early intervention in EDs must become a research priority if we are ever to better understand its role in treatment and recovery in this complex and commonly poorly served population.

References

1. Knapp M and Parsonage M. (2011). Mental health promotion and mental illness prevention. In: Do Health (ed.), *The Economic Case*. London: Department of Health.
2. Joseph R and Birchwood M. (2005). The national policy reforms for mental health services and the story of early intervention services in the United Kingdom. *Journal of Psychiatry and Neuroscience* **30**(5): 362–365.
3. Singh SP and Fisher HL. (2005). Early intervention in psychosis: obstacles and opportunities. *Advances in Psychiatric Treatment* **11**(1): 71–78.
4. Birchwood M, Todd P and Jackson C. (1998). Early intervention in psychosis. The critical period hypothesis. *British Journal of Psychiatry. Supplement* **172**(33): 53–59.
5. Treasure J and Russell G. (2011). The case for early intervention in anorexia nervosa: theoretical exploration of maintaining factors. *British Journal of Psychiatry* **199**: 5–7.
6. Perkins DO, Gu H, Boteva K, et al. (2005). Relationship between duration of untreated psychosis and outcome in first-episode schizophrenia: a critical review and meta-analysis. *American Journal of Psychiatry* **162**(10): 1785–1804.
7. Compton MT, Carter T, Bergner E, et al. (2007). Defining, operationalizing and measuring the duration of untreated psychosis: advances, limitations and future directions. *Early Intervention in Psychiatry* **1**(3): 236–250.
8. Norris M, Bondy S and Pinhas L. (2011). Epidemiology of eating disorders in children and adolescents. In: D Le Grange, J Lock, (eds), *Eating Disorders in Children and Adolescents: A Clinical Handbook*. New York: Guilford Press.
9. American Psychiatric Association. (2000). *Diagnostic and Statistical Manual of Mental Disorders: DSM-IV-TR*, 4th edition. Washington, DC: American Psychiatric Association.
10. Pagsberg AK and Wang AR. (1994). Epidemiology of anorexia nervosa and bulimia nervosa in Bornholm County, Denmark, 1970-1989. *Acta Psychiatrica Scandinavica* **90**(4): 259–265.
11. Currin L, Schmidt U, Treasure J, et al. (2005). Time trends in eating disorder incidence. *British Journal of Psychiatry* **186**: 132–135.
12. Joergensen J. (1992). The epidemiology of eating disorders in Fyn County, Denmark, 1977-1986. *Acta Psychiatrica Scandinavica* **85**(1): 30–34.
13. Turnbull S, Ward A, Treasure J, et al. (1996). The demand for eating disorder care. An epidemiological study using the general practice research database. *British Journal of Psychiatry* **169**(6): 705–712.
14. van Son GE, van Hoeken D, Bartelds AI, et al. (2006). Time trends in the incidence of eating disorders: a primary care study in the Netherlands. *International Journal of Eating Disorders* **39**(7): 565–569.
15. Lucas AR, Crowson CS, O'Fallon WM, et al. (1999). The ups and downs of anorexia nervosa. *International Journal of Eating Disorders* **26**(4): 397–405.
16. Keski-Rahkonen A, Bulik CM, Pietilainen KH, et al. (2007). Eating styles, overweight and obesity in young adult twins. *European Journal of Clinical Nutrition* **61**(7): 822–829.
17. Keski-Rahkonen A, Hoek HW, Linna MS, et al. (2009). Incidence and outcomes of bulimia nervosa: a nationwide population-based study. *Psychological Medicine* **39**(5): 823–831.
18. Walters EE and Kendler KS. (1995). Anorexia nervosa and anorexic-like syndromes in a population-based female twin sample. *American Journal of Psychiatry* **152**(1): 64–71.
19. Swanson SA, Crow SJ, Le Grange D, et al. (2011). Prevalence and correlates of eating disorders in adolescents. Results from the national comorbidity survey replication adolescent supplement. *Archives of General Psychiatry* **68**(7): 714–723.
20. Palla B and Litt IF. (1988). Medical complications of eating disorders in adolescents. *Pediatrics* **81**(5): 613–623.
21. Mitchell JE, Pyle RL, Eckert ED, et al. (1983). Electrolyte and other physiological abnormalities in patients with bulimia. *Psychological Medicine* **13**(2): 273–278.

22. Mehler PS and Krantz M. (2003). Anorexia nervosa medical issues. *Journal of Women's Health* **12**(4): 331–340.

23. Schneider M. (2003). Bulimia nervosa and binge-eating disorder in adolescents. *Adolescent Medicine State of the Art Reviews* **14**(1): 119–131.

24. Kohn MR, Golden NH and Shenker IR. (1998). Cardiac arrest and delirium: presentations of the refeeding syndrome in severely malnourished adolescents with anorexia nervosa. *Journal of Adolescent Health* **22**(3): 239–243.

25. Olivares JL, Vazquez M, Fleta J, et al. (2005). Cardiac findings in adolescents with anorexia nervosa at diagnosis and after weight restoration. *European Journal of Pediatrics* **164**(6): 383–386.

26. Chui HT, Christensen BK, Zipursky RB, et al. (2008). Cognitive function and brain structure in females with a history of adolescent-onset anorexia nervosa. *Pediatrics* **122**(2): e426–e437.

27. Katzman DK. (2005). Medical complications in adolescents with anorexia nervosa: a review of the literature. *International Journal of Eating Disorders* **37**(Suppl): S52–S59; discussion S87–S89.

28. Papadopoulos FC, Ekbom A, Brandt L, et al. (2009). Excess mortality, causes of death and prognostic factors in anorexia nervosa. *British Journal of Psychiatry* **194**(1): 10–17.

29. Moller-Madsen S, Nystrup J, Nielsen S. (1996). Mortality in anorexia nervosa in Denmark during the period 1970-1987. *Acta Psychiatrica Scandinavica* **94**(6): 454–459.

30. Signorini A, De Filippo E, Panico S, et al. (2007). Long-term mortality in anorexia nervosa: a report after an 8-year follow-up and a review of the most recent literature. *European Journal of Clinical Nutrition* **61**(1): 119–122.

31. Rosling AM, Sparén P, Norring C, et al. (2010). Mortality of eating disorders: A follow-up study of treatment in a specialist unit 1974–2000. *International Journal of Eating Disorders* **44**(4): 304–310.

32. National Institute for Clinical Excellence. (2004). Eating disorders: Core interventions in the treatment and management of anorexia nervosa, bulimia nervosa and related eating disorders. *National Clinical Practice Guideline* Number CG9 [serial on the Internet]: http://www.nice.org.uk/nicemedia/live/10932/29220/29220.pdf (November 2011).

33. American Psychiatric Association. American Psychiatric Association Practice Guidelines for the Treatment of Psychiatric Disorders: Compendium 2006. http://www.psychiatryonline.com/pracGuide/pracGuideHome.aspx (November 2011).

34. Eisler I, Dare C, Russell GF, et al. (1997). Family and individual therapy in anorexia nervosa. A 5-year follow-up. *Archives of General Psychiatry* **54**(11): 1025–1030.

35. Eisler I, Simic M, Russell GFM, et al. (2007). A randomised controlled treatment trial of two forms of family therapy in adolescent anorexia nervosa: a five-year follow-up. *Journal of Child Psychology and Psychiatry* **48**(6): 552–560.

36. Eisler I. (2005). The empirical and theoretical base of family therapy and multiple family day therapy for adolescent anorexia nervosa. *Journal of Family Therapy* **27**(2): 104–131.

37. Kreipe RE and Dukarm CP. (1999). Eating disorders in adolescents and older children. *Pediatrics in Review* **20**(12): 410–421.

38. Hall A, Slim E, Hawker F, et al. (1984). Anorexia nervosa: long-term outcome in 50 female patients. *British Journal of Psychiatry* **145**: 407–413.

39. Steinhausen HC. (1997). Outcome of anorexia nervosa in the younger patient. *Journal of Child Psychology & Psychiatry & Allied Disciplines* **38**(3): 271–276.

40. Steinhausen HC. (2002). The outcome of anorexia nervosa in the 20th century. *American Journal of Psychiatry* **159**(8): 1284–1293.

41. Guarda AS. (2008). Treatment of anorexia nervosa: insights and obstacles. *Physiology and Behavior* **94**(1): 113–120.

42. Eisler I, Dare C, Hodes M, et al. (2000). Family therapy for adolescent anorexia nervosa: the results of a controlled comparison of two family interventions. *Journal of Child Psychology & Psychiatry & Allied Disciplines* **41**(6): 727–736.

43. Lock J, Le Grange D, Agras WS, et al. (2010). Randomized clinical trial comparing family-based treatment with adolescent-focused individual therapy for adolescents with anorexia nervosa. *Archives of General Psychiatry* **67**(10): 1025–1032.

44. Lock J. (2011). Evaluation of family treatment models for eating disorders. *Current Opinion in Psychiatry* **24**(4): 274–279 doi: 10.1097/YCO.0b013e 328346f71e.

45. Scholz M and Asen E. (2001). Multiple family therapy with eating disordered adolescents: concepts and preliminary results. *European Eating Disorders Review* **9**(1): 33–42.

46. Rockwell RE, Boutelle K, Trunko ME, et al. (2011). An innovative short-term, intensive, family-based treatment for adolescent anorexia nervosa: case series. *European Eating Disorders Review* **19**(4): 362–367.

47. Salbach-Andrae H, Schneider N, Seifert K, et al. (2009). Short-term outcome of anorexia nervosa in adolescents after inpatient treatment: a prospective study. *European Child & Adolescent Psychiatry* **18**(11): 701–704.

48. Lock J and Litt I. (2003). What predicts maintenance of weight for adolescents medically hospitalized for anorexia nervosa? *Eating Disorders* **11**(1): 1–7.

49. Strik Lievers L, Curt F, Wallier J, et al. (2009). Predictive factors of length of inpatient treatment in anorexia nervosa. *European Child & Adolescent Psychiatry* **18**(2): 75–84.

50. Steinhausen H-C. (2009). Outcome of eating disorders. *Child & Adolescent Psychiatric Clinics of North America* **18**(1): 225–242.

51. Leggero C, Masi G, Brunori E, et al. (2010). Low-dose olanzapine monotherapy in girls with anorexia nervosa, restricting subtype: focus on hyperactivity. *Journal of Child and Adolescent Psychopharmacology* **20**(2): 127–133.

52. Boachie A, Goldfield GS and Spettigue W. (2003). Olanzapine use as an adjunctive treatment for hospitalized children with anorexia nervosa: case reports. *International Journal of Eating Disorders* **33**(1): 98–103.

53. Mehler C, Wewetzer C, Schulze U, et al. (2001). Olanzapine in children and adolescents with chronic anorexia nervosa. A study of five cases. *European Child & Adolescent Psychiatry* **10**(2): 151–157.

54. Dennis K, Le Grange D and Bremer J. (2006). Olanzapine use in adolescent anorexia nervosa. *Eating and Weight Disorders : EWD* **11**(2): e53–e56.

55. Norris ML, Spettigue W, Buchholz A, et al. (2011). Olanzapine use for the adjunctive treatment of adolescents with anorexia nervosa. *Journal of Child and Adolescent Psychopharmacology* **21**(3): 213–220.

56. Kafantaris V, Leigh E, Hertz S, et al. (2011). A placebo-controlled pilot study of adjunctive olanzapine for adolescents with anorexia nervosa. *Journal of Child and Adolescent Psychopharmacology* **21**(3): 207–212.

57. Swenne I and Rosling A. (2011). No unexpected adverse events and biochemical side effects of olanzapine as adjunct treatment in adolescent girls with eating disorders. *Journal of Child and Adolescent Psychopharmacology* **21**(3): 221–227.

58. Walsh BT, Kaplan AS, Attia E, et al. (2006). Fluoxetine after weight restoration in anorexia nervosa: a randomized controlled trial. *JAMA: The Journal of the American Medical Association* **295**(22): 2605–2612.

59. Woodside DB, Carter JC and Blackmore E. (2004). Predictors of premature termination of inpatient treatment for anorexia nervosa. *American Journal of Psychiatry* **161**(12): 2277–2281.

60. Carter JC, Blackmore E, Sutandar-Pinnock K, et al. (2004). Relapse in anorexia nervosa: a survival analysis. *Psychological Medicine* **34**(4): 671–679.

61. Bissada H, Tasca GA, Barber AM, et al. (2008). Olanzapine in the treatment of low body weight and obsessive thinking in women with anorexia nervosa: a randomized, double-blind, placebo-controlled trial. *American Journal of Psychiatry* **165**(10): 1281–1288.

62. The Royal Australian & New Zealand College of Psychiatrists. (2009). Consumer and Carer Clinical Practice Guidelines. http://www.ranzcp.org/resources/clinical-practice-guidelines.html (November 2011).

63. Hsu LK. (1996). Epidemiology of the eating disorders. *Psychiatric Clinics of North America* **19**(4): 681–700.

64. Rushing JM, Jones LE and Carney CP. (2003). Bulimia nervosa: a primary care review. *Primary Care Companion to the Journal of Clinical Psychiatry* **5**(5): 217–224.

65. Keel P and Mitchell J. (1997). Outcome in bulimia nervosa. *American Journal of Psychiatry* **154**(3): 313–321.

66. Favaro A, Caregaro L, Tenconi E, et al. (2009). Time trends in age at onset of anorexia nervosa and bulimia nervosa. *Journal of Clinical Psychiatry* **70**(12): 1715–1721.

67. Reas DL, Schoemaker C, Zipfel S, et al. (2001). Prognostic value of duration of illness and early intervention in bulimia nervosa: a systematic review of the outcome literature. *International Journal of Eating Disorders* **30**(1): 1–10.

68. le Grange D, Crosby RD, Rathouz PJ, et al. (2007). A randomized controlled comparison of family-based treatment and supportive psychotherapy for adolescent bulimia nervosa. *Archives of General Psychiatry* **64**(9): 1049–1056.

69. Schmidt U, Lee S, Beecham J, et al. (2007). A randomized controlled trial of family therapy and cognitive behavior therapy guided self-care for adolescents with bulimia nervosa and related disorders. *American Journal of Psychiatry* **164**(4): 591–598.

70. Lock J. (2005). Adjusting cognitive behavior therapy for adolescents with bulimia nervosa: results of case series. *American Journal of Psychotherapy* **59**(3): 267–281.

71. Kotler LA, Devlin MJ, Davies M, et al. (2003). An open trial of fluoxetine for adolescents with bulimia nervosa. *Journal of Child & Adolescent Psychopharmacology* **13**(3):329–335.

72. Flament MF, Bissada H, and Spettigue W. (2011). Evidence-based pharmacotherapy of eating disorders. *International Journal of neuropsychopharmacology* **18**: 1–19.

73. Carter JC, Olmsted MP, Kaplan AS, et al. (2003). Self-help for bulimia nervosa: a randomized controlled trial. *American Journal of Psychiatry* **160**(5): 973–978.

74. Agras WS, Crow SJ, Halmi KA, et al. (2000). Outcome predictors for the cognitive behavior treatment of bulimia nervosa: data from a multisite study. *American Journal of Psychiatry* **157**(8): 1302–1308.

75. Safer DL, Lively TJ, Telch CF, et al. (2002). Predictors of relapse following successful dialectical behavior therapy for binge eating disorder. *International Journal of Eating Disorders* **32**(2): 155–163.

76. Dancyger I, Fornari V, Schneider M, et al. (2003). Adolescents and eating disorders: an examination of a day treatment program. *Eating and Weight Disorders: EWD* **8**(3): 242–248.

77. Zeeck A, Herzog T, and Hartmann A. (2004). Day clinic or inpatient care for severe bulimia nervosa? *European Eating Disorders Review* **12**(2): 79–86.

78. Olmsted MP, Kaplan AS, and Rockert W. (2003). Relative efficacy of a 4-day versus a 5-day day hospital program. *International Journal of Eating Disorders* **34**(4): 441–449.

79. Bacaltchuk J and Hay P. (2003). Antidepressants versus placebo for people with bulimia nervosa. *The Cochrane Database of Systematic Reviews* (**4**): CD 003391.

80. Bacaltchuk J and Hay P. (2001). Antidepressants versus placebo for people with bulimia nervosa. *The Cochrane Database of Systematic Reviews* (**4**): CD 003391.

81. Arroll B, Elley CR, Fishman T, et al. (2009). Antidepressants versus placebo for depression in primary care. *The Cochrane Database of Systematic Reviews* (**3**): CD 007954.

82. Romano SJ, Halmi KA, Sarkar NP, et al. (2002). A placebo-controlled study of fluoxetine in continued treatment of bulimia nervosa after successful acute fluoxetine treatment. *American Journal of Psychiatry* **159**(1): 96–102.

83. Hudson JI, Hiripi E, Pope HG Jr, et al. (2007). The prevalence and correlates of eating disorders in the National Comorbidity Survey Replication. *Biological Psychiatry* **61**(3): 348–358.

84. Fichter MM and Quadflieg N. (2007). Long-term stability of eating disorder diagnoses. *International Journal of Eating Disorders* **40**(Suppl): S61–S66.

85. Johnson WG, Rohan KJ and Kirk AA. (2002). Prevalence and correlates of binge eating in white and African American adolescents. *Eating Behaviors* **3**(2): 179–189.

86. Striegel-Moore RH, Wilson GT, Wilfley DE, et al. (1998). Binge eating in an obese community sample. *International Journal of Eating Disorders* **23**(1): 27–37.
87. Carter JC and Fairburn CG. (1998). Cognitive-behavioral self-help for binge eating disorder: a controlled effectiveness study. *Journal of Consulting and Clinical Psychology* **66**(4): 616–623.
88. Wilfley DE, Welch RR, Stein RI, et al. (2002). A randomized comparison of group cognitive-behavioral therapy and group interpersonal psychotherapy for the treatment of overweight individuals with binge-eating disorder. *Archives of General Psychiatry* **59**(8): 713–721.
89. Marcus MD, Wing RR, Ewing L, et al. (1990). A double-blind, placebo-controlled trial of fluoxetine plus behavior modification in the treatment of obese binge-eaters and non-binge-eaters. *American Journal of Psychiatry* **147**(7): 876–881.
90. McElroy SL, Hudson JI, Malhotra S, et al. (2003). Citalopram in the treatment of binge-eating disorder: a placebo-controlled trial. *Journal of Clinical Psychiatry* **64**(7): 807–813.
91. Ricca V, Mannucci E, Mezzani B, et al. (2001). Fluoxetine and fluvoxamine combined with individual cognitive-behaviour therapy in binge eating disorder: a one-year follow-up study. *Psychotherapy & Psychosomatics* **70**(6): 298–306.
92. Fairburn CG and Bohn K. (2005). Eating disorder NOS (EDNOS): an example of the troublesome "not otherwise specified" (NOS) category in DSM-IV. *Behaviour Research and Therapy* **43**(6): 691–701.
93. Turner H and Bryant-Waugh R. (2004). Eating disorder not otherwise specified (EDNOS): profiles of clients presenting at a community eating disorder service. *European Eating Disorders Review* **12**(1): 18–26.
94. Norris M, Bondy S and Pinhas L. (Forthcoming). Epidemiology of eating disorders in children and adolescents. In: J Lock (ed.), *The Oxford Handbook of Child and Adolescent Eating Disorders*. Oxford: Oxford University Press.
95. Sysko R and Walsh BT. (2011). Does the broad categories for the diagnosis of eating disorders (BCD-ED) scheme reduce the frequency of eating disorder not otherwise specified? *International Journal of Eating Disorders* **44**(7): 625–629.
96. Altamura AC, Dell'osso B, D'Urso N, et al. (2008). Duration of untreated illness as a predictor of treatment response and clinical course in generalized anxiety disorder. *CNS Spectrums* **13**(5): 415–422.
97. de Haan L, Linszen DH, Lenior ME, et al. (2003). Duration of untreated psychosis and outcome of schizophrenia: delay in intensive psychosocial treatment versus delay in treatment with antipsychotic medication. *Schizophrenia Bulletin* **29**(2): 341–348.
98. Keshavan MS, Haas G, Miewald J, et al. (2003). Prolonged untreated illness duration from prodromal onset predicts outcome in first episode psychoses. *Schizophrenia Bulletin* **29**(4): 757–769.
99. Brunet K, Birchwood M, Lester H, et al. (2007). Delays in mental health services and duration of untreated psychosis. *Psychiatric Bulletin* **31**(11): 408–410.
100. Cachelin FM, Rebeck R, Veisel C, et al. (2001). Barriers to treatment for eating disorders among ethnically diverse women. *International Journal of Eating Disorders* **30**(3): 269–278.
101. Cachelin FM and Striegel-Moore RH. (2006). Help seeking and barriers to treatment in a community sample of Mexican American and European American women with eating disorders. *International Journal of Eating Disorders* **39**(2): 154–161.
102. Becker AE, Franko DL, Nussbaum K, et al. (2004). Secondary prevention for eating disorders: the impact of education, screening, and referral in a college-based screening program. *International Journal of Eating Disorders* **36**(2): 157–162.
103. Becker AE, Hadley Arrindell A, Perloe A, et al. (2010). A qualitative study of perceived social barriers to care for eating disorders: perspectives from ethnically diverse health care consumers. *International Journal of Eating Disorders* **43**(7): 633–647.
104. Whitehouse AM, Cooper PJ, Vize CV, et al. (1992). Prevalence of eating disorders in three Cambridge general practices: hidden and conspicuous morbidity. *British Journal of General Practice* **42**(355): 57–60.

105. King MB. (1989). Eating disorders in a general practice population. Prevalence, characteristics and follow-up at 12 to 18 months. *Psychological Medicine. Monograph Supplement* **14**: 1–34.
106. Ogg EC, Millar HR, Pusztai EE, et al. (1997). General practice consultation patterns preceding diagnosis of eating disorders. *International Journal of Eating Disorders* **22**(1): 89–93.
107. Herzog DB, Nussbaum KM and Marmor AK. (1996). Comorbidity and outcome in eating disorders. *Psychiatric Clinics of North America* **19**(4): 843–859.
108. Pritts SD and Susman J. (2003). Diagnosis of eating disorders in primary care. *American Family Physician* **67**(2): 297–304.
109. Morgan JF, Reid F and Lacey JH. (1999). The SCOFF questionnaire: assessment of a new screening tool for eating disorders. *BMJ: British Medical Association* **319**(7223): 1467–1468.
110. Rome ES, Ammerman S, Rosen DS, et al. (2003). Children and adolescents with eating disorders: the state of the art. *Pediatrics* **111**(1): e98–e108.

23
Early Intervention to Reduce Violence and Offending Outcomes in Young People with Mental Disorders

Rick Fraser[1], Rosemary Purcell[2] and Danny Sullivan[2,3]

[1]Early Intervention in Psychosis Service, Sussex Partnership NHS Foundation Trust, Sussex, UK
[2]Centre for Forensic Behavioural Science, Swinburne University of Technology, Melbourne, Victoria, Australia
[3]Victorian Institute of Forensic Mental Health, Clifton Hill, Victoria, Australia

Introduction

There is a well-established relationship between experiencing severe mental illness, particularly psychotic disorders such as schizophrenia, and increased rates of violence and criminal offending. Despite this association, it is important to recognise that only a minority of those with mental illness will offend as a result of their mental illness and that the vast majority of individuals with mental illness do not engage in criminal offending. Furthermore, the excess incidence of violent crime associated with mental illness is not observed across all diagnoses, but occurs within particular categories and/or circumstances that increasingly can be specified. Because of the potential to prevent or ameliorate this offending in those with mental illness, this is a vital issue to address; however, it is equally important to be mindful of the risk of stigmatising those with mental illness as 'dangerous' (or other pejorative terms) when the overwhelming majority will never engage in violence or offending.

Early Intervention in Psychiatry: EI of nearly everything for better mental health, First Edition.
Edited by Peter Byrne and Alan Rosen.
© 2014 John Wiley & Sons, Ltd. Published 2014 by John Wiley & Sons, Ltd.

Violence in those with mental illness represents a significant public health issue, given not only the substantial personal costs to the victim and patient/perpetrator, but the economic costs conferred via health services for treating physical injuries, mental health services for treating emotional harm suffered, lost productivity if the victim is unable to work due to injury or death and the involvement of the criminal justice and forensic hospital systems in cases of serious violence. In the United Kingdom, the estimated economic cost per homicide by a mentally ill offender has been calculated to be £1.72 million, equivalent to AUD $2.76M [1, 2].

A preventative or early intervention framework for reducing violence among the mentally ill is warranted and would likely be highly cost-effective. However, clinical service models for putative interventions are limited. While specialist forensic mental health services are available in some mental health catchments, these services typically become involved only *after* a patient has offended. This chapter will canvass the rationale for early intervention to reduce violence and criminal offending among the mentally ill, with an emphasis on younger patients, since the opportunities for prevention and early intervention are likely to have the greatest impact with this population. We will focus on interventions that have been used to reduce these 'forensic' outcomes and their effectiveness, including within special clinical populations prone to other problem behaviours or offending. Finally, service provision issues, including the challenge of capacity building in this field, will be reviewed, along with potential research and service reform initiatives that can further advance the critically (and chronically) overlooked agenda of early intervention in forensic mental health.

The rationale for early intervention to reduce violence and offending among people with mental disorders

The overwhelming majority of people who experience mental disorders are never violent. Nonetheless, there is a robust, well-established association between experiencing a major mental illness, particularly a psychotic or severe mood disorder and increased rates of violence and criminal offending [3–5]. Evidence of this relationship has been derived from three distinct research paradigms: (i) studies of violence and/or offending among individuals with a mental illness [e.g. 6, 7]; (ii) studies of mental illness among known offenders, such as prisoners [e.g. 8, 9] and (iii) epidemiological studies of offending and mental illness in community samples [5, 10].

In a landmark, methodologically rigorous Australian study, Wallace et al. [5] used a register which recorded all contacts with public mental health services in the state of Victoria to establish the prior psychiatric histories of over 4000 individuals convicted in the higher courts of serious offences. The results demonstrated that, compared to a general population sample matched for age, gender and area of residence (a socio-economic proxy measure), individuals with schizophrenia were 3 times more likely to be convicted of a sexual offence, 4 times more likely to be convicted of a violent personal assault, and 10 times more likely to have been convicted of homicide. These elevated rates of violence were similarly observed in patients with severe affective disorders (predominantly bipolar disorder and major depression). Analysis indicated that the rates of offending increased substantially when co-morbid substance use was included, although highly significant associations remained for all forms of offending in the absence of substance use.

Using data from 20 discrete studies ($n = 18,423$), Fazel et al. [7] conducted a meta-analysis which demonstrated that the level of association for general violence was 4–5 times greater in patients with psychosis compared to the general population and between 14–25 times higher for homicide. Consistent with earlier studies, the relationship between violence and psychosis was mediated in part by co-morbid substance abuse. There were no differences in the rates of violence between patients with schizophrenia versus other forms of psychotic illness (e.g. schizoaffective disorder, schizophreniform disorder, delusional disorder, psychotic disorder not otherwise specified) or between the study period or study location (including Scandinavia, the United States, the United Kingdom and Australia). This finding attests to both the consistency over time and across communities of the strong association[1] between psychosis and offending.

The evidence of a link between psychosis, violence and offending is compelling, and argued by one expert in the field to be similar in magnitude to the association between smoking and lung cancer [4]. What is less clear is *how* these constructs are related, despite considerable research in this regard. Conceptually, there are at least three possible mechanisms by which these constructs might be related [11]. The first (Pathway 1) asserts that violence emerges as a function of the symptoms of psychosis experienced by individuals with an otherwise unremarkable and 'unblemished' background. Within this pathway, there are three putative categories of psychotic symptoms which may play a role. Psychotic symptoms typically cluster into three domains: (i) *positive symptoms*, which are characterised by the presence of delusions and hallucinations; (ii) *negative symptoms*, which are characterised by blunted affect, poverty of speech, amotivation, anhedonia and social withdrawal and (iii) *disorganized symptoms*, which combine both positive and negative symptoms, but are characterised by thought disorder, disorientation, confusion and cognitive deficits.

The three-domain model of psychosis has been theoretically proposed to account for illness-related violence [12], although the bulk of empirical research has focused only on the relationship with positive symptoms. Evidence from clinical, prison and community-based studies support the contention that violence is significantly related to the patient's positive psychopathology [see 13–17]. This is particularly related to the experience of command auditory hallucinations, whereby 'voices' instruct the patient to harm another person; and persecutory delusions, in which the patient falsely believes that another person intends them harm. One major community study however failed to find a significant association between the patient's symptomatology and violence [18]. Negative and disorganised symptoms have also been argued to play a role in the emergence of violence via their interference with goal-directed behaviour, logical thinking and cognition. For example, it has been suggested that these symptoms may frustrate patients and increase the likelihood that they act violently in response to managing interpersonal interactions and conflicts [11, 12], however there is a lack of empirical data to support this contention.

---

[1] For a detailed review of potential *causal*, as opposed to correlational, pathways to violence among those with mental disorder, see Mullen, 2007.

The second pathway (Pathway 2) posits that behavioural and conduct difficulties, as well as offending behaviours, are evident *before* the frank emergence of psychosis or are apparent at first contact with mental health services [e.g. 19–22], and that personality disturbance and substance abuse among affected patients are influential in the expression of violence [23–25]. For example, in a study of 205 inpatients with severe mental illness, a greater number of conduct disorder symptoms prior to 15 years was found to be significantly associated with increased risk of serious assaults over the lifespan, aggressive behaviour in the past 6 months and violent crime after controlling for alcohol and illicit drug use [22].

Finally, the third pathway (Pathway 3) posits that violence may be a simple correlate of psychosis [26]. That is, violence and psychosis share a statistical relationship through their links with other mediating variables, such as younger age, poverty, low socio-economic status, or co-morbid substance abuse. If this were the case, no clear temporal relationship would exist between violence and psychosis, after controlling for confounding factors.

The lack of consensus regarding the temporal relationship between psychosis and offending mainly reflects disparities, and in some cases major limitations, in study methodologies. This is not to say that each route to violence may not operate, but that it cannot be discerned on the basis of the extant research *which pathway is particularly influential for which patients*. Research limitations include sampling (e.g. Pathway 1 studies that include a high proportion of non-psychotic patients who are violent – such as prisoners or general community samples – are unlikely to find associations with the positive symptoms of psychosis); the assessment of violence (relying on self-reported violence being the most obvious weakness) and the methods of assessing pre-morbid behavioural or conduct difficulties (which in most 'Pathway 2' studies has been retrospective – often 2 to 3 decades after the events – and subject to biases in recall or reporting). Furthermore, studies reporting the existence of prior offending at 'first contact with mental health services' have typically taken 'first contact' to mean the onset of psychosis. However, psychotic disorders are often episodic and may have an insidious onset, such that the person may experience months or years of deteriorating functioning before the onset of acute positive symptoms that usually precipitate help-seeking and psychiatric treatment. It may be that the observed offending in these studies in fact occurred during the prolonged period of illness onset and *does* reflect an illness-related outcome, rather than reflecting a general disposition to antisocial conduct.

Populations at risk for offending
Psychosis

The latter point is salient, particularly as a more thorough analysis of the literature on violence among the mentally ill indicates that a significant proportion of offending occurs during the *first episode* of psychosis. Several studies and reports focusing on homicide as the outcome have found that between 38 [27] and 61% [28] of individuals were experiencing their first episode of psychosis at the time they committed the offence. These findings were subsequently confirmed by a systematic review and meta-analysis, which estimated the rate of homicide during the first episode of psychosis to be approximately 15 times higher compared to the rate of homicide *after* the initiation of treatment [29]. Another systematic review by these authors also demonstrated a significant association between the duration of untreated psychosis (DUP) and homicide, such that patients who experienced a longer period of untreated illness were more likely to have killed [30]. There is a growing literature to suggest that a significant minority of patients experiencing their first episode of psychosis demonstrate aggression and violent behaviour prior to first psychiatric admission [20%; 31] or at first presentation to mental health services [40%; 32].

In light of the research demonstrating the relationship between severe mental disorder and violence and offending, particularly in those with emerging and first-episode psychosis, it has been suggested that early intervention may be critical to preventing or reducing these outcomes among the mentally ill, and thereby ultimately saving lives [33, 34].

Post-traumatic stress disorder (PTSD)

Research indicates that there is an association between traumatic experiences and later offending [35]. Victims of violence are at increased risk of mental health problems including depression, dissociation and PTSD, as well as substance use and offending behaviours. A study by Widom [36] demonstrated a link between early childhood trauma/abuse and antisocial behaviour. These youngsters were at greater risk of later involvement with the criminal justice system. Retrospective studies looking at criminal populations also show this association between early trauma and later offending behaviour [37]. A German study of 54 prison inmates found a lifetime prevalence of 36% for PTSD and a point prevalence of 17% [38]. There is a clear association between traumatic experiences and offending behaviours, with mental illness and/or substance abuse as links in this pathway. Early identification and treatment of these disorders in those who have been traumatised may decrease risk of future offending and violence.

Personality disorder

While there has in the past been some ambivalence about diagnosing personality disorder (PD) in young people, in recent years it has become increasingly clear that these constructs exhibit moderate–high stability over time, and that personality difficulties and vulnerabilities may be apparent well before the firm diagnosis of PD is made [39]. In particular, childhood conduct disorder is strongly correlated with adult antisocial or dissocial PD [40]. When there are concerning personality traits which may be associated with offending, early intervention could putatively reduce the rate of transition to adult PD, or might attenuate its consequences [41]. A separate debate about the pejorative effects of labelling young people with PD diagnoses may in fact reflect clinicians' (and researchers') own negative attitudes to PD. Regardless, a reluctance to make an appropriate diagnosis may reduce access to clinical services and thus be detrimental to young people who exhibit personality vulnerabilities or difficulties.

Young people displaying marked impulsivity and aggression are also at increased risk of delinquent behaviours and a progression to adult offending. Not only are there genetic [42] and familial [43] components to these traits and to cluster B PDs, but both the traits and related PDs associated with their early life manifestations are strongly correlated to adult offending [44].

Johnson et al. [45] in a longitudinal prospective study found that cluster A PD diagnoses in adolescence were associated with subsequent threat and acquisitive offences; cluster B diagnoses (except antisocial PD) were associated with arson, violence and property damage; and cluster C PD was not associated with elevated risk of violent offending.

Finally, the concept of psychopathy is increasingly extended to young populations, with the most salient differentiating factor from conduct disorder *simpliciter* being callous-unemotional traits [46]. While the prevalence of youth psychopathy appears much lower than that of conduct disorder, young offenders with psychopathic traits have more prolific and serious offending careers than those who do not exhibit these traits [47, 48]. There is limited evidence for any treatment interventions for psychopathy, and although early recognition may result in interventions which reduce the harm associated with psychopathy, there are ethical issues associated with labelling a young person with psychopathy.

Autism spectrum, developmental disorders and organic brain conditions

Media reports on rare acts of violence by people with Autism Spectrum Conditions (ASCs) create social misperceptions and potentially increase stigma. Some academic studies reveal a speculative association between violent crime and individuals with ASCs, particularly those with Asperger's Syndrome [49]. For those with ASCs, the importance of early intervention for offending behaviour is important to avoid later contacts with the criminal justice system. The difficulty for professionals is in distinguishing between potential and actual risk of violence, especially for those who have not actually committed criminal offences. A literature review [50] of 132 cases of patients with Asperger's Syndrome revealed that only three had a history of violent crime. A study of inmates at Broadmoor (high secure) Hospital in the United Kingdom [51] revealed a prevalence of ASC three times higher than in the general population. Although there is an association between ASC and violent crime, this association does not appear to be particularly strong. Contributory characteristics for offending in those with ASC include special obsessions, interpersonal naïveté, 'logical' explanations for offending and lack of empathy (including deficient 'theory of mind') [52].

Other developmental disorders such as Attention Deficit Hyperactivity Disorder (ADHD) may represent a risk factor for offending and substance use. Research has shown that 45% of youths and 24% of adults in the criminal justice system screen positive for childhood ADHD, with ADHD being the most powerful predictor of violent offending [53]. Effective and early treatment of ADHD may therefore reduce features of this disorder which act as a pathway into substance misuse and violent crime. Intellectual disability can also be associated with challenging behaviours, some of which potentially involve violence or other forms of offending. Research by Williams et al. [54] found that young offenders have an increased rate of traumatic brain injury and that this history is associated with a greater number of convictions and higher rate of violent crime. Other organic brain conditions that affect mental health, cognition, impulsivity and aggression can also potentially increase the risk of offending as well as violence, however it is beyond the scope of this chapter to examine these in more detail. A focus on early identification of those with problem behaviours should promote appropriate educational, behavioural and medical interventions and thus reduce risk and negative outcomes.

Substance abuse

Co-morbidity with substance abuse and dependence disorders in youth populations is marked. Early onset of substance abuse and adolescent substance dependence are correlated to lower IQ, harsh parenting, poor educational retention and achievement, increased subsequent psychiatry morbidity and forensic outcomes [55].

The evidence is increasingly clear that violent offending in mentally disordered people is significantly mediated through substance abuse [7]. This may relate not only to the disinhibiting effects of intoxication and withdrawal, but also to association with antisocial peers, acquisitive offending to fund substance use and the specific effects of some substances in engendering aggression. In particular, methamphetamine and high-potency benzodiazepines are associated with aggression during intoxication and possibly withdrawal; and cannabis use is associated with psychosis.

When considering interventions, it is increasingly apparent that substance abuse treatment in adolescents may differ in critical aspects from that for adults, and therefore require specialised services and specific interventions [56]. The adolescent brain is particularly vulnerable to insult and high-level use may result in risk-taking behaviour, offending and potentially to acquired brain injury.

Sexually abusive behaviours

For many adult sexual offenders, disordered behaviours and attitudes commence in youth. A significant minority of sexual offending is perpetrated by juvenile offenders, and some will be more persistent in their offending. Risk factors for sexually abusive behaviour are similar to other offending types, although there is an over-representation of youths with mild-moderate intellectual disability.

While there is limited evidence about the benefits of treatment, identification of sexual behaviour which is coercive, deviant or developmentally inappropriate is important and may result in therapeutic interventions in youth, rather than correctional interventions in adult life. The overlap between being a victim of abuse and becoming an abuser is complex but strongly associated [57]. Thus, targeted interventions in those being treated as victims may also necessitate consideration of the potential to become an abuser, as well as enhancing resilience factors.

Sadly there is a dearth of specialised treatment programs for younger children or those who might be diverted from the justice system, although potential for such interventions to preclude the later stigma of being labeled as a sexual offender is clearly evident.

Firesetting

Early recognition of those prone to firesetting is important. Although classic pyromania is uncommon, preoccupation with fire, impulsivity, social skills impairments and poor emotional regulation (especially associated with anger and boredom) may be associated with firesetting. Furthermore, family dysfunction is common. A diagnosis of conduct disorder and affiliation with antisocial peer groups appear relevant but are not specific. There may be an increase in prevalence in youth with intellectual disability although the empirical evidence is lacking. Interestingly, there is also little support for the fabled 'triad' of enure-sis, animal cruelty and firesetting [58]. Early, skilled and assertive intervention may be effective, although eclectic approaches tend to be used and there is no clear evidence base for treatment [59]. There are few established treatment programs and limited longer-term evaluation of effectiveness [60].

Stalking

Stalking is a maladaptive criminal behaviour comprising of repeated intrusions involving contacts and unwanted communications with an individual [61]. Prevention of stalking is challenging as there are multiple causes for this behaviour and specific treatments have yet to be fully evaluated. When there exists a specific psychopathology, then treatment of that psychopathology may end the stalking [62]. Addressing substance misuse and social problems may also have an impact. Because of the complexity of this behaviour and the interface between forensic and mental health services, multi-agency working is impor-tant, not only to manage risk but also to consider appropriate interventions to prevent reoffending.

Young people specifically as a risk population [63]

Independent of the presence of mental health problems, young people are at increased risk of committing criminal offences compared to older individuals. The peak rate of offend-ing is 18 years in males and 15 years in females [64]. This risk is further increased by other factors including social adversity, unemployment, homelessness and substance mis-use. Young people from certain ethnic and cultural minorities (BME groups) are over-represented in the criminal justice system [65]. This may in part be due to stigmatisa-tion/racial discrimination and social exclusion.

Service models to enhance prevention and early intervention in forensic mental health

There is growing recognition that mental health services have a critical role to play in managing the risks of violence among patients, and reducing the chances that a patient will engage in criminal behavior or, in cases of existing offending behaviour, commit fur-ther offences [34, 66]. However, evidence suggests that community mental health teams do not adjust their interventions for patients with histories of violence or offending [67]. Furthermore, detecting and intervening with violence risk or offending in mental health services can be limited by issues such as clinician discomfort and relative inexperience in working with at-risk patients or using relevant violence risk assessment tools, difficulty in engaging such patients [68], or competing demands on clinicians' time as they attempt to engage, diagnose and stabilise the patient in the early phase of mental illness.

There are limited examples of service models engaged in reducing the risk of violence or offending behaviours in those who have mental illness but have not yet committed any major crime [69]. Traditionally, assessing and managing risks of violence and offending have been viewed as the domain of specialist forensic mental health services, rather than general services. Unfortunately, specialist forensic services are not consistently available in mental health catchments, and typically become involved with an individual only *after* the offending has already occurred. In many regions, forensic mental health services will also be reluctant to deal with adolescents, despite this population having the highest rates of offending. In order to better manage, if not *prevent* the risks of violence and offending among the mentally disordered, an early intervention framework within *mainstream* mental health services is required. This pre-offending population will often fall between the gaps of traditional mental health and forensic services.

There are several potential approaches to managing the risks of violence among patients in non-forensic mental health services. One (appealing) strategy is to employ a dedicated forensic mental health specialist to provide risk assessment and management interventions for all patients within the service. However, even if such specialists were available for community mental health services, the significant downside to this approach is that responsibility for managing patient risk largely rests on a single individual, rather than being shared across the clinical service. A preferable strategy is to build the capacity of the existing workforce of mental health clinicians to assess and manage their patient's potential risks, using consultation and liaison with forensic specialists. The advantages of this approach are that it allows mental health clinicians to develop skills in assessing and managing the risks of violence in the context of a mentoring relationship [70], and is likely to be more cost-effective (as the consultation service may be reduced as staff develop competency and confidence in managing the risks of violence among their patients). Based on these perceived benefits, this approach was utilised in the development of the Orygen-Forensicare Satellite Clinic (O-FSC).

The O-FSC was developed within a youth mental health service in Melbourne, Australia to implement such a model of specialist in-reach [see 69 for a full description of this service]. Similar programmes have been developed elsewhere such as the Youth First initiative in Birmingham, United Kingdom where the drive is to prevent recidivist crime in those young people who have mental health and substance use disorders. Ultimately, the service model needs to allow for a collaborative approach between forensic and mental health services with a drive to upskill existing mental health clinicians, promote early referral of those with offending behaviours or at risk of offending and provide a framework in which to assess and manage risk *before* offending becomes more serious or recidivist. The first step remains an acceptance of the associations between nascent mental disorder and offending risk, and the belief that intervention geared to reducing future offending risk is part of core business.

Conclusions

Good clinical care in general mental health services emphasises assessing and managing the risk of patients harming themselves (e.g. via suicidal ideation or behaviour), but rarely emphasises assessing and managing a patient's risk of harm *to others* through violence. Even in forensic psychiatry, efforts to *prevent* first incidents of violence or offending are rare, if not absent. We believe that prevention and early intervention for risks of violence and offending should be a clinical priority within the hundreds of early psychosis services operating worldwide [71], given the elevated risks of violence among those with first-episode psychosis. The opportunities for *prevention* of violence and offending may also be amplified in the increasing number of youth mental health services being established internationally, including the 60 *headspace* centres currently operating in Australia [see 72], as these services are primarily designed for 12–25-year olds with sub-threshold or emerging mental health problems, who, while frequently presenting with anger or aggression management difficulties, rarely present with established histories of serious criminal offending. The overview and service models described here provide some guidance as to how such prevention and early intervention for violence may be achieved, although more research, innovative service design and evaluation are needed.

References

1. McCrone P, Park A-L and Knapp M. (2010). Economic evaluation of early intervention services: Phase iv report. London School of Economics: Personal Social Services Research Unit. http://www.iris-initiative.org.uk/silo/files/cost-impact-of-ei-psychosis-report-phase-4-mccrone-knapp-park-oct-2010.pdf (accessed 30 April 2014).
2. Home Office. (2004). The economic and social costs of crime against individuals and households 2003/2004: *Online Report 30/05*. London: Home Office.
3. Mullen P. (2001). A review of the relationship between mental disorders and offending behaviours and on the management of mentally abnormal offenders in the health and criminal justice services. *Canberra: Criminology Research Council*. http://www.criminologyresearch council.gov.au/reports/mullen.html (accessed 30 April 2014).
4. Maden A. (2007). *Treating Violence: A Guide to Risk Management in Mental Health*. Oxford: Oxford University Press.
5. Wallace C, Mullen P, Burgess P, et al. (1998). Serious criminal offending and mental disorder – case linkage study. *British Journal of Psychiatry* **172**: 477–484.
6. Steadman H, Mulvey E, Monahan J, et al. (1998). Violence by people discharged from acute psychiatric inpatient facilities and by others in the same neighbourhoods. *Archives of General Psychiatry* **55**(5): 393–401.
7. Fazel S, Gulati G, Linsell L, et al. (2009). Schizophrenia and violence: Systematic review and meta-analysis. *Plos Medicine* **6**: e1000120.
8. Gottlieb P, Gabrielsen G and Kramp P. (1987). Psychotic homicide in Copenhagen from 1959 to 1983. *Acta Psychiatrica Scandinavica* **76**(3): 285–292.
9. Fazel S and Danesh J. (2002). Serious mental disorder in 23,000 prisoners: a systematic review of 62 surveys. *Lancet* **359**: 545–550.
10. Swanson J, Holzer C, Ganju V, et al. (1990). Violence and psychiatric disorder in the community - evidence from the epidemiologic catchment area surveys. *Hospital and Community Psychiatry* **41**(7): 761–770.
11. Douglas KS, Guy LS and Hart SD. (2009). Psychosis as a risk factor for violence to others: A meta-analysis. *Psychological Bulletin* **135**(5): 679–706.
12. Baxter R. (1997). Violence in schizophrenia and the syndrome of disorganisation. *Criminal Behaviour and Mental Health* **7**(2): 131–139.
13. Taylor P. (1985). Motives for offending among violence and psychotic men. *British Journal of Psychiatry* **147**: 491–498.
14. Hellerstein D, Frosch W and Koenigsberg HW. (1987). The clinical significance of command hallucinations. *American Journal of Psychiatry* **144**(2): 219–221.
15. Swanson J, Borum R, Swartz M, et al. (1996). Psychotic symptoms and disorders and the risk of violent behaviour in the community. *Criminal Behaviour and Mental Health* **6**: 309–329
16. Rudnick A. (1999). Relation between command hallucinations and dangerous behavior. *Journal of the American Academy of Psychiatry and the Law* **27**(2): 253–257.
17. Teasdale B, Silver E and Monahan J. (2006). Gender, threat/control-override delusions and violence. *Law and Human Behaviour* **30**(6): 649–658.

18. Swanson J, Swartz M, Van Dorn R, et al. (2006). A national study of violent behaviour in persons with schizophrenia. *Archives of General Psychiatry* **63**(5): 490–499.
19. Munkner R, Haastrup S, Joergensen T and Kramp P. (2003). The temporal relationship between schizophrenia and crime. *Social Psychiatry and Psychiatric Epidemiology* **38**(7): 347–353.
20. Fresan A, Apiquian R, de la Fuente-Sandoval C, et al. (2004). Premorbid adjustment and violent behavior in schizophrenic patients. *Schizophrenia Research* **69**(2–3): 143–148.
21. Laajasalo T and Hakkanen H. (2005). Offence and offender characteristics among two groups of Finnish homicide offenders with schizophrenia: Comparison of early- and late-start offenders. *Journal of Forensic Psychiatry and Psychology* **16**(1): 41–59.
22. Hodgins S, Cree A, Alderton J, et al. (2008). From conduct disorder to severe mental illness: associations with aggressive behaviour, crime and victimization. *Psychological Medicine* **38**(7): 975–987.
23. Moran P, Walsh E, Tyrer P, et al. (2003). Impact of comorbid personality disorder on violence in psychosis – Report from the UK700 trial. *British Journal of Psychiatry* **182**: 129–134.
24. Elbogen EB and Johnson SC. (2009). The intricate link between violence and mental disorder. *Archives of General Psychiatry* **66**(2): 152–161.
25. Jones R, Van den Bree M, Ferriter M, et al. (2010). Childhood risk factors for offending before first psychiatric admission for people with schizophrenia: a case-control study of high security hospital admissions. *Behavioural Sciences and the Law* **28**(3): 351–365.
26. Walsh E, Buchanan A and Fahy T. (2002). Violence and schizophrenia: examining the evidence. *British Journal of Psychiatry* **180**: 490–495.
27. Appleby L, Shaw J, and Amos T. (1997). National confidential inquiry into suicide and homicide by people with mental illness. *British Journal of Psychiatry* **170**: 101–102.
28. Nielssen OB, Westmore BD, Large MMB and Hayes RA. (2007). Homicide during psychotic illness in New South Wales between 1993 and 2002. *Medical Journal of Australia* **186**(6): 301–304.
29. Nielssen O and Large M. (2010). Rates of homicide during the first episode of psychosis and after treatment: A systematic review and meta-analysis. *Schizophrenia Bulletin* **36**: 702–712.
30. Large M and Nielssen O. (2008). Evidence for a relationship between the duration of untreated psychosis and the proportion of psychotic homicides prior to treatment. *Social Psychiatry and Psychiatric Epidemiology* **43**: 37–44.
31. Humphreys MS, Johnstone EC, Macmillan JF, et al. (1992). Dangerous behavior preceding first admissions for schizophrenia. *British Journal of Psychiatry* **161**: 501–505.
32. Dean K, Walsh E, Morgan C et al. (2007). Aggressive behaviour at first contact with services: Findings from the AESOP first episode psychosis study. *Psychological Medicine* **37**: 547–557.
33. Large M and Nielssen O. (2007). Treating the first episode of schizophrenia earlier will save lives. *Schizophrenia Research* **92**: 276–277.
34. Mullen P. (2009). Facing up to unpalatable evidence for the sake of our patients. *PLOS Medicine* **6**: e1000112.
35. Ardino V. (2012). Offending behaviour: the role of trauma and PTSD. *European Journal of Psychotraumatology* **3**: 18968.
36. Widom C. (1989). Child abuse, neglect and adult behaviour: research design and findings on criminality, violence and child abuse. *American Journal of Orthopsychiatry* **59**(3): 355–367.
37. Vermeiren R. (2003). Psychopathology and delinquency in adolescents: a descriptive and developmental perspective. *Clinical Psychology Review* **23**(2): 277–318.
38. Spitzer C, Dudeck M, Liss H, et al. (2001). Post traumatic stress disorder in forensic inpatients. *Journal of Forensic Psychiatry* **12**(1): 63–77.
39. Grilo C, McGlashan T and Quinlan D. (1998). Frequency of personality disorders in two age cohorts of psychiatric inpatients. *American Journal of Psychiatry* **155**: 140–142.
40. Bernstein D, Cohen P, Skodol A, et al. (1996). Childhood antecedents of adolescent personality disorders. *American Journal of Psychiatry* **153**: 907–913.

41. Chanen A, Jackson H and McCutcheon L, et al. (2008). Early intervention for adolescents with borderline personality disorder using cognitive analytic therapy: randomised controlled trial. *British Journal of Psychiatry* **193**(6): 477–484.

42. McGuffin P and Thapar A. (1992). The genetics of personality disorder. *British Journal of Psychiatry* **160**: 12–23.

43. Silverman J, Pinkham L, Horvath T, et al. (1991). Affective and impulsive personality disorder traits in the relatives of patients with borderline personality disorder. *American Journal of Psychiatry* **148**: 1378–1385.

44. Caspi A, McClay J, Moffitt TE et al. (2002). Role of genotype in the cycle of violence in maltreated children. *Science.* **297**(5582): 851–854.

45. Johnson J, Cohen P, Smailes E, et al. (2000). Adolescent personality disorders associated with violence and criminal behaviour during adolescence and early adulthood. *American Journal of Psychiatry* **157**: 1406–1412.

46. Frick P and White S. (2008). Research Review: The importance of callous-unemotional traits for developmental models of aggressive and antisocial behavior. *Journal of Child Psychology and Psychiatry* **49**: 359–375.

47. Forth A and Burke H. (1998). Psychopathy in adolescence: assessment, violence and developmental precursors. In: DJ Cooke, AE Forth and RD Hare (eds), *Psychopathy: Theory, Research and Implications for Society*, pp. 205–229. Klower Academic Publishers.

48. Spain S, Douglas K, Poythress N, et al. (2004). The relationship between psychopathic features, violence and treatment outcome: the comparison of three youth measures of psychopathic features. *Behavioral Sciences and the Law* **22**: 85–102.

49. Långström N, Grann M, Ruchkin V, et al. (2009). Risk factors for violent offending in autism spectrum disorder: a national study of hospitalized individuals. *Journal of Interpersonal Violence* **24**: 1358–1370.

50. Ghaziuddin M, Tsai L and Ghaziuddin N. (1991). Violence in Asperger's syndrome: a critique. *Journal of Autism and Developmental Disorders* **21**: 349–354.

51. Scragg P and Shah A. (1994). Prevalence of Asperger's syndrome in a secure hospital. *British Journal of Psychiatry* **165**: 679–682.

52. Barry-Walsh JB and Mullen PE. (2004). Forensic aspects of Asperger's syndrome. *Journal of Forensic Psychiatry and Psychology* **15**(1): 96–107.

53. Young SJ, Adamou M, Bolea B et al. (2011). The identification and management of ADHD offenders within the criminal justice system: a consensus statement from the UK Adult ADHD Network and criminal justice agencies. *BMC Psychiatry* **11**: 32.

54. Williams H, Cordan G, Mewse AJ, et al. (2010). Self-reported traumatic brain injury in male young offenders: a risk factor for re-offending, poor mental health and violence? *Neuropsychological Rehabilitation* **20**(6): 801–812.

55. Lader D, Singleton N and Meltzer H. (2003). Psychiatric morbidity among young offenders in England and Wales. *International Review of Psychiatry* **15**: 144–147.

56. Brown S and Ramo D. (2006). Clinical course of youth following treatment for alcohol and drug problems. In: Liddle H and Rowe C. (eds), *Adolescent Substance Abuse: Research and Clinical Advances*, pp. 79–103. Cambridge: Cambridge University Press.

57. Ogloff J, Cutajar M, Mann E, et al. (2012). Child sexual abuse and subsequent offending and victimisation: A 45 year follow-up study. *Trends and Issues in Crime and Criminal Justice* 421–440. http://www.aic.gov.au/publications/current%20series/tandi/421-440/tandi440.html (accessed 30 April 2014).

58. Dolan M, McEwan T, Doley R, et al. (2011). Risk factors and risk assessment in juvenile firesetting. *Psychiatry, Psychology and Law* **18**(3): 378–394.

59. Repo E and Virkkunen M. (1997). Young arsonists: History of conduct disorder, psychiatric diagnoses and criminal recidivism. *Journal of Forensic Psychiatry* **8**: 311–320.

60. Fritzon K, Dolan M, Doley R, McEwan T, et al. (2011). Juvenile fire-setting: A review of treatment programs. *Psychiatry, Psychology and Law* **18**(3): 395–408.

61. Mullen P, Pathé M and Purcell R. (2000). *Stalkers and Their Victims*. Cambridge: Cambridge University Press.
62. Mullen P, Pathé M and Purcell R. (2001). The management of stalkers. *Advances in Psychiatric Treatment* **7**: 335–342.
63. Farrington D. (1986). Age and crime. In: M Tonry and N Morris (eds), *Crime and Justice: An Annual Review of Research*. Chicago: University of Chicago Press 189–250.
64. Home Office. (2006). Crime in England and Wales 2005/6. *Home Office Statistical Bulletin 12/06*. London: Home Office.
65. Youth Justice Board. (2010). Exploring the needs of young Black and Minority Ethnic offenders and the provision of targeted interventions. *Youth Justice Board*, http://www.justice.gov.uk/downloads/youth-justice/yjb-toolkits/disproportionality/Exploring-needs-young-bme-offenders.pdf (accessed 30 April 2014).
66. Mullen P. (2000). Forensic mental health. *British Journal of Psychiatry* **176**: 307–311.
67. Hodgins S, Cree A, Khalid F et al. (2009). Do community mental health teams caring for severely mentally ill patients adjust treatments and services based on patients' antisocial or criminal behaviours? *European Psychiatry* **24**: 373–379.
68. Lamb HR and Weinberger LE. (2002). A call for more program evaluation of forensic outpatient clinics: The need to improve effectiveness. *Journal of the American Academy of Psychiatry and the Law* **30**: 548–552.
69. Purcell R, Fraser R, Greenwood-Smith C, et al. (2012). Managing risks of violence in a youth mental health service: a service model description. *Early Intervention in Psychiatry* **6**: 469–475.
70. Snowden P. (1997). Practical aspects of clinical risk assessment and management. *British Journal of Psychiatry* **170**(Suppl 32): 32–34.
71. International Early Psychosis Association Writing Group. (2005). International clinical practice guidelines for early psychosis. *British Journal of Psychiatry* **187**(Suppl 48): s120–s124.
72. McGorry PD, Tanti C, Stokes R, et al. (2007). headspace: Australia's National Youth Mental Health Foundation – where young minds come first. *Medical Journal of Australia* **187**: S68–S70.

24
Early Intervention for Borderline Personality Disorder

Andrew M. Chanen[1,2] and Louise McCutcheon[1,2]
[1]*Orygen Youth Health Research Centre & Centre for Youth Mental Health, The University of Melbourne, Melbourne, Australia*
[2]*Orygen Youth Health Clinical Program, Northwestern Mental Health, Melbourne, Australia*

Introduction

Borderline personality disorder (BPD) is a severe mental disorder that is characterised by a pervasive pattern of impulsivity, emotional instability, interpersonal dysfunction and disturbed self-image [1]. BPD affects 0.7–2.7% of the general adult population [2, 3], 9.3–22.5% of psychiatric outpatients, and in some settings, over 40% of inpatients [4].The outcome for BPD in adulthood is now reliably characterised by attenuation of diagnostic criteria over time but severe and continuing functional disability across a broad range of domains that is comparable to or greater than that associated with many mental state disorders [5]. Patients with BPD also have continuing high rates of health service utilisation [6] and a suicide rate of around 8% [7]. Although effective interventions exist for adults with BPD [1], the overall outcomes from such interventions are modest and their availability is limited.

Borderline personality disorder in young people

Despite longstanding general agreement that personality disorders (PDs) have their roots in childhood and adolescence [8], diagnosing PDs prior to age 18 years has been more controversial than diagnosing PDs in adults [9], but this is no longer justified [10]. BPD is increasingly seen as a lifespan developmental disorder [11] that is just as reliable and valid

Early Intervention in Psychiatry: EI of nearly everything for better mental health, First Edition.
Edited by Peter Byrne and Alan Rosen.
© 2014 John Wiley & Sons, Ltd. Published 2014 by John Wiley & Sons, Ltd.

in adolescence as it is in adulthood [12], is not reducible to Axis I diagnoses [13], and can be identified in day-to-day clinical practice [14].

When the diagnosis is applied, BPD occurs in approximately 3% of community-dwelling adolescents and young adults [15, 16]. Indeed, BPD might be better considered as a disorder of younger people, with a rise in prevalence from puberty and a steady decline with each decade from young adulthood [17, 18]. Over 3% of the population will meet BPD diagnostic criteria between ages 14 and 22 years [18]. Limited data suggest that BPD occurs in up to 22% of outpatient adolescents and young adults [14, 19].

BPD (or dimensional representations of BPD) in young people demarcates a group with high morbidity and a particularly poor outcome. BPD uniquely and independently predicts current psychopathology, general functioning, peer relationships, self-care and family and relationship functioning [13]. It also uniquely predicts poor outcomes up to 2 decades into the future, such as a future BPD diagnosis, increased risk for axis I disorders (especially substance use and mood disorders), interpersonal problems, distress and reduced quality of life [20–22].

Prevention and early intervention

The above data suggest that BPD is a leading candidate for developing empirically based prevention and early intervention programs because it is common in clinical practice, it is among the most functionally disabling of all mental disorders, it is often associated with help-seeking (*cf.* schizotypal or antisocial PDs) and it has been shown to respond to intervention, even in those with established disorder. Moreover, BPD can be reliably diagnosed in its early stages and it demarcates a group with high levels of current and future morbidity and mortality. Data also suggest considerable flexibility and malleability of BPD traits in youth [23], making this a key developmental period during which to intervene, and adolescent BPD features have been shown to respond to intervention [24, 25].

Aims of prevention and early intervention

Prevention and early intervention for BPD should primarily aim to alter the life-course trajectory of young people with borderline personality pathology by attenuating or averting associated adverse outcomes and promoting more adaptive developmental pathways. It should not be narrowly focussed upon the diagnostic features of BPD, as these naturally attenuate over time. Such objectives might be realised through identifying appropriate risk factors and antecedents for intervention.

Risk factors

Evidence supports both gene–environment interaction and correlation in the development of BPD [26]. This means that individuals with a 'sensitive' genotype are at greater risk of BPD in the presence of a predisposing environment. Furthermore, the genes that influence BPD features also increase the likelihood of being exposed to certain adverse life events. Overall, the findings regarding neurobiological risk factors for BPD (summarised in [27]) are preliminary and do not provide clear and consistent targets for preventive interventions. For some findings, such as frontolimbic network abnormalities in adults with BPD

[1], it is unclear whether these findings are a cause, an effect, or an epiphenomenon of BPD [28] and their specificity for BPD appears to be limited [29].

Prospective, longitudinal data are more consistent in demonstrating that a range of childhood and parental demographic characteristics, adverse childhood experiences, early relational difficulties, parental problems and forms of maladaptive parenting are risk factors for adolescent and adult BPD.

Although there is a strong association between BPD and adverse childhood experiences, the precise role of childhood adversity in the aetiology of BPD remains unclear because putative risk factors, such as childhood abuse, adverse familial environment and a family history of psychopathology are highly intercorrelated [30]. One study has demonstrated that shared genetic influences, causal effects and an interaction between genes and environment, can explain the association between life events and BPD features, depending on the type of life event [26].

Specific data on prospectively assessed risk factors for BPD are scarce, with the Children in the Community (CIC) study [20] being the only study to have published prospective risk factors over multiple waves from childhood through to adulthood. A series of CIC publications (summarised in [20, 31]) report childhood abuse or neglect, childhood and parental demographic characteristics, maladaptive parenting and maladaptive school experiences as risk factors for adolescent and adult PD.

Prospective longitudinal data have found that childhood physical abuse, sexual abuse and neglect [32], along with low family of origin socio-economic status [33] are independently associated with elevated features of BPD up to two decades later. Also, maternal inconsistency in child rearing in the presence of high maternal over-involvement [34];maladaptive parenting behaviour present during the child-rearing years [35]; early separations of offspring from their mothers before age 5 [36] and early relational experiences including attachment disorganization and maltreatment, maternal hostility and boundary dissolution, family disruption related to father's presence and family life stress [37] all predict elevations in BPD features from 2 to 30 years later.

Precursor signs and symptoms

Prospective longitudinal data indicate that certain temperamental characteristics and early onset mental state or behavioural problems that are analogous to characteristics of BPD are precursors to the emergence of the BPD phenotype but do not predict its onset with certainty. These include attention deficit hyperactivity disorder (ADHD), oppositional defiant disorder (ODD), conduct disorder (CD), substance use, depression and deliberate self-harm (DSH), along with the actual features of BPD. However, it is technically imprecise to refer to many of these phenomena as 'risk factors' [38], as these same phenomena are mostly trait-like and are later used to define PD. Eaton et al. [39] refer to the signs and symptoms from a diagnostic cluster that precede a disorder but do not predict its onset with certainty as *precursor signs and symptoms*.

Maternal reports of childhood temperament are related to BPD in adolescence or adulthood, up to 30 years later [36, 37]. Substance use disorders during adolescence, particularly alcohol use disorders, also specifically predict young adult BPD [40, 41] and there are strong prospective data that disturbances in attention, emotional regulation and behaviour, especially the disruptive behaviour disorders (CD, ODD and ADHD) in childhood or adolescence, are independent predictors of young adult BPD [37, 42, 43]. Moreover, in one study, the rate of growth in ADHD scores from age 10 to 13 and the rate of growth in ODD scores from 8 to 10 uniquely predicted higher BPD symptoms at age 14, suggesting that for adolescent BPD symptoms, difficulties with emotion regulation and relationships might precede problems with impulse control [42].

DSH is a core feature of BPD [1] and retrospective reports from adults with BPD indicate childhood-onset of DSH in more than 30% and adolescent-onset in another 30% [44]. However, DSH is surprisingly under-researched as a potential precursor to BPD. Although DSH is relatively common among adolescents and young adults [45] and is associated with a range of clinical syndromes, there is evidence that repetitive DSH, which is less frequent, might differ from occasional DSH [46]. BPD can be diagnosed in the majority of female adolescent inpatients with DSH [47] and the likelihood of meeting the diagnosis of BPD is greater in adolescents endorsing both DSH and suicide attempts, compared with individuals reporting DSH or suicide attempts alone [48]. Also, the number of BPD criteria met is predictive of whether or not an adolescent has engaged in DSH or attempted suicide [49].

There is now clear evidence that dimensional representations of BPD features have similar stability in adolescence and adulthood [12]. Evidence is emerging that the underlying dimensions of BPD features (conceptualized as impulsivity, negative affectivity and interpersonal aggression) are also stable in children [50, 51]. Only the CIC has specifically measured childhood or adolescent PD features as a predictor of later PD over multiple assessments from childhood to adulthood [20]. PD symptoms in childhood or adolescence were the strongest long-term predictors, over and above disruptive behaviour disorders and depressive symptoms [20, 52–54] of later DSM-IV cluster A, B or C PD. Overall, the CIC data support a normative increase in BPD traits after puberty, perhaps bringing the problems associated with BPD to clinical attention. As this wanes in early adulthood, partly due to maturational or socialization processes [20], a group is revealed that is increasingly deviant compared with their peers [55] and perhaps conforms more to the 'adult' BPD phenotype. This suggests that young people displaying BPD features are a major group from which the adult BPD phenotype arises.

In short, signs and symptoms might appear from childhood through to adolescence that resemble aspects of the BPD phenotype and presage its later appearance in adolescence or emerging adulthood. Certain early temperamental and personality features, internalizing and externalizing psychopathology, and specific BPD criteria are all candidate precursor signs and symptoms. However, more work needs to be done to gain a better understanding of the role these factors play in the developmental pathways to BPD and to increase their specificity for BPD.

What form should intervention take?

Stand-alone universal (whole population) prevention of BPD is not currently feasible because BPD is not sufficiently prevalent to justify whole population approaches and it is unclear what form or 'dose' of intervention would be appropriate. Similarly, selective prevention (targeting those with risk factors for BPD) is currently impractical because many of the risk factors for BPD (particularly environmental factors) are non-specific and more commonly lead to, or are associated with, outcomes other than BPD. This should not diminish the importance of intervention for some risk factors (e.g., child abuse and neglect) as primary objectives because they are undesirable, immoral or unlawful. However, many factors (e.g. poverty) require major social and political change and are unlikely to have a major impact on BPD prevention in the near future. Also, it is difficult to design studies with adequate statistical power to demonstrate the efficacy or effectiveness of universal and selective prevention [56]. Some of these problems would be overcome if current universal and selective programs (e.g., parent training programs) were to measure multiple syndromes as outcomes, and the above data constitute a strong case for including BPD as one of these syndromes.

The data reviewed above suggest that 'indicated prevention' [12] is currently the 'best bet' for prevention of BPD. This targets individuals displaying precursor (i.e., early) signs and symptoms of BPD. Although the BPD phenotype is not clearly identifiable in children, its underlying dimensions can be measured, appear to be relatively stable and could be directly targeted. Moreover, typical child and adolescent psychopathology (e.g., disruptive behaviour disorders, DSH, substance use and depressive disorders) might additionally be regarded as targets for indicated prevention of BPD, rather than separate domains of psychopathology that might then be renamed in adulthood. Two programs, described below, have been developed that directly target sub-syndromal borderline pathology in adolescents [24, 25, 57], while concurrently targeting syndromal BPD.

Early detection and intervention

Early detection and intervention for BPD is now justified and practical in adolescence and emerging adulthood [10, 14] and consequently, novel early intervention programs have been developed and researched in Australia [24, 57] and the Netherlands [25]. Such programs should be differentiated from conventional BPD treatment programs that are applied to individuals who have established, complex and severe BPD but happen to be less than 18-years old. Intervention for this latter group should now be considered part of routine clinical practice in adolescent mental health [10].

Indicated prevention and early intervention also offer a unique platform for investigating BPD earlier in its developmental course, where duration of illness factors that complicate the psychopathology and neurobiology of BPD can be minimised [28].

Principles of early intervention

The Australian Helping Young People Early (HYPE) and Dutch Emotion Regulation Training (ERT) treatment programs have several features in common. They have broad inclusion criteria, with limited exclusions for co-occurring psychopathology (which is common in BPD). They view BPD dimensionally, combining sub-syndromal (indicated prevention) and syndromal (early intervention) BPD. BPD and other personality pathology are carefully diagnosed, often supported by semi-structured interview. Both HYPE and ERT are time-limited, being 16–24 and 17 sessions, respectively. Both have adapted interventions designed for adults with BPD to make them developmentally suitable. HYPE uses Cognitive Analytic Therapy (CAT) [58], whereas ERT uses Systems Training for Emotional Predictability and Problem Solving (STEPPS) [59].

The major difference between these programs is that ERT is delivered in a group for-mat as an adjunct to treatment as usual (TAU), whereas HYPE employs a comprehensive, team-based integrated intervention. In a randomised controlled trial (RCT), ERT + TAU was not substantially different to TAU alone [25]. In contrast, a quasi-experimental com-parison of the HYPE intervention and TAU [60] found that HYPE achieved faster rates of improvement in internalising and externalising psychopathology and lower levels of psychopathology at 2-year follow-up. This suggests that some or all of the elements of a team-based, integrated intervention (outlined in Box 24.1) might be important for early intervention and matches clinical experience working with this population.

Box 24.1 Additional elements of the HYPE team-based, integrated intervention program

- Assertive, 'psychologically informed' case management integrated with the delivery of individual psychotherapy

- Active engagement of families or carers, with psychoeducation and time-limited family intervention, using the same model as individual psychotherapy

- General psychiatric care by the same team, with specific assessment and treatment of co-occurring psychiatric syndromes ('co-morbidity'), including the use of phar-macotherapy, where indicated for such syndromes

- Capacity for 'outreach' care in the community

- Flexible timing and location of intervention

- Crisis team and inpatient care, with a clear model of brief and goal-directed inpa-tient care

- Access to a psychosocial recovery program that is shared with other programs at Orygen Youth Health

- Individual and group supervision of staff

- A quality assurance program.

Applied indicated prevention and early intervention: the HYPE program

Service context

The HYPE program [57] is part of Orygen Youth Health [61], the government-funded youth mental health service in western and north-western metropolitan Melbourne, Aus-tralia. Orygen services a catchment population of approximately 160,000 15–25-year olds and offers a comprehensive mental health service for severe mental disorders.

Referral and initial assessment

Youth with BPD commonly seek clinical help but opportunities for early intervention are frequently missed [13]. Referrals are made to Orygen's single point of entry and are usually precipitated by a mental state disorder (e.g., major depression), not BPD *per se*. First-episode psychosis patients are always allocated to Orygen's Early Psychosis Prevention and Intervention Service, regardless of co-morbidity.

Selection of patients

The primary inclusion criterion for HYPE is having three or more DSM-IV BPD criteria. Previously published data [14] indicate that 39% of non-psychotic patients assessed at Orygen meet this threshold. This threshold reflects HYPE's mixed indicated prevention and early intervention mission [12], recognizes the dimensional nature of BPD [62] and reduces practical disputes about 'eligibility' when there is a clear clinical need for intervention, such as when there is prominent parasuicidal behaviour, impulsivity and affective instability, without meeting the threshold for a categorical diagnosis of BPD.

HYPE has no specific exclusion criteria for other forms of psychopathology because co-morbidity is the norm in BPD at any age [13]. Also, as described above, some of this psychopathology represents precursor signs and symptoms for BPD. Low IQ is not a contraindication to treatment in HYPE, provided the individual has sufficient verbal skills to participate in the program.

Patients are not compelled to attend HYPE. Those with substance use problems or a history of overt aggression are asked not to attend appointments while intoxicated and to respect the safety of themselves and others while at Orygen. However, there is no 'behavioural contract' with new patients, as this is often experienced as both provocative and an invitation to a battle for control. Rather, these issues are addressed if and when they arise within the overall treatment model (described below).

Screening and assessment of BPD in young people   Despite its high prevalence in clinical services, many clinicians lack the skills or confidence to assess adolescent BPD. BPD often complicates assessment, frequently causing patients to feel intruded upon or overwhelmed. Operationally, a BPD criterion is defined as 'present' if it is displayed outside any period(s) of Axis I disorder(s) and there has been a recurrent pattern for 2 or more years (1 year longer than required for adolescents in the DSM-IV). Clearly, many PD features are exacerbated by periodic Axis I disorders but they must be present, at least to some degree, outside of these periods.

Sometimes, distinguishing state (Axis I) from trait-based (Axis II) problems can be difficult but our overall experience is that the process (described elsewhere [57]) is usually uncomplicated. Assessment can be facilitated by using a screening instrument, such as the 15 BPD items from the Structured Clinical Interview for DSM-IV Axis II disorders (SCID-II) Personality Questionnaire and its operating characteristics have been described elsewhere [14]. A score of 13–15 (out of 15) indicates a possible BPD diagnosis and 9–12 a possible sub-syndromal BPD diagnosis. Detailed clinical assessment for BPD is then conducted, supplemented by a semi-structured BPD interview (SCID-II BPD module).

Treatment model

The elements of HYPE's integrated, team-based treatment model are described above (Principles of Early Intervention). A single practitioner (called a case manager) provides both psychotherapy and case management and all patients are jointly managed with a psychiatrist (or senior psychiatric trainee) and reviewed weekly by the entire treating team. The reasoning behind this model is both pragmatic and theoretical. First, integrating therapy, case management and psychiatric care minimizes the number of clinicians involved, reducing opportunities for disputes or 'splits' among professionals. Second, combining therapy with case management provides opportunities to generalise progress in therapy to other problems and situations. Third, the costs involved in having two clinicians (therapist and case manager) per patient are relatively higher, as the work is never divided *pro rata*. Finally (and in our view most importantly), a team-based approach, provides a supportive environment for clinicians and facilitates the development of a 'common language' through a shared model of BPD and appropriate interventions for the disorder.

Although they are combined, the model clearly distinguishes between therapy and case management in order to avoid therapy sessions being 'hijacked' by day-to-day crises. Case management is defined as work that focuses upon general psychiatric care, housing, educational or vocational issues, family matters, liaison with other services and agencies and the management of suicidal crises or deliberate self-injury. Therapy is defined as time spent using the specific tools of CAT (see below), reflecting upon how and why the presenting problems have emerged and recur and the development of more adaptive ways of coping. Although sessions normally observe a 'fifty minute hour', shorter sessions are possible, depending upon the capacity of the individual to manage therapy. This allows therapists to address patients' often unpredictable needs by offering some case management in addition to the therapy within a realistic time frame. If the minimum amount of therapy (usually 25 minutes) is not achieved, another therapy session is scheduled in its place, preferably in the same week. If therapy sessions are repeatedly disrupted, this becomes a focus for the therapy itself.

Cognitive analytic therapy   CAT is the core of the HYPE therapeutic model and the *lingua franca* of the team. CAT is a time-limited, integrative psychotherapy that has been developed in the United Kingdom over the past 30 years [58]. CAT arose from a theoretical and practical integration of elements of psychoanalytic object relations theory and cognitive psychology, developing into an integrated model of development and psychopathology. The self is seen in CAT to be characterized by an 'internalized' repertoire of relationship patterns, acquired throughout early and subsequent development. When development is suboptimal (as in the development of PDs) and early care giving interactions are less nurturing or even destructive, these relationship patterns will be internalised and used inappropriately and/or inflexibly.

CAT is practical and collaborative in style, with a particular focus upon understanding the individual's problematic relationship patterns and the thoughts, feelings and behavioural responses that result from these patterns. A central feature in CAT is the joint (patient-therapist) creation of a shared understanding of the patient's difficulties and their developmental origins, using plain-language written and diagrammatic 'reformulations'. These form the basis for understanding relationship problems both outside and within therapy and assist the patient to recognize and revise their dysfunctional relationship patterns. Because of its strong relational focus, CAT has been increasingly used with more complex and relational types of disorder, especially BPD [63], where it has a specific model and intervention [64].

CAT has particular advantages for early intervention in BPD. Its integrative approach encompasses co-occurring problems (e.g., other personality pathology, mental state and substance use disorders) within the overall treatment model, rather than seeking separate interventions. Also, CAT sees 'psychological mindedness' as a goal of therapy, rather than a prerequisite. Youth, especially those with BPD, rarely present as 'therapy ready' in any traditional sense and they usually have limited and/or adverse experiences of mental health services or therapy. Finally, while CAT is essentially a talking-based therapy, the model can be modified for use with less verbal patients or those with intellectual/learning difficulties.

Routinely, 16 CAT sessions (plus whatever case management is required) are offered to each patient, with four post-therapy follow-up sessions (at 1, 2, 4 and 6 months) to monitor progress and risk. This is negotiable to a lesser amount, especially for those who are ambivalent about treatment, but can be extended up to 24 sessions, if needed.

Consent, confidentiality and 'informed refusal'   Verbal informed consent is routinely obtained from the young person, along with parental or guardian consent. The right to and limits of confidentiality are clearly outlined to all involved at the outset and a clear statement is always made that 'duty of care' will prevail and that the safety of the young person and others is paramount.

BPD directly and adversely affects young people's capacity to access and use treatment services. Failure to attend appointments and other forms of non-communicative behaviour are expected and are not immediately interpreted as refusal of treatment. HYPE emphasises engagement and outreach, initially to inform potential patients about the actual nature of the treatment program (often dispelling unfounded fears) and the risks and benefits of participating or not. Following 6 weeks of vigorous efforts to engage the young person (at least weekly phone calls, letters and home visits, where appropriate), non-attendees are discharged with an invitation for re-referral. A clear message of refusal is always respected, unless duty of care considerations must prevail.

The episode of care   Our clinical experience is that most youth drop in and out of treatment and prefer time-limited therapy contracts. This notion of 'intermittent' therapy for PDs has received some support in the literature [65]. The CAT time limit does not preclude future episodes of CAT, either completing the balance of the 16-session intervention or in the form of 'booster' sessions. The emphasis in CAT is upon providing an agreed ending, which is usually achieved. For those patients who do have a planned ending (as opposed to dropping out), the usual practice is to discharge them after their first follow-up appointment.

Family involvement   Family conflict is a prominent feature of adolescent PD and 37% of HYPE patients are not living with any biological parent by mean age 16 years [13], rising to 57% by mean age 19 years [57]. Consistent with young people's preferences, the HYPE intervention is mostly individually based but the usual practice is to at least involve family members or carers in assessment, treatment planning and psychoeducation and to provide support within the limits of confidentiality and resources. The primary aim of this involvement is to facilitate engagement and change in the patient. Where indicated, HYPE offers more formal family intervention sessions, conducted by the primary therapist and another HYPE clinician, as appropriate, within the overall CAT model.

Psychoeducation, stigma and discrimination The BPD diagnosis is communicated with cautious optimism, based upon the natural history of BPD traits being towards improvement [12] and the evidence supporting the effectiveness of the HYPE intervention [24, 60]. Education and training for patients and professionals about the nature of BPD in young people emphasises that they have infrequently entered into the mutually hostile relationship with the health system that often characterises adult BPD. There is little need to 'undo' iatrogenic complications or adopt defensive or discriminatory institutional practices, such as prohibiting inpatient care.

Pharmacotherapy There are no methodologically sound studies of pharmacotherapy for BPD in young people. Psychotherapy and case management are given primacy in the treatment model and pharmacotherapy is presented as an adjunctive collaborative endeavour for co-occurring mental state (Axis I) disorders, such as mood or anxiety disorders, within the CAT model. The potential for polypharmacy is monitored (and discouraged) through weekly clinical review meetings.

After hours response and inpatient care Written management plans are developed for all patients and made available electronically to Orygen's after hours services and inpatient unit. These outline the jointly developed formulation of the patient's difficulties, current management plan and specific recommendations for management during acute crises that are based upon the shared formulation and goals developed with the patient. HYPE's primary aim is to promote appropriate self-care and self-management skills for community living and to minimise the risk of iatrogenic harm. Inpatient care is usually only used when all options for community treatment have been exhausted. Admission is usually voluntary, infrequent and brief and has specific goals. HYPE case managers work with inpatient and crisis teams to facilitate a 'common language', to minimize collusion with patients' problems and to achieve the goals of admission.

Treatment fidelity and supervision Treatment fidelity and completion of the tasks of an episode of care (e.g., assessment, management planning, attendance, engagement and risk management) are monitored weekly. In common with many BPD treatment models, supervision is an integral part of HYPE. It aims to support clinicians, allow time for reflection and to ensure a high standard of care. CAT supervision occurs weekly in small groups (two or three participants) and there is a fortnightly peer group case discussion. Individual case management supervision occurs every 2 weeks.

Specific challenges in working with youth with BPD

Youth with BPD often have difficulty fitting in with (adult) clinicians' expectations to attend appointments regularly and on time. HYPE adopts a flexible (time and location of appointments) and transparent (processes and policies) approach to engagement. When clinicians' needs (e.g., duty of care) might be experienced as being at odds with the patient's expressed needs, this is acknowledged. The CAT model facilitates this discussion through the early establishment of common ground. Our approach to challenges to engaging and treating young people and strategies for managing these difficulties are described elsewhere [66, 67].

The very nature of BPD makes it unrealistic to demand that young people with BPD organize themselves to attend regularly in the early phase of treatment. Rather, increased capacity for self-care and self-management is a goal of treatment and responsibility for attendance is progressively handed over to the patient. Early in treatment, young people are actively followed up (e.g., telephone calls, letters and home visits) with a focus upon barriers to attendance. The early, joint development of a shared understanding of the patient's difficulties is used to promote this discussion and allows the therapist to be aware of collusion with the patient's dysfunctional relationship patterns. Early in therapy, therapist collusion might be deliberate and strategic (e.g., home visits to a passive, angry and controlling patient) to facilitate a dialogue promoting change.

Multi-agency involvement is typical of this patient group. HYPE case managers adopt the same active, open, transparent and collaborative attitude with all concerned. The jointly constructed CAT model is used (with the patient's consent) to promote a shared, plain-language understanding of the patient's difficulties that ensures all are 'singing from the same song sheet' and minimizes professional disputes or 'splits' [68]. This model also facilitates advocacy on behalf of the young person.

Discharge   An explicit aim of HYPE is to promote support networks independent of mental health services and to avert unhelpful involvement with the mental health system. However, this is at odds with BPD patients' high needs for treatment of recurrent mental state disorders [13] and their intolerance of aloneness. Referrals are often made to external, non-mental health networks for post-discharge support. Patients are also encouraged to practice what they have learned in therapy and to delay seeking further psychotherapy until their 6-month follow-up review. This does not preclude further case management or treatment of mental state disorders, as necessary. However, this is infrequently required.

Remaining barriers and potential risks

Despite evidence of sufficient reliability and validity for the BPD diagnosis in young people, stigma and discrimination are key lingering barriers to the early diagnosis of BPD in day-to-day clinical practice. BPD is highly stigmatised among professionals [69] and it is also associated with patient 'self-stigma' [70]. This fuels the perception that the diagnosis is 'controversial' [9] and clinical experience suggests that many clinicians will deliberately avoid using the diagnosis in young people with the aim of 'protecting' individuals from harsh and/or discriminatory practices.

While concerns about stigma and discrimination are genuine and the response is well intentioned, this practice runs the risk of perpetuating negative stereotypes, reducing the prospect of applying specific beneficial interventions for the problems associated with BPD and increasing the likelihood of inappropriate diagnoses and interventions and iatrogenic harm (such as polypharmacy).

The National Institute for Health and Clinical Excellence (NICE) guideline for BPD [10] supports the diagnosis of BPD in adolescents and the forthcoming revisions of the ICD and DSM classification systems are both proposing to remove age-related caveats on the diagnosis of PDs [71, 72]. Moreover, the ICD (and possibly the DSM) will include the identification of subthreshold personality pathology. These innovations foster not only the early diagnosis of BPD but also the identification of subthreshold BPD, supporting the aims of indicated prevention and early intervention. However, this will bring into the clinical realm, young people (and adults) who might once have been considered 'colourful' and potential benefits are accompanied by potential risks associated with 'medicalising' common problems; risks that are not confined to the field of BPD.

Conclusion and future perspectives

BPD should now be seen as a lifespan developmental disorder with substantial ramifications across subsequent decades. Consequently, intervention at any stage should aim to alter the life-course trajectory of borderline personality pathology, not just its diagnostic features. At present, there is sufficient evidence to support diagnosing and treating the BPD syndrome when it first appears becoming part of routine clinical practice. There are also data showing that targeting sub-syndromal borderline pathology through indicated prevention is a promising approach and that the benefits of intervention appear to outweigh the risks. However, this approach requires further development and evaluation over longer periods in order to ensure that there are no significant 'downstream' adverse effects.

Acknowledgements

Orygen Youth Health Research Centre is funded by an unrestricted philanthropic grant from the Colonial Foundation, Melbourne, Australia.

The authors report no competing financial interests.

We gratefully acknowledge the invaluable contributions made by the young people and their families who have attended the HYPE Clinic, along with those made by our HYPE colleagues and many others.

References

1. Leichsenring F, Leibing E, Kruse J, et al. (2011). Borderline personality disorder. *Lancet* **377**(9759): 74–84.
2. Coid J, Yang M, Tyrer P, et al. (2006). Prevalence and correlates of personality disorder in Great Britain. *British Journal of Psychiatry* **188**: 423–431.
3. Trull TJ, Jahng S, Tomko RL, et al. (2010). Revised NESARC personality disorder diagnoses: gender, prevalence, and comorbidity with substance dependence disorders. *Journal of Personality Disorders* **24**(4): 412–426.
4. Zimmerman M, Chelminski I and Young D. (2008). The frequency of personality disorders in psychiatric patients. *Psychiatric Clinics of North America* **31**(3): 405–420, vi.
5. Gunderson JG, Stout RL, McGlashan TH, et al. (2011). Ten-year course of borderline personality disorder: psychopathology and function from the collaborative longitudinal personality disorders study. *Archives of General Psychiatry* **68**(8): 827–837.

6. Horz S, Zanarini MC, Frankenburg FR, et al. (2010). Ten-year use of mental health services by patients with borderline personality disorder and with other axis II disorders. *Psychiatric Services* **61**(6): 612–616.

7. Pompili M, Girardi P, Ruberto A, et al. (2005). Suicide in borderline personality disorder: a meta-analysis. *Nordic Journal of Psychiatry* **59**(5): 319–324.

8. APA. (1980). *Diagnostic and statistical manual of mental disorders*, 3rd edition. Washington DC: American Psychiatric Association.

9. Chanen AM and McCutcheon LK. (2008). Personality disorder in adolescence: the diagnosis that dare not speak its name. *Personality and Mental Health* **2**(1): 35–41.

10. National Collaborating Centre for Mental Health. (2009). Borderline personality disorder: treatment and management. London: National Institute for Health and Clinical Excellence. CG78 Contract No.: 78.

11. Tackett JL, Balsis S, Oltmanns TF, et al. (2009). A unifying perspective on personality pathology across the life span: developmental considerations for the fifth edition of the diagnostic and statistical manual of mental disorders. *Development and Psychopathology* **21**(3): 687–713.

12. Chanen AM, Jovev M, McCutcheon L, et al. (2008). Borderline personality disorder in young people and the prospects for prevention and early intervention. *Current Psychiatry Reviews* **4**(1): 48–57.

13. Chanen AM, Jovev M and Jackson HJ. (2007). Adaptive functioning and psychiatric symptoms in adolescents with borderline personality disorder. *Journal of Clinical Psychiatry* **68**(2): 297–306.

14. Chanen AM, Jovev M, Djaja D, et al. (2008). Screening for borderline personality disorder in outpatient youth. *Journal of Personality Disorders* **22**(4): 353–364.

15. Bernstein DP, Cohen P, Velez CN, et al. (1993). Prevalence and stability of the DSM-III-R personality disorders in a community-based survey of adolescents. *American Journal of Psychiatry* **150**(8): 1237–1243.

16. Moran P, Coffey C, Mann A, et al. (2006). Personality and substance use disorders in young adults. *British Journal of Psychiatry* **188**(4): 374–379.

17. Ullrich S and Coid J. (2009). The age distribution of self-reported personality disorder traits in a household population. *Journal of Personality Disorders* **23**(2): 187–200.

18. Johnson JG, Cohen P, Kasen S, et al. (2000). Age-related change in personality disorder trait levels between early adolescence and adulthood: a community-based longitudinal investigation. *Acta Psychiatrica Scandinavica* **102**(4): 265–275.

19. Chanen AM, Jackson HJ, McGorry PD, et al. (2004). Two-year stability of personality disorder in older adolescent outpatients. *Journal of Personality Disorders* **18**(6): 526–541.

20. Cohen P, Crawford TN, Johnson JG, et al. (2005). The children in the community study of developmental course of personality disorder. *Journal of Personality Disorders* **19**(5): 466–486.

21. Crawford TN, Cohen P, First MB, et al. (2008). Comorbid axis I and axis II disorders in early adolescence: prognosis 20 years later. *Archives of General Psychiatry* **65**(6): 641–648.

22. Winograd G, Cohen P and Chen H. (2008). Adolescent borderline symptoms in the community: prognosis for functioning over 20 years. *Journal of Child Psychology and Psychiatry and Allied Disciplines* **49**(9): 933–941.

23. Lenzenweger MF and Castro DD. (2005). Predicting change in borderline personality: using neurobehavioral systems indicators within an individual growth curve framework. *Development and Psychopathology* **17**(04): 1207–1237.

24. Chanen AM, Jackson HJ, McCutcheon L, et al. (2008). Early intervention for adolescents with borderline personality disorder using cognitive analytic therapy: a randomised controlled trial. *British Journal of Psychiatry* **193**(6): 477–484.

25. Schuppert M, Giesen-Bloo J, van Gemert T, et al. (2009). Effectiveness of an emotion regulation group training for adolescents-a randomized controlled pilot study. *Clinical Psychology and Psychotherapy* **16**(6): 467–478.

26. Distel MA, Middeldorp CM, Trull TJ, et al. (2011). Life events and borderline personality features: the influence of gene-environment interaction and gene-environment correlation. *Psychological Medicine* **41**(4): 849–860.

27. Chanen AM and Kaess M. (2012). Developmental pathways toward borderline personality disorder. *Current Psychiatry Reports* **14**(1): 45–53.

28. Chanen AM, Velakoulis D, Carison K, et al. (2008). Orbitofrontal, amygdala and hippocampal volumes in teenagers with first-presentation borderline personality disorder. *Psychiatry Research Neuroimaging* **163**(2): 116–125.

29. Brunner R, Henze R, Parzer P, et al. (2010). Reduced prefrontal and orbitofrontal gray matter in female adolescents with borderline personality disorder: is it disorder specific? *Neuroimage* **49**(1): 114–120.

30. Bradley R, Jenei J and Westen D. (2005). Etiology of borderline personality disorder: disentangling the contributions of intercorrelated antecedents. *Journal of Nervous and Mental Disease* **193**(1): 24–31.

31. Cohen P. (2008). Child development and personality disorder. *Psychiatric Clinics of North America* **31**(3): 477–493.

32. Johnson JG, Cohen P, Brown J, et al. (1999). Childhood maltreatment increases risk for personality disorders during early adulthood. *Archives of General Psychiatry* **56**(7): 600–606.

33. Cohen P, Chen H, Gordon K, et al. (2008). Socioeconomic background and the developmental course of schizotypal and borderline personality disorder symptoms. *Development and Psychopathology* **20**(2): 633–650.

34. Bezirganian S, Cohen P and Brook JS. (1993). The impact of mother-child interaction on the development of borderline personality disorder. *American Journal of Psychiatry* **150**(12): 1836–1842.

35. Johnson JG, Cohen P, Chen H, et al. (2006). Parenting behaviors associated with risk for offspring personality disorder during adulthood. *Archives of General Psychiatry* **63**(5): 579–587.

36. Crawford TN, Cohen PR, Chen H, et al. (2009). Early maternal separation and the trajectory of borderline personality disorder symptoms. *Development and Psychopathology* **21**(3): 1013–1030.

37. Carlson EA, Egeland B and Sroufe LA. (2009). A prospective investigation of the development of borderline personality symptoms. *Development and Psychopathology* **21**(4): 1311–1334.

38. Kraemer HC, Kazdin AE, Offord DR, et al. (1997). Coming to terms with the terms of risk. *Archives of General Psychiatry* **54**(4): 337–343.

39. Eaton WW, Badawi M and Melton B. (1995). Prodromes and precursors: epidemiologic data for primary prevention of disorders with slow onset. *American Journal of Psychiatry* **152**(7): 967–972.

40. Rohde P, Lewinsohn PM, Kahler CW, et al. (2001). Natural course of alcohol use disorders from adolescence to young adulthood. *Journal of the American Academy of Child and Adolescent Psychiatry* **40**(1): 83–90.

41. Thatcher DL, Cornelius JR and Clark DB. (2005). Adolescent alcohol use disorders predict adult borderline personality. *Addictive Behaviors* **30**(9): 1709–1724.

42. Stepp SD, Burke JD, Hipwell AE, et al. (2011). Trajectories of attention deficit hyperactivity disorder and oppositional defiant disorder symptoms as precursors of borderline personality disorder symptoms in adolescent girls. *Journal of Abnormal Child Psychology* **40**(1): 7–20.

43. Burke JD and Stepp SD. (2011). Adolescent disruptive behavior and borderline personality disorder symptoms in young adult men. *Journal of Abnormal Child Psychology* **40**(1): 35–44.

44. Zanarini MC, Frankenburg FR, Ridolfi ME, et al. (2006). Reported childhood onset of self-mutilation among borderline patients. *Journal of Personality Disorders* **20**(1): 9–15.

45. Nock MK. (2010). Self-injury. *Annual Review of Clinical Psychology* **6**: 339–363.

46. Brunner R, Parzer P, Haffner J, et al. (2007). Prevalence and psychological correlates of occasional and repetitive deliberate self-harm in adolescents. *Archives of Pediatrics and Adolescent Medicine* **161**(7): 641–649.

47. Nock MK, Joiner JTE, Gordon KH, et al. (2006). Non-suicidal self-injury among adolescents: diagnostic correlates and relation to suicide attempts. *Psychiatry Research* **144**(1): 65–72.
48. Muehlenkamp JJ, Ertelt TW, Miller AL, et al. (2011). Borderline personality symptoms differentiate non-suicidal and suicidal self-injury in ethnically diverse adolescent outpatients. *Journal of Child Psychology and Psychiatry, and Allied Disciplines* **52**(2): 148–155.
49. Jacobson CM, Muehlenkamp JJ, Miller AL, et al. (2008). Psychiatric impairment among adolescents engaging in different types of deliberate self-harm. *Journal of Clinical Child and Adolescent Psychology* **37**(2): 363–375.
50. Stepp SD, Pilkonis PA, Hipwell AE, et al. (2010). Stability of borderline personality disorder features in girls. *Journal of Personality Disorders* **24**(4): 460–472.
51. Crick NR, Murray-Close D and Woods K. (2005). Borderline personality features in childhood: a short-term longitudinal study. *Development and Psychopathology* **17**(4): 1051–1070.
52. Cohen P. (1996). Childhood risks for young adult symptoms of personality disorder: method and substance. *Multivariate Behavioral Research* **31**(1): 121–148.
53. Bernstein DP, Cohen P, Skodol A, et al. (1996). Childhood antecedents of adolescent personality disorders. *American Journal of Psychiatry* **153**(7): 907–913.
54. Kasen S, Cohen P, Skodol AE, et al. (1999). Influence of child and adolescent psychiatric disorders on young adult personality disorder. *American Journal of Psychiatry* **156**(10): 1529–1535.
55. Crawford TN, Cohen P, Johnson JG, et al. (2005). Self-reported personality disorder in the children in the community sample: convergent and prospective validity in late adolescence and adulthood. *Journal of Personality Disorders* **19**(1): 30–52.
56. Cuijpers P. (2003). Examining the effects of prevention programs on the incidence of new cases of mental disorders: the lack of statistical power. *American Journal of Psychiatry* **160**(8): 1385–1391.
57. Chanen AM, McCutcheon L, Germano D, et al. (2009). The HYPE clinic: an early intervention service for borderline personality disorder. *Journal of Psychiatric Practice* **15**(3): 163–172.
58. Ryle A and Kerr IB (eds). (2002). *Introducing Cognitive Analytic Therapy*. John Wiley & Sons Ltd. Chichester.
59. Blum N, St John D, Pfohl B, et al. (2008). Systems training for emotional predictability and problem solving (STEPPS) for outpatients with borderline personality disorder: a randomized controlled trial and 1-year follow-up. *American Journal of Psychiatry* **165**(4): 468–478.
60. Chanen AM, Jackson HJ, McCutcheon L, et al. (2009). Early intervention for adolescents with borderline personality disorder: a quasi-experimental comparison with treatment as usual. *Australian and New Zealand Journal of Psychiatry* **43**(5): 397–408.
61. McGorry PD, Parker AG and Purcell R. (2007). Youth mental health: a new stream of mental health care for adolescents and young adults. In: G Meadows, B Singh and M Grigg (eds), *Mental Health in Australia: Collaborative Community Practice*, 2nd edition, pp. 438–449. Cambridge: Cambridge University Press.
62. Zimmerman M, Chelminski I, Young D, et al. (2012). Does the presence of one feature of borderline personality disorder have clinical significance? implications for dimensional ratings of personality disorders. *The Journal of Clinical Psychiatry* **73**(1): 8–12.
63. Ryle A. (2004). The contribution of cognitive analytic therapy to the treatment of borderline personality disorder. *Journal of Personality Disorders* **18**(1): 3–35.
64. Ryle A (ed.). (1997). *Cognitive Analytic Therapy of Borderline Personality Disorder: The Model and The Method*. New York, John Wiley & Sons.
65. Paris J. (2007). Intermittent psychotherapy: an alternative to continuous long-term treatment for patients with personality disorders. *Journal of Psychiatric Practice* **13**(3): 153–158.
66. McCutcheon LK, Chanen AM, Fraser R, et al. (2007). Tips and techniques for engaging and managing the reluctant, resistant or hostile young person. *Medical Journal of Australia* **187**(7): S64–S7.
67. Chanen AM and McCutcheon LK. (2008). Engaging and managing an unwilling or aggressive young person. *Medicine Today* **9**(6): 81–83.

68. Kerr IB. (1999). Cognitive-analytic therapy for borderline personality disorder in the context of a community mental health team: Individual and organizational psychodynamic implications. *British Journal of Psychotherapy* **15**(4): 425–438.

69. Aviram RB, Brodsky BS and Stanley B. (2006). Borderline personality disorder, stigma, and treatment implications. *Harvard Review of Psychiatry* **14**(5): 249–256.

70. Rusch N, Holzer A, Hermann C, et al. (2006). Self-stigma in women with borderline personality disorder and women with social phobia. *Journal of Nervous and Mental Disease* **194**(10): 766–773.

71. Skodol AE, Bender DS, Morey LC, et al. (2011). Personality disorder types proposed for DSM-5. *Journal of Personality Disorders* **25**(2): 136–169.

72. Tyrer P, Crawford M, Mulder R, et al. (2011). The rationale for the reclassification of personality disorder in the 11th Revision of the International Classification of Diseases (ICD-11). *Personality and Mental Health* **5**(4): 246–259.

V
Conclusions

25

Early Intervention and the Power of Social Movements: UK Development of Early Intervention in Psychosis as a Social Movement and its Implications for Leadership

David Shiers[1,2,3] and Jo Smith[1,4,5]

[1] National Early Intervention Programme, England
[2] Leek, North Staffordshire, UK
[3] National Mental Health Development Unit, London, UK
[4] Worcestershire Health and Care NHS Trust, Worcester, UK
[5] University of Worcester, Worcester, UK

"*More powerful than the march of mighty armies is an idea whose time has come.*"

Victor Hugo 1852 [1]

Declaration of interests:
[1] DS is a clinical advisor to the National Audit of Schizophrenia (paid consultancy); a board member of the National Mental Health Collaborating Centre (NCCMH); a member of the Quality Standards group of the National Institute for Health and Clinical Excellence (NICE); the views expressed are not those of either NCCMH or NICE.
[2] JS is a Consultant Clinical Psychologist and Early Intervention Clinical Development Lead with Worcestershire Health and Care NHS Trust, Worcester, UK and an external consultant for the Catalyst Individual Placement Support Programme with Janssen-Cilag, UK; the views expressed are not those of either Worcestershire Health and Care NHS Trust or Janssen-Cilag.

An international context

Although this chapter will focus on how these changes came about in England, it is important to appreciate this in the context of a growing international early psychosis movement. From early collaborations in 1992/3 between service innovations such as Early Psychosis Prevention and Intervention Centre (EPPIC) and Psychosis and Crisis Evaluation Clinic (PACE) in Melbourne, Australia, and the Archer Centre in North Birmingham, England, an international community of interest emerged initially drawing in developments such as Norway's Treatment and Early Intervention in Psychosis Programme (TIPS), Amsterdam with its family intervention programmes; Denmark's OPUS, a psychiatric service for patients experiencing a first episode of psychosis (FEP) and a number of Early Intervention in Psychosis (EIP) services in Canada, United States and Singapore. Subsequently, these pioneering services have formalised their mutually supportive relationship by the creation of the International Early Psychosis Association (IEPA) (www.iepa.org.au). This was further enhanced by the creation of an international consensus statement, the Early Psychosis Declaration (EPD) endorsed by the IEPA and the World Health Organisation (WHO) in 2004. Within that international context, England has arguably enjoyed the most uniform EIP service implementation and our chapter explores how this transformation came about.

Early intervention in psychosis: *'developing the head'* – the knowledge base

The idea that it was desirable to treat conditions like schizophrenia earlier in their course is not new. Radical thinkers such as Harry Sullivan challenged (and may still challenge) traditionalists, convinced by Kraepelin's [2] original description of 'dementia praecox' as a single disease entity (schizophrenia) with a universally poor outcome.

> *"I feel certain that any incipient cases might be arrested before the efficient contact with reality is completely suspended, and a long stay in institutions made necessary."*
>
> Sullivan [3]

However, Kraepelin's dismal construction continued to dominate the values and principles of treatment for much of the twentieth century. It was not until 1977 that this pessimistic mindset was discredited by Manfred Bleuler's [4] classic description, developed from observations of the course of schizophrenia in 208 patients and families collected over 20 years. Bleuler concluded of the dementia praecox model:

> *"It seems almost incredible how one-sided theories on the schizophrenias, upheld entirely by wishful thinking and unsupported by empirical fact, could propagate themselves."*
>
> Bleuler [4]

Further meticulous long-term studies would reveal that even the most severely affected could achieve positive outcomes amounting to partial or even complete recovery [5, 6]. Subsequently, the Northwick Park study found that individuals with a FEP taking longer than 1 year to access services had threefold more relapse in the following 2 years than those accessing services in under 1 year [7]. This study sparked intense research and clinical interest in the early phase of psychosis. This phase became conceptualised by Birchwood [8] as a *'critical period'* with major implications for secondary prevention of impairments and disabilities and a rationale for intervening intensively and early, heralding the emergence of a range of new evidence-based treatments for these young people and their families. The initial Northwick Park findings would in time be further reinforced by an important meta-analysis which showed that longer duration of untreated psychosis (DUP) predicted more toxic pathways linked to poor response to treatment, recovery and long-term outcome [9].

Professor Fiona Macmillan, co-author of the Northwick Park study, helped develop the first UK EIP service in North Birmingham with her colleague Professor Max Birchwood mirroring similar service innovation in Melbourne [10]. Thus were laid the modern foundations for EIP service development in the United Kingdom.

EIP: *'developing the heart'* – the right to social justice

"Obsolete theories on schizophrenia without empirical foundations were not merely harmless assertions; they caused a great deal of harm."

Bleuler 1977 [4]

Bleuler's conclusions highlighted what was driving an increasingly politicised reaction against psychiatry. Dissent began to be voiced by people describing themselves as *survivors* of hospitalisation in overcrowded institutions where they had endured coercive treatments and a range of indignities, deprivations and abuses. Psychiatric institutions and professionals stood criticised for performing social control, rather than providing clinical support. This became a civil rights issue. Moreover, many professionals were disillusioned with the prevailing system even if they were unsure of what would work better. The century closed with UK political sensitivity heightened by high-profile media concerns for public safety (e.g. the tragic killing of Jonathan Zito by Christopher Clunis) [11]. The prevailing UK policy of 'Care in the Community' became severely criticised for neglect of individuals by overburdened community mental health teams (CMHTs) that relied excessively on crisis hospital admission and medication.

Important in this dissent was a small group from the West Midlands region (population 5.2 million) in the 1990s, which formed following a complaint about local services by co-author Dr. David Shiers (DS) after his 16-year-old daughter had developed a psychosis. A 3-year journey through various hospital settings left his daughter effectively 'written-off' at the age of 19 in an antiquated asylum, situated where DS worked as a GP [12]. Professor Antony Sheehan, Regional Director of Mental Health, responded to David's complaint by encouraging a small group to come together to improve services for young people. Some early proponents of EIP were identified: Professor Birchwood, clinical psychologist and researcher and service developer in schizophrenia; Dr Jo Smith, clinical psychologist from Worcestershire, who established one of the first UK family services for people with

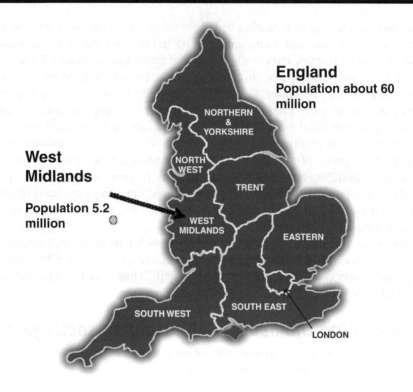

psychosis and their families; Professor Macmillan, the psychiatrist responsible for DS's daughter's care and co-author of the Northwick Park study. Identifying themselves as Initiative to Reduce the Impact of Schizophrenia (IRIS), (IRIS Guidelines 1999, [13]) and (website www.iris-initiative.org.uk), the group began to mobilise support for EIP. Their influence subsequently evolved from its original West Midlands base to become a coordinated national network. IRIS has supported four particularly influential steps in the EIP journey from margin to mainstream:

1. 1997/8: Several pathways to care audits within the West Midlands

2. 1998: IRIS regional service guidelines

3. 2002-4: Early Psychosis Declaration

4. 2004-10: National Early Intervention Development Programme

We shall explore how these four initiatives synergised the 'head' and the 'heart'.

1. *1997/8: West Midlands pathways to care audits.* Several audits revealed typically *late intervention in crisis* reflecting problematic interfaces, for example primary/specialist interface and Child and Adolescent Mental Health Services (CAMHS)/Adult service interface. Although not unique to the United Kingdom [14], these audits provided hard evidence of *local* service experience with which to confront *local* health systems (Box 25.1) [15].

Box 25.1   Audit of pathways to care for 45 people with first-episode psychosis in the West Midlands

- Fifty percent developed psychosis under the age of 24 and 20% under the age of 18.

- Duration of untreated psychosis (DUP) was 7–15 months.

- Only 20% were engaged via community mental health services without recourse to hospitalisation.

- For 80% their first experience of mental health services was hospitalisation.

- Fifty-two percent required use of the Mental Health Act (1983).

- Forty-five percent of these involved the police or criminal justice system.

- Only one person engaged services via psychiatric outpatients.

IRIS collaborated with voluntary sector consumer organisations such as Rethink, whose campaign *'Getting help early'* had highlighted negative attitudes held by people with early psychosis and their carers towards traditional CMHTs. Thus, the 'head' provided the audit evidence and the 'heart' spoke out of its injustice. The stage was set for challenging the 'one size fits all' CMHT approach, as this campaign message captured:

When your car breaks down
you can get help within **60 minutes**.

When your mind breaks down
you may not get help for **18 months**.

rethink severe mental illness · www.rethink.org

2. *1998: IRIS regional guidelines.* (IRIS guidelines 1999, [13]. As a consequence of those initial audits, and with the established North Birmingham EIP service as a practice exemplar, IRIS created a network for service innovation. The regional mental health lead asked IRIS to develop clinical guidelines from best available evidence. Importantly,

this drew on experiences from similar EIP service innovations in Australia, Scandinavia, Canada and the United States. The IRIS guidelines described ten core service features:

- *Early detection and assessment of frank psychosis*

- *Early and sustained case manager engagement*

- *A comprehensive, collaborative and shared assessment plan*

- *Low-dose pharmacotherapy and cognitive therapy*

- *A family approach to care*

- *Relapse prevention and treatment resistance strategies*

- *Access to work and valued occupation*

- *Assessment of basic needs for everyday living*

- *Assessment and treatment of co morbid difficulties*

- *Public education strategy*

IRIS also set out some key service principles:

- **A youth and user focus.** EIP services should be youth-friendly, reflecting youth culture and young people's aspirations concerning the importance of work and autonomy.

- **Early, proactive and sustained engagement**. Engagement, via an identified, named case manager, seeks common ground, builds on their personal strengths and offers flexible access in low-stigma settings for example, home, cafes and college. Interventions offer practical assistance to resolve identified problems important to the individual. Failure to take prescribed medication, illicit drug use and non-attendance do not lead to discharge: instead the service uses an assertive outreach model to maintain client contact. Where insight is poor, the team will work with and support the family.

- **Embrace diagnostic uncertainty:** referral is based on suspicion rather than certainty of diagnosis. The service adopts low thresholds for reassessment, avoids premature diagnosis until symptom stability is achieved and adopts symptom-based approaches to treatment. Psycho-education is based on risk/vulnerability factors for psychosis. The term 'psychosis' is favoured rather than specific diagnoses like Schizophrenia, given its diagnostic unreliability in emerging psychosis and to avoid negative stereotypes and low expectations for recovery.

- **Treat in the least restrictive and stigmatised setting**: avoid crisis admissions by home treating whenever possible to minimise disruption, stigmatisation and trauma, with systems in place for out of hours cover over evenings and weekends. Where admission is considered necessary to achieve symptom stabilisation, effect medication changes or manage risk (where home treatment and community management is not feasible) admission is ideally to age appropriate, youth friendly and inpatient environments.

- **Emphasis on social roles:** individualised care plans develop individual activity programs designed to enable individuals to sustain and access main stream community educational, vocational, social and leisure pursuits. Interventions are informed by evidence-based practice models including individual placement support (IPS), client-centred practice, occupational therapy and solution-focused approaches.

- **Family-orientated approach:** family interventions aim to provide hope, optimism and respect for the family. Care plans foster partnership with families in supporting recovery while addressing family (and sibling) support needs. Intervention is geared to the specific needs of any given family and informed by an understanding of family adaptation to early psychosis. For example, addresses burden, uncertainty, stigma, loss, intrusion and desire for independence while preventing unhelpful entrenchment patterns of interaction such as criticism, rejection and emotional over-involvement by tackling their precursors notably, feelings of loss, guilt and shame appraisals.

The IRIS guidelines offered a service response to the very issues raised by Rethink's *'Getting help early'* campaign and the IRIS audit findings. They became the blueprint for the policy implementation guide [16], underpinning the subsequent national EIP reform. The 'heart' was being supported by an evidence-based 'head'. And EIP was moving from the margins to the mainstream.

3. *Early Psychosis Declaration* (www.iris-initiative.org.uk). As part of creating pressure for political reform, IRIS embarked on an initiative to generate a consensus about the standards of care that those developing early psychosis and their families should expect. A model was used that had successfully transformed diabetes care 10 years previously – the St. Vincent Declaration for Diabetes [17]. Initiated by IRIS, with support from Rethink and the National Institute Mental Health in England (NIMHE), a consensus was developed into the Newcastle Declaration for early psychosis over two days by a group of 30 people from across England with particular interest in early psychosis, which included users, carers, practitioners and senior civil servants [18]. These people from apparently diverse perspectives were able to agree a platform of shared dissatisfaction from which to establish a common positive purpose. This remarkable meeting was to shift the whole focus of EIP service development towards *improvement of health* rather than *reduction in illness*. Supported by the IEPA and WHO as an international consensus [19], this became known as the EPD and was formally launched at the UK national EIP conference in Bristol in 2004 by WHO mental health director, Benedetto Saraceno. Subsequently, IRIS produced a practical toolkit to support EPD implementation, enabling services to benchmark and plan development [20].

International consensus statement [19]

- Establish a clear vision, some core values and some actions required to achieve early intervention and recovery for all young people experiencing psychosis.

- Generate optimism and raise expectations from young people experiencing psychosis and their families that will influence the development of better services.

- Provide a framework for enabling those young people and their families to work alongside practitioners and services to:
  - Acknowledge the key shared concerns
  - Develop a set of jointly agreed, valued and measurable goals
  - Jointly commit to a set of strategic actions to achieve these goals
- Attract and encourage practitioners from a wide range of health, social, educational and employment services to contribute by working in partnership to support these young people and their families.

The 'heart' in seeking *health improvement* rather than *disease reduction*, and the 'head' in setting evidence-based and measurable standards, had combined to create a compelling vision for change which now transcended national boundaries.

4. A National EIP Development Programme– 'The head and heart deliver.' The next piece in our 'head' and 'heart' narrative is how the informal systems that had driven change were beginning to consolidate and stabilise.

An emergent direction was clear – the EPD as a value-base, a policy priority established, a strengthening evidence-base and the service model agreed. A structure was needed that could organise the various elements – the National EIP Development Programme. Established by NIMHE and Rethink in 2004, this initiative would support National Service Framework (NSF) implementation until its conclusion in 2010. The authors, as a small central hub, linked closely with nine regional EIP lead to support a coordinated EIP movement which embraced three synergistic elements – policy, research and practice. Programme friend, Dr. Glenn Roberts, likened these elements to wind vectors that filled the sails to drive the craft forward (Roberts G, personal communication, 2006). We have described these elements below as single entities. The reality was a complex blend, sometimes one and sometimes another vector would assume the main driving force. Pushed on by these forces, the programme learnt how to navigate the complex waters of change.

Policy. Responding to groups like IRIS and Rethink in the late 90s and influenced by the IRIS guidelines and the EPD, policymakers developed the NSF for adult mental health [21], the NHS Plan [22] and the Policy Implementation Guide [16]. These drew upon the evidence base to specify, bottom-up (i.e. on the basis of population and individual need), team case loads, the full range of effective interventions for psychosis to be provided and the service configurations necessary to deliver them. Designed to deliver a more intensive and person-centred approach, these aimed to break the cycle of crisis response and hospitalisation by offering a 3-year package of evidence-based interventions, sensitive to age and phase of illness. EIPs priority status has remained undiminished from 1999, supported by the national programme's successful interweaving of policy, research and practice.

Research. The 'heart's' dissatisfaction with traditional services underpins this whole narrative. The policymakers had responded as Box 25.2 shows. Could the 'head' come up with the evidence?

Box 25.2 Policy development to support early intervention in the United Kingdom

National Service Framework Adult Mental Health [21] Outlining a 10-year policy commitment. EIP service development now becomes a firm policy intention.

NHS Plan [22] Mental health sits as a top priority within the wider plan for modernisation of the entire NHS. For EIP the NHS Plan gave specific commitment to:

- Fifty new teams will ensure *'all young people who experience a first episode of psychosis, such as schizophrenia will receive the early and intensive support they need'.*

- Reduce the DUP to a service average of 3 months (maximum individual 6 months) and continuous service support for the first 3 years.

Priorities and planning framework 2003 – 2006 [23] Set out the NHS plan objectives against timelines, reaffirming EIP as a priority with its own targets.

Policy implementation guide [16]. The 'PIG' gave detailed service specifications: The EIP model should provide care for 3 years for those aged 14–35 with emerging psychosis.

Core interventions in the treatment and management of schizophrenia [24] Values EIP's role within the care pathway, supported by an evidence base of treatments

NSF for children, young people and maternity services [25] Reinforces the commitment to ensure seamless provision of EIP for those young people in transitional age.

2006 EIP Recovery Plan 2006/7 [26] *required* EIP provision to 7500 new patients in 06/07 in order to put EIP development back on target *(after slippage on original target was acknowledged)*

2007–2012 NHS operating framework EIP [27]: continuing priority to put EIP services in all areas

2011 No Health Without Mental Health [70]: EIP continues as a national policy priority

---

The National Institute for Health and Clinical Excellence in its review of evidence for treating schizophrenia agreed there was a problem with generic CMHTs [24]:

> *"Despite the fact that CMHT's remain the mainstay of community mental health care (for psychosis), there is surprisingly little evidence to show that they are an effective way of organising services (for psychosis)."*
>
> NICE 2014 [24]

When even good quality 'standard' CMHTs are compared with EIP services: the latter report improved clinical outcomes: shorter DUP, lower use of legal detention, reduced hospital admissions [28]; lower-relapse rates, improved medication adherence [29]; better service engagement, consumer satisfaction and lower-suicide rates [30]; gains in functional and social aspects in terms of educational or vocational pursuits [31]; better able to establish or re-establish relationships [30] greater rates of independent living and reduced

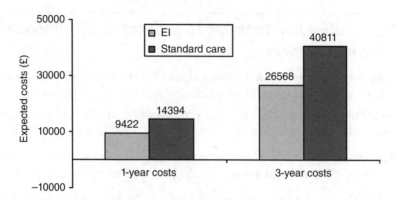

Figure 25.1   EI cost impact of early intervention. McCrone et al. 2009. Early Intervention in Psychiatry 2009; **3**: 266–273. Reproduced with permission of John Wiley & Sons

homelessness; lower levels of substance misuse and better overall global functioning. Two randomised controlled trials showed advantages of EIP for up to 2 years following intervention [29, 32, 33], with some effects persisting at 5-years follow-up [29, 34]. For comprehensive evidence, see reviews by Addington [35] and McGorry et al. [36, 37].

And the National Institute for Health and Clinical Excellence again [24]:

> *"The Guideline Development Group recognised that the rationale for an early intervention service is powerful, both ethically (helping people with serious mental health problems at an early stage to reduce distress and possibly disability) and in terms of flexibility and choice (service users and carers want help sooner than is usually available). New evidence from the clinical review clearly demonstrates that early intervention can be effective with benefits lasting at least 2 years."*

NICE 2014 [24]

Cost benefits of EIP. In the first UK economic impact analysis, McCrone and Knapp modelled the costs associated with EIP and standard CMHT care over a 1-year and a 3-year period. The overall costs strongly favoured EIP care. Over 3 years, the cost per case estimated £26,568 for EIP against £40,816 for CMHT care, a saving of £14,248 per case, reflecting mainly reductions in admission and readmission rates – see Figure 25.1 [38, 39].

The Kings Fund report, 'Paying the Price' predicted potential annual savings of £60 million (2008 prices) from full EIP service coverage in England over the next 20 years [40]. Moreover, recent cost modelling suggests that these figures are an underestimate when the impact of improved employment and educational attainment are factored in; saving another £2000 per client per year widening the cost-effectiveness gap yet further in favour of EIP [41].

A national study of service implementation evaluated the views of service users [42]. Most (24 of the 36 interviewed) described EIS in positive terms, for instance, offering activities and services that were youth friendly and made sense; helping them come to terms with their illness; understanding why they had become unwell; and working with them over time to identify triggers and early warning signs. Of their families, many said

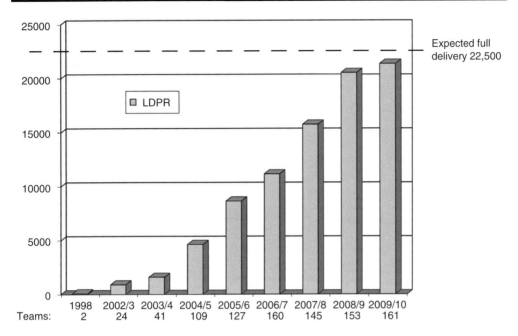

Figure 25.2   Growth in EIP cases and services 1998–2010 (21,372 cases March 2010)

family support had increased and they felt closer to their families. Families were described as supportive in the care process by advocating for treatment, helping them cope with symptoms, and helping develop and use relapse plans.

Practice and service development. From 1998, as the NSF got underway, just two teams provided care for about 80 people. Department of Health estimates of Local Delivery Plan Returns (LDPR) at March 2010 revealed 161 teams serving 21,372 people, within a positive trajectory towards full-policy implementation (Figure 25.2) [43].

However, service capacity in terms of numbers of teams or cases *on-the-books* is necessary but not sufficient of itself. The ultimate test of whether this policy is improving peoples' lives is to assess how the service experience has changed. Informing the NICE schizophrenia review [24], an important systematic review examined the nature of the early intervention service provision [44]. This study specifically examined the characteristics of early intervention services designed to provide multimodal psychosocial interventions, pharmacotherapy and some form of case management with lower case-loads and an assertive approach to treatment, all within the context of intervening as early as possible. The authors concluded: 'Early intervention services are an effective way of delivering care for people with early psychosis and can reduce hospital admission, relapse rates and symptom severity, while improving access to and engagement with a range of treatments' [44].

And one aspect common to many EIP services is the commitment to evaluating services against quality standards. Table 25.1 illustrates Worcestershire EIP Service audits data, a nonresearch-based EIP service, and whose outcomes are replicable by many EIP services across England:

Table 25.1   Worcestershire EIS outcome data

DUP (median)	National audit data 12–18m	2006 (*n* = 78) (22% 14–18 years) 6m	2008 (n + 106) (18% 14–18 years) 5m
Percent admitted with FEP (entry point to EI)	80%	41%	17.5%
Percent admitted on Mental Health Act (MHA)	50%	27%	10%
Readmission	50% (in 2 years)	28%	17%
Percent engaged at 12m	50%	100% (79% well engaged)	99% (70% well engaged)
Family involved (satisfied)	49% (56%)	91% (71%)	84%
Employment (education and training)	8–18%	55%	56%
Suicide attempted completed	48% 6% (in first 5 year)	21% 0%	7% 0%

Source: Smith et al. 2009 [45].

Uptake of audit standards was explored by the National EIP Programme service mapping exercise: [46]

• Majority of EIP services measure DUP (79%), readmission (68%), employment (71%) and educational outcomes (68%)

• Fewer measure service engagement (59%), relapse (51%) and parasuicide (47%)

This illustrates how the EPD could inspire local services to evaluate quality standards routinely. The 'heart' raised its expectations and the 'head' responded by embracing these aspirations as hard measures which would ultimately transform services.

This section has illustrated how the National EI Programme learned to harness the three elemental vectors of policy, research and policy to move EIP forward, always guided by a narrative understanding of the impact of emerging psychosis on these young people and their families.

"You don't need an engine when you have wind in your sails."

Bate, Robert, Bevan, 2004 [47]

EIP as a social movement

The following section will explore the process of change. We have organised our discussion into two sections: firstly (section A) **Social movement: a radically different approach to health care reform**) which explores the general principles behind social movement; and then (section B) **EIP as a Social Movement: why it happened, where it happened and**

when it happened – which considers how this can apply to EIP development in the United Kingdom.

We have drawn heavily from the work of Dr. Helen Bevan and colleagues (NHS Institute for Innovation and Improvement) with Professor Paul Bate and Dr. Glenn Robert (University College London). Their application of social movements literature to health care reform has guided our consideration of the EIP health care reform. In doing so, we have extracted key elements from their two major publications:

Towards a Million Change Agents. A review of the social movements literature; implications for large scale change in the NHS (53 Bate, Bevan, Robert 2004) and The Power of One, the Power of Many (54 Bibby et al 2008).

A. Social movement: a radically different approach to health care reform.

The conventional wisdom is that most health care improvement initiatives are derived from planned or 'programmatic' approaches. However, another less used concept holds a different perspective about how large-scale change occurs – that of social movements theory.

"Social movements can be viewed as collective enterprises seeking to establish a new order of life. They have their inception in a condition of unrest, and derive their motive power on one hand from dissatisfaction with the current form of life, and on the other, from wishes and hopes for a new system of living. The career of a social movement depicts the emergence of a new order of life."

Blumer 1969 [48]

Well-known examples include the Civil Rights movement in the United States, Apartheid in South Africa, feminism and the women's movements, lesbian and gay rights campaign, Campaign for Nuclear Disarmament (CND)/peace movement and the green parties/environmental movement. These movements benefitted from a network of leaders at multiple levels to guide and mobilise a successful social movement. The key leadership task is to frame the proposition of joining the movement in a way that makes irresistible, emotional and logical arguments to ignite collective action, mobilise people and inspire change.

"People change what they do less because they are given analysis that shifts their thinking than because they are shown a truth that influences their feelings."

Kotter 2002 [49]

To mobilise movements out of these early interactions, leaders offer frames, tactics and organisational vehicles that allow participants to construct a collective identity and participate in collective action at various levels [47]. It is through the collective narratives and scripts then that leaders weave and make meaning for others [50]. A movement must have its own form of narrative which acts as the 'hook' for new recruits. The story has to grab them, make sense and reinforce self-identity and personal biography. Narrative is the entry point into the practices through which people make choices, shape action and form into social movements:

"Social movements ... are constituted by the stories people tell to themselves and to one another. They reflect the deepest ways in which people understand who they are and to whom they are connected ... they are constructed from the interweaving of personal and social biographies – from the narratives people rehearse to themselves about the nature of their lives."

Kling 1995 [51]

The role of leaders, therefore is to assemble, craft and hone the narrative script for the movement. The extent of mobilisation of others to join a movement is a function of the degree of overlap or alignment between the individual and the narrative in terms of ideas, interests and sentiments.

"Leadership is the art of mobilising others to want to struggle for shared aspirations."

Kouzes 2003 [52]

Influencing factors include the extent to which the 'movement' is perceived to address a grievance, problem or moral imperative, people believe the situation is actually changeable/mutable (i.e. worth doing/can actually be done/will make a difference, it is seen to serve an interest or rationale, and it is perceived to carry risk and cost.

B. EIP as a Social Movement: why it happened, where it happened and when it happened.

The possibility that major health care change may be generated by similar sociopolitical processes to these civil movements has attracted attention from Dr Helen Bevan and colleagues from the NHS Institute for Innovation [47, 53, 54]. In the Table 25.2 they contrast the radically different assumptions that distinguish a social movement approach from the more traditional programmatic approach. Dr Bevan concluded that EIP development was an exemplar of major health care change achieved through social movement [54].

The social movement narrative for EIP began to emerge in the late 90s. When UK Health Minister, Frank Dobson directed his contention that *'Care in the community has*

Table 25.2   Health care improvement through social movement

Project/programme approach	Social movements approach
A planned programme of change with goals and milestones (centrally-led)	Change is about releasing energy and is largely self-directing (bottom-up)
'Motivating' people	'Moving' people
Change is driven by an appeal to the 'what is in it for me'	There may well be personal costs involved
Talks about 'overcoming resistance'	Insists change needs opposition – it is the friend not enemy of change
Change is done 'to' people or 'with' them – leaders and followers	People change themselves and each other – peer to peer
Driven by formal systems change: structures (roles, institutions) lead the change process	Driven by informal systems: structures consolidate, stabilise and institutionalise emergent direction

Source: Bate et al. 2004 [47].

failed' [55] at beleaguered psychiatric services, he was exposing a system of care that felt out of touch with what its users and families sought.

"A reformation means a mass of people have reached the point of disillusionment with past ways and values. They recognise the prevailing system is self-defeating, frustrating and hopeless. They won't act for change but won't strongly oppose those who do. The time is ripe for revolution."

Alinsky 1971 [56]

Arguably, such a reformation was the backdrop to our growing dissent in the late 90s. Resistance from local services and planners in the West Midlands to acknowledge the problem fed that dissent:

"Only in the face of opposition has significant social change been achieved."

Palmer 1997 [57]

For social movements to catch hold the cause must appeal as much to *emotion* as to *reason*. The emerging narrative began to connect with people outside the West Midlands as for instance we joined forces with Rethink Mental Illness, a national mental health charity. The commitment for change became not an option but an imperative, and by doing so strengthened commitment to overcome uncertainty and difficulties [54].

"Contentious politics occur when ordinary people, often in league with more influential citizens, join forces in confrontation with elites, authorities and opponents ... when backed by dense social networks and galvanised by culturally resonant, action-oriented symbols, contentious politics leads to sustained interaction with opponents. The result is the social movement."

Tarrow 1998 [58]

The early 2000s saw this epidemic of ideas and possibilities spreading between people striving for similar changes to the United Kingdom, particularly from Australia, North America and Scandinavia.

"Something that has sprouted legs and run all over the place."

Holt 1920 [59]

There was a need to channel this collective energy:

"Get organised. Build power and work within the system. Frankin D Roosevelt's response to a reform delegation 'Okay you have convinced me. Now go out and bring pressure on me!' Action comes from keeping the heat on."

Alinsky 1971 [56]

Echoing Alinsky's words, our previously informal systems were consolidating into more stable arrangements *to build power and to work within the system* like the UK's mental health reforms and its National EIP Programme, and the IEPA with its emerging international collaborations.

Alignment in social movements depends on how the case is framed and presented by the leaders – that is, the script will be decisive in capturing people's attention and intention. The EPD demands '*an ordinary life for all young people with emerging psychosis and their families*'. Securing the initial involvement is the crucial issue since, once individuals have joined, the interactions and relationships they build tend to ensure they stay with the movement. Subsequent sustainability becomes a social issue – fostering solidarity through collective identity, commitment and purpose [54].

The impact of NIMHE at the 'centre' should not be underestimated. NIMHE was created to support the implementation of the NSF. Its CEO, Professor Sheehan (and a co-founder of IRIS) stated '*NIMHE is a relationship organisation*'. This organisation was able to identify and create the receptive environment (organisational, structural, political and cultural) and to trigger conditions that helped bring the EIP movement to life. The centre consistently responded with support; for instance listening to and acting on complaint, encouraging us to *keep the heat on*, building a policy context, facilitating creation of the EPD, forming and supporting the national EIP programme.

At its heart, this has been a story of grass roots people, particularly at the level of local practitioners and managers. Paul Bate [47] describes grass roots change or local mobilisation as the concrete actions taken by an individual in the direction of change; at an organisational level the rallying and propelling of a segment of the organisation to realise common change goals. Perhaps the greatest achievement of this social movement has been to change the dominant service culture:

> "*The key is to recognize and respect the person as a person first, and only secondarily to view him or her as having a mental illness.*"
>
> Davidson 2010 [60]

Thus, EIP development in the United Kingdom can be seen within the wider context of the recovery movement, which has challenged and continues to challenge the traditional culture and practice of psychiatry.

Where next?

Fifteen years on from when IRIS first voiced its dissent, we can recognise remarkable change. Few could have anticipated the extraordinary shift in how we would understand and treat psychosis, particularly the early phase, bringing with it new hope for young people with emerging psychosis and their families. Alongside these treatment advances, major investment and redesign of community-based specialist mental health provision has established EIP services in many countries. That investment has been rewarded by better clinical outcomes, increased consumer satisfaction and reduced downstream health utilisation.

> "*I have seen how much progress early intervention teams have made, how innovative they have been and the impact they are having. I now believe that early intervention*

will be the most important and far reaching reform of the NSF era... I think early intervention will have the greatest effect on people's lives."

Professor Louis Appleby
UK National Director for
Mental Health October 10th 2008
Policies and Practice for Europe (DH/WHO Europe
Conference attended by 35 countries)

Much of the transformation has come not through securing new investment but by invoking a new mindset which challenges *Treatment as Usual* by seeing different ways of doing things. Moreover, this has not just been about achieving a narrow EIP service development; it is about moving a whole system towards a different ethos built on hope and recovery. And whilst we argue this journey should commence from the start we recognise that even with good EIP provision, many of these young people remain needy, vulnerable and with persistent symptoms/distress beyond the current tenure of typical services (1.5–3 years, internationally). Reductions in suicide rates in the initial 3 years of an EIP service can be lost by a rebound in the immediate period afterwards [61], a reminder of how fragile gains from EIP can be and the importance of considering what happens across the whole care pathway, including the rehabilitation and recovery phases. Nor are these young people just at high risk of death from suicide. Ultimately, more will die from physical disorders, often cardiovascular, and the result of smoking, obesity, lack of exercise and diabetes. A widening mortality gap, currently 20 years for men and 15 years for women, caused Professor Thornicroft to recently conclude this a

"... scandal of premature mortality that contravenes international conventions for the right to health."

Thornicroft 2011 [62]

Behind this *'scandal of premature mortality'* lies an inescapable truth, that mental and physical disorders invariably coexist, often exacerbated by social deprivation.

This 'triple whammy' of adversity patients is too often compounded by inadequate access to health care, poor organisation of health services and a failure by doctors across the primary/specialist interface to agree responsibility [63] It is now clear that many of the precursors of future physical ill-health have their origins in the first few years of psychosis [64]. The realisation that problematic weight gain and its potential cardiac and metabolic effects can be observed within weeks of antipsychotic treatment initiation [65] is beginning to stimulate new models of EIP service which actively intervene to promote physical well-being and protect cardiometabolic health in the early critical period [66]. Such developments herald the start of a new era for *early intervention* which embraces a body and mind approach [67], and encapsulated in the recent international declaration, Healthy Active Lives (HeAL) [68]. Launched in June 2013 as an issue of social justice, HeAL sets out clear principles, goals and processes including five-year targets that emphasise the importance of cardiometabolic risk prevention to avoid future physical health complications.

These and other current challenges, along with some yet to define themselves, means the EIP service innovation should be viewed as the beginning of a mental health service transformation rather than an endpoint. Indeed, perhaps our most important discovery has been about learning how to do things differently rather than arriving at some final destination. The principles and practices of EIP, with interventions directed towards more individually focused and hopeful ways of working and towards as complete a recovery as possible over whatever time it takes, should set ripples flowing out to all phases of care, for mental health teams of all age groups and in all sub-specialties of psychiatry [69].

Useful resources

- Birchwood M, Fowler D and Jackson C. (2000) (eds). *Early Intervention in Psychosis. A Guide to Concepts, Evidence and Interventions.* John Wiley and Sons Ltd., Chichester.

- Edwards J and McGorry PD. (2002). *Implementing Early Intervention in psychosis. A guide to Establishing Early Psychosis Services.* Martin Dunitz Ltd., London.

- IRIS Guidelines Update. (2014). IRIS Initiative Ltd. www.iris-initiative.org.uk

- NICE (NHS National Institute for Health and Clinical Excellence). (2013). *Psychosis and Schizophrenia in Children and Adolescents CG 155.* http://nice.org.uk/CG155

- NICE (NHS National Institute for Health and Clinical Excellence). (2014). *Psychosis and Schizophrenia in Adults (Update) CG 178.* http://nice.org.uk/CG178.

Useful websites

www.iris-initiative.org.uk — UK site promoting good practice in EIP services.
www.iepa.org.au International Early Psychosis Association website

References

1. Victor Hugo. A loosely translated quote from *HISTOIRE D'UN CRIME* – First published 1st October 1877.
2. Kraepelin E. (1896) *Psychiatrie: Ein Lehrbuch fur Studierende und Aerzte. Funfte. Funfte, vollstandig umgearbeitete Auflage.* Leipzig.
3. Sullivan HS. (1927). Tentative criteria for malignancy in schizophrenia. *American Journal of Psychiatry* **84**: 759–782.
4. Bleuler M. (1977). The schizophrenic disorders. Translated by Siegfried M. In: M. Clemens (ed.), New Haven and London: Yale University press.
5. Strauss JS and Carpenter WT. (1974). Characteristic symptoms and outcomes in schizophrenia. *Archives of General Psychiatry* **30**: 429–434.
6. Chompi L. (1980). The natural history of schizophrenia in the long term. *British Journal of Psychiatry* **136**: 413–420.
7. Johnstone EC, Crow TJ, Johnson AL, Macmillan JF. (1986). The northwick park study of first episodes of schizophrenia I. Presentation of the illness and problems relating to admission. *British Journal of Psychiatry* **148**: 115–120.
8. Birchwood M, Todd P and Jackson C. (1998). Early intervention in psychosis. The critical period hypothesis. *British Journal of Psychiatry. Supplement* **172**: 53–59.
9. Marshall M, Lewis S, Lockwood A, et al. (2005). Systematic review of the association between duration of untreated psychosis and outcome in cohorts of first episode patients. *Archives of General Psychiatry* **62**; 975–983.

10. Birchwood M and Macmillan F. (1993). Point of view: early intervention in schizophrenia. *Australian and. New Zealand Journal of Psychiatry* **27**: 374–378.
11. Coid J. (1994). The Christopher Clunis enquiry. *Psychiatric Bulletin* **18**: 449–452.
12. Shiers D and Shiers A. (1998). Who cares?. *BMJ : British Medical Association* **316**: 785.
13. IRIS Initiative to Reduce the Impact of Schizophrenia. (1999). *Early Intervention in Psychosis: Clinical Guidelines and Service Frameworks.* Birmingham: West Midlands Partnership for Mental Health.
14. Johannessen JO. (2004). The development of early intervention services. In: J. Read, L. Mosher and R. Bentall (eds), *Models of Madness.* London: ISPS and Brunner-Routledge.
15. Macmillan F, Ryles D, Shiers D, et al. (1999). *Audit of care pathways in North Staffordshire.* Unpublished.
16. Department of Health. (2001). *The Mental Health Policy Implementation Guide.* London: Department of Health.
17. WHO/IDF Saint Vincent Declaration Working Group. (1990). Diabetes mellitus in europe: A problem at all ages in all countries. A model for prevention and self care. *Acta Diabetologica* **27**: 181–183.
18. IRIS, NIMHE, Rethink. (2002). *Newcastle Declaration for Early Psychosis* Newcastle-Upon- Tyne: National Institute for Mental Health in England (NIMHE) Conference, June 2002.
19. Bertolote J and McGorry P. (2005). Early intervention and recovery for young people with early psychosis: consensus statement. *British Journal of Psychiatry* **187**(48): 116–119.
20. The Early Psychosis Declaration self-assessment toolkit. (2005). National Institute for Mental Health in England. http://www.iris-initiative.org.uk/the-early-psychosis-declaration/early-psychosis-declaration/early-psychosis-declaration-selfassessment-toolkit/ (accessed 23 April 2014).
21. Department of Health. (1999). *National Service Framework for Mental Health.* London: Department of Health.
22. Department of Health. (2000). *NHS Plan.* London: Department of Health.
23. Department of Health. (2002). *Improvement, Expansion and Reform: The Next 3 Years. Priorities and Planning Framework 2003 - 2006.* London: Department of Health.
24. NICE: NHS National Institute for Health and Clinical Excellence. (2009). *Schizophrenia Guidance (Update) CG 82.* http://www.nice.org.uk/CG82 (accessed 23 April 2014).
25. Department of Health. (2004). *The National Services Framework for Children, Young People and Maternity Services: the Mental Health and Psychological Wellbeing of Children and Young People.* London: Department of Health.
26. Department of Health. (2006). *EI Recovery Plan.* London: Department of Health.
27. Department of Health. (2007, 2008, 2009, 2010, 2011). Consecutive annual publications in years 2007, 2008, 2009, 2010, 2011. *NHS Operating Frameworks* London: Department of Health.
28. Yung AR, Organ BA and Harris MG. (2003). Management of early psychosis in a generic adult mental health service. *Australian and New Zealand Journal of Psychiatry* **37**(4): 429–436.
29. Craig T, Garety P, Power P, et al. (2004). The Lambeth Early Onset (LEO) Team: randomised controlled trial of the effectiveness of specialised care for early psychosis. *British Medical Journal* **329**: 1067–1073.
30. Power P. (2004). Suicide prevention in first episode psychosis. In: P. McGorry and John Gleeson (eds), *Psychological Interventions in Early Psychosis.* Oxford: Wiley Press.
31. McGorry PD. (2005). Evidence based reform of mental health care. *British Medical Journal* **331**: 586–587.
32. Garety PA, Craig TK, Dunn G, et al. (2006). Specialised care for early psychosis: symptoms, social functioning and patient satisfaction: randomised controlled trial. *British Journal of Psychiatry* **188**: 37–45.

33. Petersen L, Jeppesen P, Thorup A, et al. (2005). A randomised multicentre trial of integrated versus standard treatment for patients with a first episode of psychotic illness. *BMJ: British Medical Association* **331**: 602.
34. Bertelsen M, Jeppesen P, Petersen L, et al. (2008). Five-year follow-up of a randomized multi-center trial of intensive early intervention vs. standard treatment for patients with a first episode of psychotic illness: the OPUS trial. *Archives of General Psychiatry* **65**: 762–771.
35. Addington J. (2007). The promise of early intervention. *Early Intervention in Psychiatry* **1**: 294–307.
36. McGorry P, Killackey E and Yung A. (2007). Early intervention in psychotic disorders: detection and treatment of the first episode and the critical early stages. *Medical Journal of Australia supplement* **187**(7): 8–10.
37. McGorry P, Killackey E and Yung A. (2008). Early intervention in psychosis. *World Psychiatry* **7**(3): 148–156.
38. McCrone P, Knapp M and Dhanasiri S. (2009). Economic impact of services for first-episode psychosis: a decision model approach. *Early Intervention in Psychiatry* **3**: 266–273.
39. McCrone P, Craig TKJ, Power P, et al. (2010). Cost-effectiveness of an early intervention service for people with psychosis. *British Journal of Psychiatry* **196**: 377–382.
40. McCrone P, Dhanasiri S, Patel A, et al. (2008). Paying the Price: The Cost of Mental Health Care in England in 2026. King's Fund, London.
41. McCrone P, Park A-La and Knapp M. (2010). Economic Evaluation of Early Intervention (EI) Services: Phase IV Report. PSSRU Discussion Paper 2745. http://www.pssru.ac.uk/pdf/dp2745.pdf (accessed 23 April 2014).
42. Lester HE, Birchwood M, Jones P, et al. (2011). The views of young people on early intervention services in England. *Psychiatric Services* **62**: 882–887.
43. Community mental health activity. Annual Return Recorded as of March 2010. NHS Information Centre, London.
44. Bird V, Premkumar P, Kendall T, et al. (2010). Early intervention services, cognitive behavioural therapy and family intervention in early psychosis: systematic review. *British Journal of Psychiatry* **197**: 350–356.
45. Smith J. (2009). Worcestershire Early Intervention Service 2006 and 2008 EIP cohort data. Worcester: Worcestershire Mental Health Partnership NHS Trust, unpublished.
46. Smith J. and Shiers D. (October 2007). *National EI Programme Service Mapping Exercise*, National Institute for Mental Health in England, London, unpublished.
47. Bate P, Robert G and Bevan H. (2004). The next phase of healthcare improvement: what can we learn from social movements? *Quality and safety in health care* **13**: 62–66.
48. Blumer H. (1969). Symbolic Interactionism, Englewood Cliffs, NJ; Transition.
49. Kotter J and Cohen D. (2002). *The Heart of Change: Real-life Stories of How People Change Their Organizations*. Boston: Harvard Business School Press.
50. Morgan G and Smircich L. (1980). The case for qualitative research. *Academy of Management Review* **5**: 491–500.
51. Kling J. (1995). 'Narratives of possibility: social movements, collective stories and the dilemmas of practice.' Paper presented at the 'New Social Movement and Community Organising Conference', University of Washington School of Social Work, November 1–3, 1995.
52. Kouzes JM and Posner BZ. (2003). *The Leadership Challenge*, 3rd edition. San Francisco: Jossey-Bass.
53. Bate SP, Bevan H and Robert G. (2004). Towards a million change agents a review of the social movements literature; implications for large scale change in the NHS. NHS Modernisation Agency; London.
54. Bibby J, Bevan H, Carter E, et al. (2008). The power of one, the power of many', Bringing social movement theory to healthcare practice. In: J Banaszak-Holl, SR Levitsky and M Zald (eds), *Social Movements and the Transformation of Health Institutions*. Oxford: Oxford University Press.

55. Warden J. (1998). England abandons care in the community for the mentally ill. *BMJ: British Medical Association* **317**: 1611.

56. Alinsky S. (1971). *Rules for Radicals. A Practical Primer for Realistic Radicals.* New York: Vintage Books.

57. Palmer P. (1997). *The Courage to Teach. Exploring the Inner Landscape of a Teacher's Life.* San Francisco: Jossey Bass.

58. Tarrow S. (1998). *Power in Movement: Social Movements, Collective Action and Politics*, 2nd edition. New York: Cambridge University Press.

59. William (Billy) Holt. (1897–1977). A quote attributed to William Holt, writer, artist, traveller and broadcaster - from his writings describing the 1920-30s mill-town environment of the Calder Valley, England. *See Professor Paul Bate.* http://eprints.ucl.ac.uk/1135/1/M7.pdf (accessed 23 April 2014).

60. Davidson L. (2010). Recovery and Medical Practice, Is Recovery Movement Anti-Professional? Oct 8th 22 Recovery to Practice (RTP) Weekly Highlights. http://www.samhsa.gov/recoverytopractice/WeeklyHighlights.aspx?Volume=1 (accessed 23 April 2014).

61. Harris GH, Burgess PM, Chant DC, et al. (2008). Impact of a specialized early psychosis treatment programme on suicide. Retrospective cohort study. *Early Intervention in Psychiatry* **2**: 11–21.

62. Thornicroft G. (2011). Physical health disparities and mental illness: the scandal of premature mortality. *British Journal of Psychiatry* **199**: 441–442.

63. Leucht S, Burkard T, Henderson J, et al. (2007). Physical illness and schizophrenia. *Acta Psychiatrica Scandinavia* **116**: 317–333.

64. Tiihonen J, Lönnqvist J, Wahlbeck K, et al. (2011). No mental health without physical health. *Lancet* **377**: 611.

65. Foley D and Morley KI. (2011). Systematic review of early cardiometabolic outcomes of the first treated episode of psychosis. *Archives of General Psychiatry* **68**: 609–616.

66. Curtis J, Newall H and Samaras K. (2012). The heart of the matter: cardiometabolic care in youth with psychosis. *Early Intervention in Psychiatry.* doi:10.1111/j.1751-7893.2011.00315.x

67. Shiers D, Jones P and Field S. (2009). Early intervention in psychosis: keeping the body in mind. *British Journal of General Practice* **59**: 395–396.

68. Healthy Active Lives (HeAL). (2013). International physical health in youth (iphYs) group. www.iphYs.org.au.

69. Shiers D, Rosen A and Shiers A. (2009). Beyond early intervention: can we adopt alternative narratives like 'Woodshedding' as pathways to recovery in schizophrenia? *Early Intervention in Psychiatry* **3**: 163–171.

70. Department of Health. (2011). *No Health Without Mental Health.* London: Department of Health.

26
Challenging Stigma

Amy C. Watson[1], Patrick Corrigan[2] and Kristin Kosyluk[2]

[1]Jane Addams College of Social Work, University of Illinois at Chicago, Chicago
[2]Illinois Institute of Technology, Chicago

In western cultures, stereotypes and attitudes about persons with psychiatric disorders are widely shared and overwhelmingly negative. Common themes suggest that they are dangerous, incompetent, unable to care for themselves and childlike [1–7]. This kind of stigma blocks individuals from opportunities for full inclusion in community life and can greatly exacerbate the negative impact of mental illness. Stigma may also prevent or delay people from seeking and engaging in mental health treatments that could significantly mitigate the impact and course of their illness. Thus, when considering the promise of early intervention in psychiatry (EI), we must be mindful of the impact of stigma on persons who may benefit from EI and the potential for EI to cue stigma processes. Additionally, we must actively employ strategies to reduce stigma.

In this chapter, we define stigma, examine its consequences for persons with mental illnesses and discuss its implications for EI. We then describe approaches to reduce stigma that can be implemented by local communities. By incorporating stigma reduction strategies into EI efforts, we can maximise their benefit and support recovery and opportunities for full inclusion.

Mental illness stigma: its definition and consequences

Erving Goffman defined stigma as 'an attribute that is deeply discrediting' and reduces the bearer from 'a whole and usual person to a tainted discounted one' [8]. Building on the work of Goffman [8] as well as others [9], Link and Phelan [10] defined stigma as a *process* consisting of five interrelated components that, when they converge, result in status loss and discrimination for members of stigmatised groups. The process begins with the recognition, labelling, categorising and associating of human difference with negative meanings through stereotypes or cognitive linkages to undesirable qualities. Next, is the separation

---

Early Intervention in Psychiatry: EI of nearly everything for better mental health, First Edition.
Edited by Peter Byrne and Alan Rosen.

of 'us' from 'them,' with 'them' being the stigmatised and 'us' being the stigmatisers. This results in status loss and discrimination for those who have been stigmatised. Underlying this process is the exercise of power that allows the process to unfold. Without the exercise of power, labelling, stereotyping and separating 'us' from 'them' will not produce status loss and discrimination.

When powerful others engage in the process of stigmatisation, they possess the capacity to deny opportunities to stigmatised persons to participate fully in community life and citizenship [10]. For persons with mental illnesses, this may result in barriers to social relationships; discrimination in employment, education and housing; disparities in access to quality health care and blocked opportunities for full civic engagement. It may lead to label avoidance, in which people delay or opt to not seek mental health services when distressed in order to avoid the egregious effects of public stigma [11].

Three 'types' of stigma

The stigma of mental illness may appear in interactions *between people and groups* (public stigma), within *stigmatised persons themselves* (internalised stigma or self-stigma); and in *institutional and social structures* (structural stigma).

Public Stigma. Public stigma has been the focus of social cognitive models and researchers and advocates are working to understand and reduce mental illness stigma [12]. In these models, the stigma process is understood in terms of four cognitive structures: cues, stereotypes, prejudice and discrimination. The process begins with cues from which members of the public infer that a person has a mental illness. Cues that identify a person as a member of the group 'mentally ill' may be related to psychiatric symptoms, social skill deficits, physical appearance and labels [13, 14]. Research has shown that many of the symptoms of severe mental illness – inappropriate affect, bizarre behaviour, language irregularities and talking to self aloud – tend to produce stigmatising reactions from the public [7, 15, 16]. Likewise, social skill deficits present in some psychiatric disorders [15, 17–19] potentially mark a person as having a mental illness and cue the stigma process. Moreover, poor hygiene or other aspects of appearance may be assumed to indicate mental illness and lead to stigmatising responses [20, 21]. Even prodromal symptoms (of psychosis) may cue stigma, long before a person is clinically labelled. Finally, people may be publicly labelled as having a mental illness if others are aware of their diagnosis, psychiatric hospitalisation or see them entering or leaving a facility that provides psychiatric treatment. (Locating EI services in 'neutral' settings may therefore reduce the risk of cueing stigma for those accessing services).

These cues activate stereotypes, which are knowledge structures that are learned by most members of society [22–27]. Stereotypes are especially efficient means of categorising information about social groups. Not everyone with the knowledge of stereotypes about a group agrees with them [28–30]. People who are prejudiced, however, endorse these negative stereotypes (e.g. I agree, I think people with mental illnesses are dangerous) and generate negative emotional reactions as a result (e.g. I am afraid to have them live in my neighbourhood) [26, 31–35]. Prejudice, which is fundamentally a cognitive and affective response, leads to discrimination, the behavioural reaction [36]. Discriminatory behaviour manifests itself as negative action against members of the stigmatised group. For example, if I believe that people with mental illnesses are dangerous and I am afraid to be near them, I may protest supportive housing in my neighbourhood. I may also advocate for more coercive commitment laws and take other action to keep them out of my community.

Self-Stigma. Self-stigma includes the same components as public stigma, although, the components interact within the stigmatised person him or herself [37–39]. First, long before the onset of symptoms, individuals are fully aware of cultural stereotypes about mental illness and may even endorse them. Thus, with the onset of illness, these stereotypes become self-relevant. For example, a college student experiencing a first episode of schizophrenia may tell himself: 'people assume I am incompetent and cannot finish college because of my illness.' Second, prejudice consists of individuals agreeing and internalising stereotypes: 'they are right, I cannot accomplish anything.' Third, discrimination includes individuals reacting to prejudice with a behavioural response. In the case of our example, 'there is no point in even trying to go back to school – I just cannot do it.'

Just like public stigma, self-stigma negatively impacts individuals in many aspects of life. Specifically, individuals engaging in self-prejudice and self-discrimination may avoid pursuing employment, housing, political, education, relationship and health care goals. By being continually bombarded with stigmatising images and behaviours, individuals may endorse these notions and experience reduced self-esteem, self-efficacy and confidence, which may lead to the lack of drive to pursue life goals [40]. Moreover, even if they do not fully endorse stigmatised views of themselves, individuals who are aware of negative stereotypes may feel less valued in society and withdraw in order to shield themselves from negative and discriminatory responses from others. Stigma may result in *not* pursuing social, educational, vocational and civic opportunities, often out of self-protection.

Structural Stigma. At the societal level, political, economic and historical forces create stigmatising social barriers that restrict life opportunities for individuals with mental illnesses. Structural stigma consists of two levels: institutional policies and social structures. Examples of institutional policies, based on the prejudice of leaders, include laws and regulations that discriminate against individuals with mental illnesses. For example, some states in the United States maintain laws and administrative rules that restrict the rights of individuals with mental illnesses in the areas of jury service, voting, holding public office, marriage, parenting, and professional licensures. When government entities develop these laws and rules based on the label of mental illness rather than the severity of disability resulting from the impact of psychiatric symptoms on functioning, they are institutionalising structural stigma [41].

Second, structural stigma develops historically through economic and political injustices wrought by prejudice and discrimination. The essential aspect of this type of structural stigma is not direct intent but rather the effect of keeping individuals with mental illness in subordinate positions. There is not a specific prejudicial group in power maintaining structural stigma; rather, it is the product of historical trends in mental illness discrimination. For example, in the United States, structural stigma long maintained a political and economic environment which made it very difficult to achieve parity between mental and physical health insurance coverage (parity of esteem). For decades, insurance benefits for treatment of somatic illnesses were less restrictive than benefits for treatment of mental illnesses. Another example of structural stigma includes mental illness research, which receives minimal federal dollars when compared to other health care research. Since agencies fund physical health research at a much higher rate, knowledge that reduces mental illness stigma and enlightens mental health policies cannot match the same rate of knowledge growth in physical health conditions.

The consequences for people with mental illnesses

Numerous studies have documented the public's widespread endorsement of stigmatising attitudes [35, 42, 43–46]. While recent studies suggest that the publics' understanding of mental illnesses may have become more nuanced, perceptions of dangerousness and fear have increased [7] and the desire for social distance from persons with mental illnesses remains strong [35, 42, 43]. Thus, social attitudes may be moving further away from social inclusion and community integration.

The consequences of public mental illness stigma are severe and touch all aspects of a person's life. Here, we briefly discuss three critical life domains, education, employment and housing, however, it is important to keep in mind that stigma has the potential to invade and negatively impact all facets of the lives of persons with mental illnesses (e.g. relationships, health care, interactions with the justice system and participation in civic groups). Education is critical to the pursuit of many life goals and is related to a myriad of health and mental health outcomes [44]. Post-secondary education is also a prerequisite for many jobs with reasonable benefits and adequate salary. Because the onset of severe mental illness often occurs during the late teens and early 20s, completion of high school and the pursuit of higher education may be disrupted. Individuals that experience educational disruptions due to illness may be discouraged from returning. Those who persevere in their pursuit of college education report that they experience significant stigma in the college environment [45, 46].

Work provides a vehicle for social integration and a sense of self-worth and social identity. For people with mental illness, employment provides structure, social connections, goals and income – essential components of recovery [47]. Unfortunately, research confirms that stigma creates barriers to obtaining and keeping good jobs [48–53], when employers refuse to hire a person with a mental illness or to provide reasonable accommodations that allow that person to be successful in the job. It is not only employer stigma that creates barriers to employment for persons with mental illness. Competitive employment has not traditionally been a focus of the mental health system [47] and clinicians have discouraged individuals from considering employment for fear that the stress of employment would exacerbate the illness.

Another life domain key to recovery (and to general healthy living in the community) is access to safe and affordable housing. A safe place to live is an important goal for all of us. Here again, research confirms that stigma blocks opportunities to lease safe housing [54, 55] and site groups homes and other types of housing for persons with mental illnesses [56]. As a result, persons with mental illnesses may end up living in substandard units in unsafe neighbourhoods, isolated from family and positive social activities. This puts them at risk for a variety of negative outcomes, including victimisation, substance misuse and criminal activity.

As discussed above, stigma processes may also occur within the individual who is stigmatised in the form of self- and perceived stigma. Both self- and perceived stigma lead to a loss of self-esteem and self-efficacy and limit prospects for recovery as individuals constrict their social networks and opportunities in anticipation of rejection [57–61]. For example, college students experiencing mental illness may withdraw from academic settings for fear of loss of confidentiality and discrimination [62]. Likewise, adults with mental illness may also choose not to pursue intimate relationships to avoid rejection due to their mental illness [59, 63].

Stigma also creates barriers to accessing mental health services, preventing some people from accessing or fully participating in effective treatments. In fact, up to 40% of people with severe mental illnesses do not receive treatment in a given year [64]. While many factors may prevent people from obtaining services, stigma plays a role. Research indicates that people who are concerned about what others would think and those with more stigmatising attitudes themselves are less likely to seek care [65, 66]. Stigma may increase delays in seeking treatment [67, 68]. Additionally, stigma may affect participation once people enter care in terms of reducing adherence to treatment [61].

Stigma and early intervention

Given the wide-ranging negative impacts of stigma, it is not surprising that some people may choose not to access services and supports in an effort to avoid being labelled and experiencing the sometimes devastating consequences. However, in doing so, they forgo the benefits of effective treatments and support that could alleviate some of the distress associated with psychiatric disorders. They may also miss the opportunity to prevent or at least mitigate more serious disability. Thus, stigma has significant implications for EI services. Regardless of how promising they may be, people may be very hesitant to access treatments. Thus, it behoves EI programs to engage communities they serve in anti-stigma campaigns.

EI programs also have implications for stigma, both positive and negative. On the positive side, EI interventions may reduce 'cues' that initiate the stigma process. Early intervention may reduce the severity of symptoms that signal to others that a person has a mental illness, thereby reducing stigma [69]. It may also prevent stigmatising events such as hospitalizations, job loss and other crisis situations.

Negative implications may result from extending mental illness related labels sooner and to a larger group of people. Writing about the potential stigma associated with the proposed 'high risk for psychosis' category for the DSM-V, Yang et al. [70] caution that we do not yet fully understand what the effects will be. They note that as this high-risk designation will most likely be given to young adults who are in the early stages of identity development, concerns about stigma are heightened. The label may be understood as a pre-diagnosis and exert negative effects similar to a label of psychosis on family and community reactions as well as initiate self-stigma processes. Even in the most controlled clinical settings, over 50% of individuals identified as 'at-risk' do not progress to psychosis [71]. In the specialised clinical research programs currently using this designation and providing EI services, great care is taken to mitigate the impact of stigma. For example, McGorry et al. [69] located their service in a non-psychiatric setting and gave the programme a generic name. Patients and families are provided with information to decatastrophise psychotic disorders. Yang et al. [70] expressed concern that in more common community use, the rate of false positives may be even higher, with less attention to curtailing stigma. Thus, we must remain vigilant to the potential stigma consequences of EI and work tirelessly to reduce mental illness stigma. In the next section, we discuss approaches for doing just that.

Challenging mental illness stigma

Given the potential impact of stigma on EI service participation and EI interventions on stigma experienced by service users, it is critical that EI programs incorporate strategies to reduce both public- and self-stigma. First, we consider public stigma. Advocacy groups, government agencies and professional associations have launched campaigns employing a range of strategies, targeting various audiences and components of public stigma. These approaches can be categorised into three paradigms based on social psychological research: protest, education and contact [72]. We discuss each in turn followed by a discussion of effective messaging and targeting of campaigns.

Protest. Protest strategies identify specific instances of stigma and discrimination and highlight the injustice; the goal here is to shame those who are responsible [73]. Advocacy groups have used this approach to address stigmatising images in the media. For example, an organisation may identify that a television programme perpetuates a stigmatising image of mental illness, organise a letter writing campaign to the media outlet urging a boycott of the program's advertisers. In the United States, groups such as National Alliance on Mentally Illness (NAMI) Stigmabusters and Mental Health America report some successes using protest strategies. For example, in 2010, they were successful in getting a television advertising campaign for the fast food chain *Burger King* discontinued. The commercials, presumably set in psychiatric hospitals, featured the 'Crazy King' who is described by medical types as 'crazy' and 'insane' because he wants to give away his meat for the low, low price of $3.99! While such protests may be effective for eliminating offensive representations or behaviours, they may not improve the attitudes of the people promoting them. Additionally, protest approaches risk producing rebound effects with the consequence that prejudices about a group remain unchanged or possibly, get worse [74–76]. Despite the potential for attitude rebound, protest strategies may be useful for changing behaviours. When successful, they may reduce the number of stigmatising messages the public is bombarded with and thus have a place in our arsenal of strategies.

Education. Educational approaches to stigma reduction challenge inaccurate stereotypes about mental illnesses, replacing them with factual information (e.g., contrary to the myth that people with mental illnesses do not recover, many people with even the most severe illnesses improve and live productive lives in the community). Public service announcements, lectures and presentations, web pages, books, flyers, movies, videos and other audio-visual aids are utilised to disseminate accurate information and educate the public [77–79]. Given the many options for electronic communication, education campaigns can be disseminated to large audiences at relatively low costs. Research supports that people with a better understanding of mental illnesses are less likely to endorse stigma and discrimination [32, 74, 80]. However, research on educational interventions for stigma reduction suggests that the magnitude and duration of these improvements is quite limited [81] and the impact on subsequent behaviours questionable.

Contact. Interpersonal contact is the most promising approach to challenging mental illness stigma. In contact interventions, members of the general population meet and interact with people with mental illnesses. Contact has long been considered an effective means for reducing intergroup prejudice [82–84]. In formalising the 'contact' hypothesis, Allport [83] contended, and more recent research supports [84–86] that 'optimal' contact interventions contain four elements: equal status between groups; a common goal that members of both groups are working on; no competition between groups; and (higher) authority sanction for the contact. Contact conditions that more closely approximate the four 'optimal' conditions appear to produce the largest reductions in stigmatising attitudes [86]. However, even brief, less interactive contact strategies have produced promising results. For example, strategies that employ a brief presentation by a person with mental illness who tells of his or her experiences with mental illnesses have produced attitude and behaviour improvements superior to those seen with educational interventions alone [32, 74]. Additionally, the impact of contact interventions appears to be more durable over time. A recently completed meta-analysis uncovered 79 studies that examined anti-stigma programs yielding more than 600 effect sizes [86]. Two results were especially relevant: contact yields significantly greater effects on attitudes and behavioural intentions than education and *in vivo* contact seems to have greater impact than video-based approaches.

The primary drawback to contact approaches is that they are difficult and resource intensive to disseminate widely. One example of a contact-based program that has been successfully disseminated in the United States is the NAMI program *In Our Own Voice: Living with Mental Illness* (IOOV). In this structured program, persons in recovery from mental illness share their personal stories and interact with their audience. The IOOV program has been provided to law enforcement, schools, businesses and other community groups. As of spring 2007, the IOOV program was active in 38 states and had been provided to over 200,000 people [87]. The three studies of IOOV published to date suggest that it is effective for reducing stigma and improving knowledge about mental illness [88–90].

In reality, we are not limited to selecting a single approach. Many of the existing anti-stigma campaigns utilise an educational approach, either by itself or in conjunction with protest or contact. Regardless of the approach selected, it is important to consider that message, as not all anti-stigma messages have the same impact. For example, in an effort to reduce blame associated with mental illnesses, many of campaigns have focused on the biological model of mental illness. Research suggests that 'brain disease,' 'illness like any other' and 'genetic' messages may reduce blame for psychiatric illness [32, 91–94]. However, framing mental illness solely in biological terms may inadvertently exacerbate other components of stigma [93–97]. While improving some aspects of stigma, biologically based messages have been shown to increase perceptions of unpredictability and dangerousness, increase desire for social distance and invoke harsher treatment [93–97]. Biological explanations may further promote the idea that persons with mental illnesses are fundamentally different from everyone else [97], solidifying the distinction between 'us' and 'them' – a key component in the stigma process [10]. Focusing solely on biologically based messages may also increase the benevolence stigma, the belief that persons with mental illness are innocent and childlike and, as such, must be taken care of and supervised by a more responsible party [39]. This can be particularly disempowering, as people with mental illnesses may be treated (or view themselves) as incompetent and unable to pursue goals and opportunities important to their recovery.

In contrast, framing mental illness in psychosocial terms has been shown to increase positive perceptions of persons with mental illnesses and reduce fear [97]. Psychosocial explanations of mental illness focus on environmental stressors and trauma as causal factors. The idea is to normalise psychiatric symptoms as understandable reactions to difficult life events. This may reduce perceptions of otherness, or the distance between 'us' and 'them.' Finally, several studies have examined approaches focusing specifically on providing accurate information about the risk of violence among persons with mental illnesses, which tends to be grossly overestimated by most members of the public. Such messages appear to reduce fear and desire for social distance, but may also increase blame, as people are viewed as in more control of their behaviour [32, 98].

Each message has potential to improve some aspects of stigma and make others worse. Given what we have learned, framing mental illness as a disorder with both biological and psychosocial components exacerbated by stressful life events from which people can and do recover seems most effective. Addressing perceptions of violence is also important, as dangerousness is one of the most pernicious stereotypes about persons with mental illnesses and is often the basis for social exclusion at both interpersonal and policy levels. Such a combined approach more accurately reflects our current understanding of mental illness and has potential to address multiple components of public stigma. The particular balance of information should be tailored to the specific components of stigma, behaviours and groups being targeted [99].

Targeted stigma strategies

While we certainly would like to reduce public stigma in the population as a whole, targeting everyone makes it very difficult to develop an effective strategy. It may be more effective to target our anti-stigma resources to specific groups, particularly those who have power to promote or limit opportunities in domains important to recovery [100]. This allows us to identify specific behaviours that need to be changed or barriers that need to be removed. Once we have identified the 'problem,' we can identify the groups that are responsible, the specific attitudes or components of stigma likely underpinning the problem and the specific behaviours we want to eliminate and those we want to promote. With these in mind, we can select the strategies and messages to be used.

For example, imagine that parents of patients in a clinic have been complaining that teachers and school administrators have been giving their children a hard time and have not been very willing to provide supports. An anti-stigma advocate decides to hold a couple of focus groups with parents, patients in your program and teachers/school personnel. From these focus groups, the advocate learns more about what difficulties students are encountering and what type of understanding and assistance they would find useful. The advocate also discovers that teachers and school administrators hold some serious misconceptions about psychiatric disorders (e.g., students with mental illnesses, come from bad homes, are lazy, unintelligent and not likely to attend college) and, while many would like to be supportive of students, they are unsure as to how to be of help. With this information, the advocate develops a 90-minute intervention that includes educational content on mental illness and relevant educational and social supports. The advocate determines a balanced message that includes both biological and psychosocial themes is most appropriate. He or she also incorporates contact by inviting families to participate and share their experiences. The advocate works with local school districts to schedule time during faculty and staff meetings and training days to present the program. Additional written materials are disseminated along with contact information for a person at the agency who can provide ongoing support to school social workers, teachers and administrators who have questions about how to best support their students. In addition to improving the school climate for patients, the advocate finds that schools are now referring students to the agency.

Another example of targeting high schools (and colleges) to reduce stigma, increase knowledge and enhance help-seeking to support early intervention is the 'On the Edge' program being implemented in schools and colleges in the United Kingdom [101]. The program, using an applied drama model, has three phases implemented over a 3-week period. In the engagement phase, students are presented with a shoebox containing items belonging to a fictional young man in order to stimulate their curiosity. A week later, the evocation phase involves a visit from a drama company that presents the story of the young man, who is experiencing early psychosis. The audience interviews the characters in role to learn more about their experiences. Then, the audience breaks into discussion groups facilitated by one of the actors, before reconvening for a concluding presentation and take away message about early psychosis and sources for information and help. The third and final phase, educational consolidation, occurs one week later. In this teacher-led session, students reflect on their experience of the play. Teachers are provided with a 'Back from the Edge' educational support pack. An evaluation of the program suggests improvements in knowledge, attitudes and awareness of sources of help.

As stigma and discrimination are ubiquitous in the lives of persons with mental illnesses, there are likely ample additional problems and groups to target with anti-stigma programs. These may include employers who discriminate in hiring decisions or refuse to provide accommodations to qualified individuals; peer groups that may exclude persons with mental illnesses from social opportunities (or even worse, bully them); law enforcement agencies that fail to provide officers with appropriate training in recognising and responding to mental health crisis; media outlets that promote stigmatising portrayals of mental illnesses; etc. Local efforts can be tailored to address the issues most important to stakeholders in a particular community and are flexible enough to respond to emerging issues. Here, it is important that these efforts are carefully tailored, multifaceted and ongoing [100].

These approaches for dealing with public stigma are also applicable for institutional and structural discrimination. By definition, institutional discrimination is the intentional result of policies and practices that aim to restrict the rights and opportunities of persons with mental illnesses [102]. Once the individuals with the power to change the targeted policies and practices are identified (not always an easy task), specific strategies and messages can be developed. Often, combined or multiple parallel or serial approaches are required.

Mitigating the impact of self-stigma

While the problem of stigma is clearly located in society and should be addressed at that level, people with mental illnesses may need some immediate strategies to deal with its demoralizing impact. Two specific strategies may be useful for attenuating the personal impact of stigma: cognitive reframing of the negative self-statements that result from stigma and strategies that enhance the person's sense of empowerment, thereby countering self-stigma. Cognitive reframing provides a mechanism to change negative self-thoughts related to stigmatising stereotypes. When self-stigmatising, people internalise self-statements representing the negative stereotype, and may engage in very negative self-talk. For example, they may tell themselves: 'no one will want to date a crazy person like me, and I don't blame them', or 'I am just not smart enough or together enough to finish college.' Cognitive reframing teaches the person to identify and challenge these harmful self-statements. Here, the person may seek feedback from trusted others on the accuracy of these statements or look for other information that challenges the assumptions. For example, the person may interpret their college entrance exam scores as evidence that he or she is indeed smart enough to finish college.

Strategies employing cognitive techniques have shown promise for reducing internalised stigma and improving self-esteem [103, 104]. These approaches can be implemented individually or in group settings and can be professionally or peer facilitated [105]. Group interventions may have the benefit of addressing an important aspect of internalised stigma-alienation-by increasing sense of belonging through positive social connections with others.

Research suggests that empowerment is at the opposite end of a continuum anchored by self-stigma [106]. Thus, strategies supporting empowerment have the potential to move people away from the self-stigma end of the continuum. Treatment providers and programs can align themselves to promote empowerment. For example, recovery-oriented services are collaborative rather than based in adherence frameworks. In collaborative exchanges, individuals and practitioners view each other as peers and work together to understand the illness and develop a treatment plan; this gives the person control over an important part of their life. Providing services that are responsive to service user satisfaction or lack thereof can also promote empowerment, as the service user has a voice in shaping programs. Coaching-based psychosocial services can also facilitate empowerment. Coaches provide services and support that help people be successful in various important settings: work, housing, education and health settings. This can be particularly empowering when coaches are peer providers who have lived experience of mental illness themselves. Additional opportunities for peer support may also enhance empowerment by providing social connections, positive group awareness and an arena for group advocacy.

Conclusion

The goal of EI programs is engage the person into treatment quickly to forestall greater exacerbation of symptoms leading to a worse disease course. Stigma will interfere with this goal. Ironically, EI efforts may also increase people's exposure to stigma. The mental health community needs to be exquisitely sensitive to the two-headed monster that is stigma. And, just as EI researchers and advocates continue to develop interventions to improve the prognosis of people first suffering the challenges of severe mental illness, so must researchers and advocates partner to understand stigma's egregious impact and continue to identify innovative and effective ways to interdict it.

Acknowledgements

This work was supported by grant number P20 MH 085981 from the National Institute of Mental Health. The contents are solely the responsibility of the authors and do not necessarily represent the official views of NIH.

References

1. Brockington IF, Hall P, Levings J, et al. (1993). The community's tolerance of the mentally ill. *British Journal of Psychiatry* **162**: 93–99.
2. Corrigan PW. (1998). The impact of stigma on severe mental illness. *Cognitive and Behavioral Practice* **5**: 201–222.
3. Watson AC, Corrigan PW and Ottati V. (2004). Police officers' attitudes toward and decisions about people with mental illness. *Psychiatric Services* **55**: 49–53.
4. Wahl OF. (1992). Media images of mental illness: a review of the literature. *Journal of Community Psychology* **20**: 343–352.
5. Crisp AH, Gelder MG, Rix S, et al. (2000). Stigmatization of people with mental illnesses. *The British Journal of Psychiatry* **177**: 4–7.
6. Pescosolido BA, Monahun J, Link BG, et al. (1999). The public's view of the competence, dangerousness, and need for legal coercion of persons with mental health problems. *American Journal of Public Health* **89**(9): 1339–1345.
7. Phelan JC, Link BG, Stueve A, et al. (2000). Public conceptions of mental illness in 1950 and 1996: what is mental illness and is it to be feared? *Journal of Health and Social Behavior* **41**(2): 188–207.
8. Goffman E (ed.). (1963). *Stigma: Notes on the Management of a Spoiled Identity*. New York: Simon & Schuster, Inc.
9. Jones EE, Farina A, Hastorf AH, et al. (1984). *Social Stigma: The psychology of Marked Relationships*. New York: Freeman.
10. Link BG and Phelan JC. (2001). Conceptualizing stigma. *Annual Review of Sociology* **27**: 363–385.
11. Corrigan PW. (2004). How stigma interferes with mental health care. *American Psychologist* **59**(7): 614–625.
12. Corrigan PW, Markowitz FE and Watson AC. (2004). Structural levels of mental illness stigma and discrimination. *Schizophrenia Bulletin* **30**(3): 481–491.
13. Corrigan PW. (2000). Mental health stigma as social attribution: implications for research methods and attitudes change. *Clinical Psychology: Science and Practice* **7**(1): 48–67.
14. Sartorius N. (2002). Iatrogenic stigma of mental illness. *The British Journal of Psychiatry* **324**(7352): 1470–1471.
15. Penn DL, Kohlmaier JR and Corrigan PW. (2000). Interpersonal factors contributing to the stigma of schizophrenia: social skills, perceived attractiveness, and symptoms. *Schizophrenia Research* **45**(1–2): 37–45.
16. Schumaker M, Corrigan PW and Dejong T. (2003). Examining cues that signal mental illness stigma. *Journal of Social and Clinical Psychology* **22**(5): 467–476.
17. Bellack AS, Morrison RL, Wixted JT, et al. (1990). An analysis of social competence in schizophrenia. *The British Journal of Psychiatry* **156**: 809–818.
18. Muser KT, Bellack AS, Douglas MS, et al. (1991). Prediction of social skill acquisition in schizophrenic and major affective disorder patients from memory and symptomatology. *Psychiatry Research* **37**(3): 281–296.
19. Ottati V, Bodenhausen GV and Newman LS. (2005). Social psycological models of mental illness stigma. In: PW Corrigan (ed.), *On the stigma of mental illness: Practical strategies for research and social change*, pp. 99–128. Washington, DC: American Psychological Association.
20. Penn DL, Mueser KT and Doonan R. (1997). Physical attractiveness in schizophrenia: the mediating role of social skill. *Behavior Modification* **21**: 78–85.
21. Day EN, Edgren K and Eshleman A. (2007). Measuring stigma toward mental illness: development and application of the mental illness stigma scale. *Journal of Applied Social Psychology* **37**(10): 2191–2219.
22. Augoustinos M, Ahrens C and Innes JM. (1994). Stereotypes and prejudice: the Australian experience. *British Journal of Psychology* **33**: 125–141.

23. Augoustinos M and Rosewarne DL. (2010). Stereotype knowledge and prejudice in children. *British Journal of Developmental Psychology* **19**(1): 143–156.

24. Ajzen I. (2001). Nature and operation of attitudes. *Annual Review of Psychology* **52**: 27–58.

25. Judd CM and Park B. (1993). Definition and assessment of accuracy in social stereotypes. *Psychological Review* **100**: 109–128.

26. Krueger J. (1996). Personal beliefs and cultural stereotypes about racial characteristics. *Journal of Personality and Social Psychology* **71**: 536–548.

27. Lyons A and Kashima Y. (2003). How are stereotypes maintained through communication? the influence of stereotype sharedness. *Journal of Personality and Social Psychology* **85**(6): 989–1005.

28. Devine PG. (1989). Stereotypes and prejudice: their automatic and controlled components. *Journal of Personality and Social Psychology* **56**: 5–18.

29. Jussim L, Nelson TE, Manis M, et al. (1995). Prejudice, stereotypes, and labeling effects: sources of bias in person perception. *Journal of Personality and Social Psychology* **68**: 228–246.

30. Lepore L and Brown R. (1997). Category and stereotype activation: is prejudice inevitable? *Journal of Personality and Social Psychology* **72**(2): 275–287.

31. Angermeyer MC and Matschinger H. (2003). The stigma of mental illness: effects of labeling on public attitudes towards people with mental disorder. *Acta Psychiatrica Scandinavica* **108**: 304–309.

32. Corrigan PW, Rowan D, Green A, et al. (2002). Challenging two mental illness stigmas: personal responsibility and dangerousness. *Schizophrenia Bulletin* **28**(2): 293–309.

33. Devine PG. (1995). Prejudice and out-group perception. In: A. Tessor (ed.), *Advanced Social Psychology*, pp. 467–524. New York: McGraw-Hill.

34. Feldman DB and Crandall CS. (2007). Dimensions of mental illness stigma: what about mental illness stigma causes social rejection? *Journal of Social and Clinical Psychology* **26**(2): 137–154.

35. Martin JK, Pescosolido BA and Tuch SA. (2000). Of fear and loathing: the role of 'disturbing behavior,' labels, and causal attributions in shaping public attitudes toward people with mental illness. *Journal of Health and Social Behavior* **41**(3): 208–223.

36. Crocker J, Major B and Steele C. (1998). Social stigma. In: D Gilbert, ST Fiske, G Lindzey (eds), *The handbook of social psychology*, pp. 504–553. Boston, MA: McGraw-Hill.

37. Corrigan PW and Watson AC. (2002). The paradox of self-stigma and mental illness. *Clinical Psychology: Science and Practice* **9**: 35–53.

38. Corrigan PW, Watson AC and Barr L. (2006). The self-stigma of mental illness: implications for self esteem and self efficacy. *Journal of Social and Clinical Psychology* **25**(8): 875–884.

39. Watson AC, Corrigan PW, Larson JE, et al. (2007). Self stigma in people with mental illness. *Schizophrenia Bulletin* **33**(6): 1312–1318.

40. Corrigan PW, Larson JE and Rösch N. (2009). Self-stigma and the "why try" effect: impact on life goals and evidence-based practices. *World Psychiatry* **8**(2): 75–81.

41. Corrigan PW, Watson AC, Heyrman ML, et al. (2005). State legislation as proxies of structural stigma. *Psychiatric Services* **56**(5): 557–563.

42. Brockington IF, Hall P, Levings J, et al. (1993). The community's tolerance of the mentally ill. *British Journal of Psychiatry* **162**: 93–99.

43. Pescosolido BA, Monahan J, Link BG, et al. (1999). The publics' view of the competence, dangerousness, and need for legal coercion of persons with mental health problems. *American Journal of Public Health* **89**(9): 1339–1345.

44. Bijl RV, Ravelli A and van Zessen G. (1998). The Netherlands Mental Health Survey and Incidence Study (NEMESIS): objectives and design. *Social Psychiatry and Psychiatric Epidemiology* **33** (12): 581–586.

45. Austin T. (1999). The role of education in the lives of people with mental health difficulties. In: C Newnes, G Holmes and C Dunn (eds), *This is Madness*, pp. 253–262. Wiltshire, England: Redwood Books.

46. Weiner E and Wiener J. (1996). Concerns and needs of university students with psychiatric disabilities. *Journal of Postsecondary Education and Disability* **12**: 2–9.

47. Stuart H. (2006). Mental illness and employment discrimination. *Current Opinion in Psychiatry* **19**(5): 522–526.

48. Baldwin ML and Marcus SC. (2006). Perceived and measured stigma among workers with serious mental illness. *Psychiatric Services* **57**(3): 388–392.

49. Brohan E and Thornicroft G. (2010). Stigma and discrimination of mental health problems: workplace implications. *Occupational Medicine* **60**: 414–420.

50. Corrigan PW and Kleinlein P. (2004). The impact of mental illness stigma. In: PW Corrigan (ed.), *On the Stigma of Mental Illness: Practical Strategies for Research and Social Change*, pp. 11–44. Washington, DC: American Psychological Association.

51. Krupa T, Kirsh B, Cockburn L, et al. (2009). Understanding the stigma of mental illness in employment. *Work: A Journal of Prevention. Assessment, and Rehabilitation* **33**(4): 413–425.

52. Wahl OF. (1999). *Telling Is Risky Business: The Experience of Mental Illness Stigma*. New Brunswick, NJ: Rutgers University Press.

53. Stuart H. (2007). Employment equity and mental disability. *Current Opinion in Psychiatry* **20**(5): 486–490.

54. Forchuk C, Nelson G and Hall B. (2006). "It's important to be proud of the place you live in": housing problems and preferences of psychiatric survivors. *Perspectives in Psychiatric Care* **42**(1): 42–52.

55. Page S. (1977). Effects of the mental illness label in attempts to obtain accommodation. *Canadian Journal of Behavioral Science* **9**: 85–90.

56. Zippay A. (2007). Psychiatric residences: notification, NIMBY, and neighborhood relations. *Psychiatric Services* **58**: 109–113.

57. Kahng SK and Mowbray CT. (2005). What affects self-esteem of persons with psychiatric disabilities: the role of causal attributions of mental illness. *Psychiatric Rehabilitation Journal* **28**(4): 354–360.

58. Link BG, Struening EL, Neese-Todd S, et al. (2001). Stigma as a barrier to recovery: the consequences of stigma for the self-esteem of people with mental illnesses. *Psychiatric Services* **52**: 1621–1626.

59. Markowitz FE. (1998). The effects of stigma on the psychological well-being and life satisfaction of persons with mental illness. *Journal of Health and Social Behavior* **39**: 335–348.

60. Perlick DA, Rosenheck RA, Clarkin JF, et al. (2001). Stigma as a barrier to recovery: adverse effects of perceived stigma on social adaptation of persons diagnosed with bipolar affective disorder. *Psychiatric Services* **52**: 1627–1632.

61. Sirey JA, Bruce ML, Alexopoulos GS, et al. (2001). Stigma as a barrier to recovery: perceived stigma and patient-rated severity of illness as predictors of antidepressant drug adherence. *Psychiatric Services* **52**: 1615–1620.

62. Mowbray CT, Mandiberg JM, Stein CH, et al. (2006). Campus mental health services: recommendations for change. *American Journal of Orthopsychiatry* **76**(2): 226–237.

63. Wright ER, Wright DE, Perry BL, et al. (2007). Stigma and the sexual isolation of people with serious mental illness. *Social Problems* **54**(1): 78–98.

64. Wang PS, Lane M, Olfson M, et al. (2005). Twelve-month use of mental health services in the United States. *Archives of General Psychiatry* **62**(6): 629–640.

65. Cooper AE, Corrigan PW and Watson AC. (2003). Mental illness stigma and care seeking. *Journal of Nervous and Mental Disease* **191**(5): 339–341.

66. Kessler RC, Berglund PA, Bruce ML, et al. (2001). The prevelance and correlates of untreated serious mental illness. *Health Services Research* **36**(6 Pt 1): 987–1007.

67. McGorry PD and Killackey EJ. (2002). Early intervention in psychosis: a new evidence based paradigm. *Epidemiologia e Psichiatria Sociale* **11**(4): 237–247.

68. Compton MT and Esterberg ML. (2005). Treatment delay in first-episode non-affective psychosis: a pilot study with African American family members and the theory of planned behavior. *Comprehensive Psychiatry* **46**: 291–295.

69. McGorry PD, Yung A and Phillips L. (2001). Ethics and early intervention in psychosis: keeping up the pace and staying in step. *Schizophrenia Research* **51**(1): 17–29.

70. Yang LH, Wonpat-Borja AJ, Opler MG, et al. (2010). Potential stigma associated with inclusion of the psychosis risk syndrome in the DSM-V: An empirical question. *Schizophrenia Research* **120**(1–3): 42–48.

71. Cannon TD, Cadenhead K, Cornblatt B, et al. (2008). Prediction of psychosis in youth at high clinical risk: a multisite longitudinal study in North America. *Archives of General Psychiatry* **65**(1): 28–37.

72. Corrigan PW and Penn DL. (1999). Lessons from social psychology on discrediting psychiatric stigma. *American Psychologist* **54**(9): 756–776.

73. Watson AC and Corrigan PW. (2005). Changing public stigma: a targeted approach. In: PW. Corrigan (ed.), *A Comprehensive Review of the Stigma of Mental Illness: Implications for Research and Social Change*, pp. 281–295. Washington DC: American Psychological Association.

74. Corrigan PW, River LP, Lundin R, et al. (2001). Three strategies for changing attributions about severe mental illness. *Schizophrenia Bulletin* **27**(2): 187–195.

75. Macrae CN, Bodenhausen GV, Milne AB, et al. (1994). Out of mind but back in sight: stereotypes on the rebound. *Journal of Personality and Social Psychology* **67**(5): 808–817.

76. Penn DL and Corrigan PW. (2002). The effects of stereotype suppression on psychiatric stigma. *Schizophrenia Research* **55**(3): 269–276.

77. Active Minds. (2011). http://www.activeminds.org/ (accessed 12 October 2011).

78. Pate GS. (1988). Research on reducing prejudice. *Social Education* **52**: 287–289.

79. SAMHSA. (2011). Mental illness: what a difference a friend makes, (n.d.). http://www.whatadifference.samhsa.gov/ (accessed 12 October 2011).

80. Brockington IF, Hall P, Levings J, et al. (1993). The community's tolerance of the mentally ill. *The British Journal of Psychiatry* **162**: 93–99.

81. Corrigan PW and McCracken SG. (1997). Intervention research: integrating practice guidelines with dissemination strategies–a rejoinder to paul, stuve, and cross. *Applied and Preventive Psychology* **6**: 205–209.

82. Alexander LA and Link BG. (2003). The impact of contact on stigmatizing attitudes toward people with mental illness. *Journal of Mental Health* **12**(3): 271–289.

83. Allport G. (1954). *The Nature of Prejudice*. Reading, MA: Addison-Wesley.

84. Pettigrew TF and Tropp LR. (2000). Does intergroup contact reduce prejudice: recent meta-analytic findings. In: S. Oskamp (ed.), *Reducing Prejudice and Discrimination*, pp. 93–114. Mahwah, NJ: Lawrence Erlbaum & Assoc.

85. Cook SW. (1985). Experimenting on social issues: The case of school desegregation. *American Psychologist* **40**: 452–460.

86. Gaertner SL, Dovidio JF and Bachman BA. (1996). Revisiting the contact hypothesis: the induction of a common ingroup identity. *International Journal of Intercultural Relations* **20**(3): 271–290.

87. National Alliance on Mental Illness. (2009). In Our own Voice. http://www.nami.org/Template .cfm?Section=In_Our_Own_Voice&Template=/ (accessed 1 June 2009).

88. Corrigan PW, Rafacz JD, Hautamaki J, et al. (2010). Changing stigmatizing recollections about mental illness: the effects of NAMI's in our own voice. *Community Mental Health Journal* **46**: 517–522.

89. Wood AL and Wahl OF. (2006). Evaluating the effectiveness of a consumer-provided mental health recovery education presentation. *Psychiatric Rehabilitation Journal* **30**(1): 46–52.

90. Rusch L, Kanter J, Angelone A, et al. (2008). The impact of in our own voice on stigma. *American Journal of Psychiatric Rehabilitation* **11**(4): 373–389.

91. Farina A, Fisher JD, Getter H, et al. (1978). Some consequences of changing people's views regarding the nature of mental illness. *Journal of Abnormal Psychology* **87**: 272–279.

92. Fisher JD and Farina A. (1979). Consequences of beliefs about the nature of mental disorders. *Journal of Abnormal Psychology* **88**: 320–327.

93. Lincoln TM, Arens E, Berger C, et al. (2008). Can antistigma campaigns be improved? a test of the impact of biogenetic vs. psychosocial causal explanations on implicit and explicit attitudes to schizophrenia. *Schizophrenia Bulletin* **34**: 984–994.

94. Phelan J. (2002). Genetic bases of mental illness–a cure for stigma? *Trends in Neuroscience* **25**: 430–431.

95. Mehta S and Farina A. (1997). Is being "sick" really better? effect of the disease view of mental disorders on stigma. *Journal of Social and Clinical Psychology* **16**: 405–419.

96. Read J, Haslam N, Sayce L, et al. (2006). Prejudice and schizophrenia: a review of the 'mental illness is an illness like any other' approach. *Acta Psychiatrica Scandinavica* **114**: 303–318.

97. Read J and Law A. (1999). The relationship of causal beliefs and contact with users of mental health services to attitudes to the mentally ill. *International Journal of Social Psychiatry* **45**: 216–229.

98. Penn DL, Lommana S, Mansfield M, et al. (1999). Dispelling the stigma of schizophrenia: II. the impact of information on dangerousness. *Schizophrenia Bulletin* **25**(3): 437–446.

99. Hinshaw SP and Stier A. (2008). Stigma as related to mental disorders. *Annual Review of Clinical Psychology* **4**: 367–393.

100. Corrigan PW. (2011). Best practices: strategic stigma change (SSC): five principles for social marketing campaigns to reduce stigma. *Psychiatric Services* **62**: 824–826.

101. Roberts G, Somers J, Dawe J, et al. (2007). On the edge: a drama-based mental health education programme on early psychosis for schools. *Early Intervention in Psychiatry* **1**: 168–176.

102. Pincus FL. (1996). Discrimination comes in many forms: individual, institutional, and structural. *American Behavioral Scientist* **40**: 186–194.

103. Knight MTD, Wykes T and Hayward P. (2006). Group treatment of perceived stigma and self-esteem in schizophrenia: a waiting list trial of efficacy. *Behavioral and Cognitive Psychotherapy* **34**: 1–14.

104. Macinnes DL and Lewis M. (2008). The evaluation of a short group programme to reduce self-stigma in people with serious and enduring mental health problems. *Journal of Psychiatric and Mental Health Nursing* **15**(1): 59–65.

105. Lucksted A, Drapalski A, Boyd J, et al. (2009). *Resisting Internalized Stigma: A Nine Session Class for Individuals Receiving Mental Health Services*. Baltimore, MD: VA VISN-5 MIRECC.

106. Corrigan PW and Watson AC. (2002). Understanding the impact of stigma on people with serious mental illness. *World Psychiatry* **1**(1): 16–20.

27

Conclusion: Towards Standards for Early Prevention and Intervention of Nearly Everything for Better Mental Health Services

Alan Rosen[1,2,3] and Peter Byrne[4,5]

[1] School of Public Health, University of Wollongong
[2] Brain and Mind Research Institute, University of Sydney
[3] Mental Health Commission of New South Wales, Australia
[4] Homerton University Hospital, London
[5] Royal College of Psychiatrists, UK

Introduction

In recent years, there has been an explosion of interest in the possibility of early intervention (EI) in mental health care, with the ultimate aim of preventing the onset of severe mental illness, or at the very least, preventing or reducing the secondary morbidity and impaired functioning associated with these illnesses. This has been largely driven by advances in our understanding of the early stages of the psychotic disorders, which have led to the identification of modifiable risk/protective factors that can be targeted by appropriate therapeutic interventions, leading to much better outcomes for affected individuals and their families. EI represents a key shift in theoretical perspective, providing a coherent focus for the timely prevention, detection and intervention in mental illnesses, and opens the way for a more congenial, pre-emptive or timely and ultimately, more personalised and preventive psychiatry. This shift in focus and perspective must be reflected in the timing,

Early Intervention in Psychiatry: EI of nearly everything for better mental health, First Edition.
Edited by Peter Byrne and Alan Rosen.
© 2014 John Wiley & Sons, Ltd. Published 2014 by John Wiley & Sons, Ltd.

pattern and tenure of service delivery, as well as in service structures themselves. In this chapter, we review the EI paradigm as a rationale and framework for improving the systematising of evidence-based primary to tertiary preventive efforts and the responsiveness of mental health services for individuals with many types of significant psychiatric disorders and their families, in most age-groups and settings. We address some key questions: Is EI anything really new? Should it only be for young people with psychosis? Should the work of EI teams be time-limited? Can there be an EI approach to long-term or persistent disorders? Can EI be applied to enhancing wellness and wellbeing? We also address the need for and uses of tools of EI service quality, from values and principles to standards, accreditation, best practice and implementation guidelines and similar applications of fidelity criteria. We finally summarise the overall benefits of taking an EI approach, as potentially one of the most important advances in mental health care made in recent years.

The definition of and rationale for early intervention across the disorder, stage of life and phases of care spectra

Early interventions seek to reduce the impact of a clinical or behavioural condition or disability for individuals and the wider community, for example, by mitigating or alleviating the impact of a developing, a newly established or an existing disability, and/or preventing a further deterioration in an existing disability. They may be invoked as soon as the condition or disability is first identified or appears, where there is a discrete change in the condition or disability, or at particular lifetime transition points (widening and paraphrasing the definition of Productivity Commission of Australia [1]).

Early intervention is defined in multifaceted ways: 'In relation to EI, 'early' can broadly be understood in two ways – namely, early in the life of a person (for example, newborns, children and youth – sometimes also described as early childhood intervention or support for children) or early relative to the identification or appearance of the disability' [1]. EI should be *timely*, (as perceived by service-users rather than providers) in the sense of being as soon as the person presenting wants it, and as soon as all key resource people for example, close family, can be gathered, but not an emergency "here and now" response if it can be avoided. This is opposed to late intervention, and not subject to delays, rationing or waiting lists for urgent or pressing care, which would not be tolerated in the care of many other emerging, severe and acute clinical conditions, for example, in cardiac or cancer care.

Early intervention is closely linked to and intertwined with frameworks of prevention [2, 3]. Primary prevention is performed before a clinical condition has emerged. It involves anticipating the onset of a condition which can be completely avoided, or is amenable to reversal, substantive remission or considerable amelioration if picked up early. It includes genetic counselling, replacement of a missing nutrient or hormone and careful monitoring and counselling through potentially prodromal states. Secondary prevention includes EI once a clinical condition clearly exists. In early secondary prevention, early detection of a clinical condition is a prelude to effective EI to improve immediate clinical outcomes and prevent any continuing disability setting in, if possible. Tertiary prevention involves the restoring of a purposeful existence and restoration of functional competencies from disability, or the prevention or minimisation of permanent disability, even once chronicity has been established.

Is early intervention really a new idea?

Is EI a relatively new idea or a trajectory that always made sense to reflective and practical clinicians, their clientele and their family carers?

Pioneers such as Pat McGorry in Australia, Max Birchwood in the United Kingdom and Tom McGlashan in the United States explicitly led the charge to systematically research, systematise and roll out EI services for young people struggling with their first episodes of psychosis on a national basis. However, as they would readily acknowledge, there were many forebears promoting this trajectory. McGorry and colleagues [4] credit Harry Stack Sullivan (1927), Ewen Cameron (1938) and Ainslie Meares (1959) as key ancestors in their views that 'if prepsychotic states could be recognised and if the person could receive help at this early stage, then the psychosis, with all its psychologically and socially disruptive effects, could be prevented or at least minimised.' Many of us would join them in still citing Ian Falloon and Grainne Fadden [5] as developing and piloting county-wide, early prevention and intervention teams in the United Kingdom, which were not yet termed 'early intervention' teams but which functioned approximately as such. They operated closely with general practitioners, regularly working from and engaging their clientele in primary health settings. They provided timely psychosocial, evidence-based interventions and medications relatively sparingly only when necessary, for all psychiatric disorders and all age-groups. They appeared to reduce the emergence and incidence of severe psychiatric disorders. Other pioneering clinicians and researchers and a selection of their key contributions have been listed and referenced in Rosen et al. [6] (see extract in Table 27.1).

Should access to early intervention teams be time-limited?

No: the concept and practice should not be restricted by diagnosis, symptomatic presentation, age-group or phase of care. The most urgent priority for early prevention and intervention has been and will continue to be young people on the brink or threshold of severe mental illness. However, while the bulk of the action in research and dissemination has occurred in younger people with psychosis, and has been more recently applied more widely to young people with all mental conditions (www.headspace.org.au) many of the concepts, frameworks, access strategies and practices have much relevance to many age-groups, psychiatric conditions and phases of care [7].

Shiers, Rosen and Shiers [7] argue against strictly applied or automatic discharge or transfer from early intervention in psychosis teams to another team within 1.5 to 3 years, which has become the norm for many mental health services which operate them. They advocate for the intensity and elements of this approach continuing for 10 years or more, but only if required, for those individuals who are still buffeted in their lives by persisting or intermittent episodes of severe mental illness.

Table 27.1   Some pioneering EI researchers and clinicians and selected key contributions

Country	Investigators	Key contributions
Australia	Mario Alvarez-Jimenez Jackie Curtis Jane Edwards John Gleeson Eoin Killackey Henry Jackson Patrick McGorry Alison Yung	Developed the EPPIC and PACE early psychosis and prodromal services; developed a national youth mental health service stream, 'headspace'; recognised the importance of physical health care in early psychosis; the EPPIC and PACE long-term studies; ACT and family intervention for EI; developed a vocational rehabilitation model for young people with first-episode psychosis; developed an innovative social media platform specifically to support recovery in early psychosis
Canada	Don Addington Jean Addington Lili Kopala Ashok Malla Bob Zipursky	Developed family interventions for early psychosis; developed the PRIME early psychosis service in Canada; contributed to the NAPLS study
Denmark	Merete Nordentoft	Developed an early psychosis service in Denmark; the OPUS study; Suicide prevention and EI.
Germany	Joachim Klosterkotter Stephan Ruhrmann Frauke Schultze-Lutter	Developed the basic symptoms criteria; contributed to the EPOS study
Hong Kong	Eric Chen	Developed the EASY early intervention service
Norway	Jan Olav Johannessen Tor K. Larsen Tom McGlashan	TIPS early detection and intensive community-based treatment study and service
Singapore	Siow Ann Chong	Developed the EPIP early intervention service
The Netherlands	Llewe der Haan Don Linzen Jim van Os	Investigation of the development of prodromal psychopathology, contributed to the EPOS study
United Kingdom	Max Birchwood Tom Craig Grainne Fadden Ian Falloon Paul French Peter Jones Helen Lester Shon Lewis Tony Morrison Paddy Power David Shiers	Developed family interventions; the Buckinghamshire study; the concept of the 'critical period'; developed early intervention services in London, Birmingham and Manchester; developed CBT for psychotic symptoms; the EDIE trial; the EPOS study; physical health monitoring in early psychosis; family intervention for EI; EI in primary care
United States	Ty Cannon Barbara Cornblatt MatcheriKeshavan Jeffrey Lieberman Tom McGlashan Larry Seidman Richard J Wyatt	Developed early psychosis programmes in the United States; contributed to the CATIE trial and the NAPLS trial; Neurobiology of early psychosis

We expect flexibility too. As in Hickam's Dictum (http://en.wikipedia.org/wiki/Hickam%27s_dictum), we commonly see a second common mental disorder in a person treated for something else. In this setting, we expect secondary prevention of (say) psychosis to run alongside primary prevention (sometimes secondary too) of problems with anxiety, depression and/or substances.

Is early prevention and intervention just for young people with first episode psychosis?

Shiers, Rosen and Shiers [7] maintain that 'from our national perspectives, we are aware that other parts of the service can sometimes perceive EI teams as being or behaving as elitist. EI teams must respond positively by being both good service neighbours, (contributing constructively to an integrated mental health service), whilst at the same time becoming ambassadors for continuing this intensive EI type of approach for however long it takes, creating ripples into the sometimes still waters of systems of care further down the care pathway.'

For instance, they might do this by promoting psychosocial interventions, family work, physical care of individuals with mental illness, lowest-possible-dose medication treatments and minimal use of hospitals and involuntary care, strictly only when necessary. Early interventionists should be engaging other providers working with other phases of care and other conditions with the idea and sentiment that: *we value and have learnt from your expertise, your commitment to your clientele and what you do. We also have something we can bring to this – which we are happy to share*.

'Maybe we need a series of pools, each drawing on a renewed wellspring of hope for different phases, and each with their own sequential spring-board of therapeutic optimism and creative inspiration. Just as 'engagement' is not solely an intervention applied at the beginning of the therapeutic encounter, but must keep being renewed throughout the therapeutic enterprise for each individual and family, so it is with (operationalising) hope-instilling and therapeutic optimism. The principles and practices of EI, with interventions directed towards more individually focused and hopeful ways of working and towards as complete a recovery as possible over whatever time it takes, should set ripples flowing out to all phases of care, and for mental health teams for all age-groups and in all sub-specialties of psychiatry' [7].

Recently the Schizophrenia Commission UK recommended: 'We want the values and ethos of EIP to spread across the entire mental health system...' (and) 'that Clinical Commissioning Groups commission services to extend the successful principles of EI to support people experiencing second and subsequent episodes...' ([8], pp. 15–16) ([9], Chapter 15 in Byrne, Rosen et al., 2014, in press).

What are the essential ingredients of an early intervention approach?....underlying principles of early intervention provision

Table 27.2 summarises some of the candidate principles of all early intervention provision. These are largely the principles of any high quality contemporary mental health service, but brought forward, made convenient and systematised, so that easy access to

Table 27.2   Underlying candidate principles of all early intervention provision

(i)   **Early prevention, detection and intervention is better than late prevention, detection and intervention**
Early prevention, detection and intervention in most mental health disorders usually provide much better recovery and outcomes much sooner for individuals and families suffering them [see below: Conclusion: The overall benefits of an EI approach: (a) the rational/logical benefit]. This implies encouraging prompt referral by community agencies, reducing treatment delays, providing low-key mobile crisis resolution services, individual and family education and minimising coercive emergency entry to mental health services.

(ii) **Taking a population/public health approach**
This entails not just resting on your laurels, your case-load or your waiting list, or just adopting a passive-response style of service, waiting for people in need to turn up. It requires an active-response anticipatory service, and being prepared to reach out, to engage people in need at home, if needed, or if invited in by the family, even by passing messages patiently beneath an isolated person's locked bedroom door on multiple occasions, if necessary. This also means estimating the likely demand or projected number of people with new, as yet undetected, undiagnosed or untreated disorders, and planning and providing enough service providers both to meet this demand and to go out of your way to raise the awareness of potential referral sources, to look for potential clientele in need and to seek appropriate referrals.

(iii) **Requiring both evidence-based interventions and efficient service delivery systems**
Public health proactive approaches to prevention, early detection and intervention, and encouraging timely help-seeking is summarised in Section 2 of Table 27.2 Early intervention and in Australian Healthcare and Hospitals Association et al. 2008. It requires both specific sets of intervention methods or contents, involving specific skills training, supervision and fidelity measurement, as well as specific service delivery systems or service delivery vehicles (see Chapter 15). Sections on Crisis, as well as consideration of the Biomedical, Psychological, Social and Cultural components of care and recovery in Table 27.2 are also relevant to early intervention services. Low profile, low impact, least invasive, voluntary, community-based interventions and service delivery systems should be chosen for early intervention wherever possible.

(iv) **Integration and balance**
Thornicroft and Tansella [10], advocate for a better balance between community-based and hospital-based mental health care. Over the last 2 decades in Australia and New Zealand, the debate over whether mental health services should be provided 'primarily or exclusively' in community or hospital settings has been exposed as a contrived battle over a non-issue. For most of this period, clinical and other expert opinion leaders and policy-makers in this field have been advocating for integrated mental health services ([11–14]).
This involves ensuring more than a balance in community and hospital service provision and resourcing, but integrating both, and a weighting of resources towards community care, with less emphasis on inpatient care, based on evidence—a necessary but insufficient precondition for effective design and delivery of mental health services. A wider integration should then be built with all-of-government and all-of-community partnerships (see Table 27.1).

(v)   **Community focussed**
The World Psychiatric Association International Guidance [14] now proposes models 'with most services... ***provided in community settings close to the populations served, (and) with hospital stays being reduced as far as possible,*** and usually located in acute wards in general hospitals.'
In middle to higher income countries, more viable community-based alternatives to long-term institutionalisation and many acute involuntary inpatient admissions can be provided by evidence-based modular mobile crisis and home treatment teams, early intervention teams,

Table 27.2   (*Continued*)

assertive community treatment teams and 24-hour staffed community-based residential respite centres [15]. The latter are voluntary and often staffed predominantly by NGOs and peer workers, with public clinical professionals visiting frequently. Specific assertive community teams and community respite houses for early intervention with young people have developed in some jurisdictions.

Current and previous National Mental Health Strategies in several developed countries (e.g. Australia, New Zealand, United Kingdom, Ireland and Canada) have made a great deal of progress towards reforming mental health services, with a greater emphasis on community care. However, they have not gone far enough in terms of defining and making specific commitments to implement the required strategies on a continuing basis. An effective method of increasing the specificity, uniformity and fidelity of nationwide implementation is to define individual service components and staffing levels required to deliver a comprehensive, locality-based continuum of community care that addresses the needs of, say, an average population of 200,000. Earlier studies [16] specified the intervention costs fairly accurately, but vastly underestimated the costs of the service delivery systems (or transmission vehicles) and management and physical infrastructure (see Table 27.2 from Australian Healthcare and Hospitals Association et al. [17]). Service models need to be clearly defined; resourcing of services must be done on a rational and equitable basis, not simply on an historical basis; quality monitoring and outcome measures and standards must be meaningful and ensure good practice across multiple providers.

(vi)   Not only community-centred but also **mobile 24-hour accessible home crisis engagement, assessment and care** in both urban, suburban and regional settings, with telehealth-based proxies in rural/remote settings. They should be provided from one-stop-shop centres located at shopping and transport hubs, providing access to psychiatric, drug and alcohol and general medical clinical support and welfare services

(vii)   **Managing clinical complexity**
Clinical complexity denotes the richness of our field and represents a pointed challenge to practitioners to widen our professional responsibilities. Most significant psychiatric disorders have multifaceted aetiologies, including genetic, developmental, psychological, social and cultural causes, precipitants and aggravating influences. This entails consideration in assessment and treatment as required, of multilayered formulations incorporating co-occurring disorders, combining psychiatric disorders with substance use disorders, physical illnesses and (e.g. cardiovascular or metabolic) sequelae of psychiatric treatment, other disabilities, transcultural or indigenous status and social determinants of disease such as poverty or homelessness. It follows that this will require a multifactorial holistic approach to intervention, encompassing biophysical, psychological, social and cultural approaches as well.

(viii)   **Developing a person-centred approach**
Conventional health care paradigms focusing just on the disease state, primary diagnosis and immediate care are increasingly regarded as inadequate.
A person-centred approach would also facilitate attention to the positive aspects of health, such as buoyancy or resilience, personal, family, social and cultural resources and quality of life. This is important for health promotion, prevention, clinical treatment, rehabilitation and recovery [18]. So services should be both service-user and family centred. Service-users are engaged in their own care and treatment. Families are engaged in the service-user's care as much as possible. Services should be age-appropriate, stage of life friendly and sensitive to gender and culture. Services support service-users in recovering and maintaining age-appropriate social roles (e.g., going to school, maintaining a job).
Services should be linked to other services and supports in the community, particularly primary care.
Treatment should be provided in the least restrictive and stigmatising setting. Home-based treatment may be appropriate for adolescents and young adults [19].

(continued)

Table 27.2 *(Continued)*

(ix) **Clinical staging determines clinical care and support strategy**
Assessment, clinical treatments, care, support and follow-up are provided and titrated according to clinical staging, which is relevant and applicable to all psychiatric disorders (see McGorry P, Afterword).

(x) **Operating in accordance with and monitoring on the basis of evidence-based fidelity criteria.**

(xi) **Fidelity monitoring** ensures that teams or services are applying the core ingredients of evidence-based service delivery systems (e.g. Assertive Community Treatment (ACT), [20], [21]), or of an Intervention (e.g. cognitive behavioural treatment (CBT) [22, 23]), and hence for these and other essential components of an early intervention service (e.g. an early intervention in psychosis service, [23]).

Adapted from Iris Guidelines 2012, Ministry of Health and Longterm Care: Early Psychosis Intervention Standards, Ontario, 2011 [19], Australian Clinical Guidelines for Early Psychosis, 2010 [24].

such services can be assured from the moment of serious concern by individuals or their families, their primary practitioners and other referring agents. They also emphasise age-appropriate and welcoming environments, located centrally in their local or regional communities, and providing a relevant multiplicity of services operated locally where possible under the one roof.

Service quality: defining a good service

Extrapolating from the AIMHS Standards [25, 26] and the National Standards for Mental Health Services [27], a comprehensive mental health service is defined as one which brings together a number of components into a unified system, ensuring continuity of care for consumers and families, with a focus on a partnership between public, NGO and fee-for-service mental health services.

These components may now often include:

– a single point (or process) of entry into a service

– specialist crisis intervention, assessment, acute care, ongoing care and rehabilitation care across the service user's lifespan [15, 28].

– a specialist EI team

– a care coordination or case management system integrating inputs from inpatient and community public mental health, NGO and fee-for-service provider services.

– the active involvement of consumers and families

– interdisciplinary mental health teams, including

– Consumer and carer peer support workers, vocational, housing, dual disorder drug and alcohol and community forensic professionals, indigenous and/or transcultural/bilingual mental health workers where relevant and sessional community pharmacists.

– a coordinated management system between all partner services on a whole-of-government and whole-of-community basis.

Quality improvement and standards, accreditation

We propose the development of a set of standards of early prevention, detection and intervention to apply to all mental health disorders in all age-groups, including co-occurring disorders.

We have been taught informally over the years that .... laws are meant to be bent, rules are meant to be broken, and guidelines are meant to be interpreted .... but standards are meant to be aspired to and independently monitored.

Adherence to laws, rules and guidelines is variable, according partly to the strength of the evidence, to how compelling is the moral case put for adherence, and especially to the negative and positive sanctions (i.e. rewards and punishments) which may be applied.

A set of standards can be used as a basis for internal calibration and improvement, or for external monitoring, surveying and accreditation. Internally, standards can be a checklist or blueprint of the generally evidence-based characteristics required for the desirable service to be established and sustained. Externally, standards provide both the current goal and the yardstick by which all similar facilities or operations are measured up. For external rating and accreditation purposes they need to be quantifiable as well as qualitative, comparable between time sampling intervals and across services. Therefore, they are often based on fidelity criteria for both the vehicle they travel in, the service delivery system and the interventions which for their contents. Or on both purposes, they should be explicitly aspirational, as well as practically achievable and understandable by all stakeholder groups. They should not be static: they should be capable of being regularly upgraded, to meet an expectation of continuous improvement, '*every ceiling in time becomes the floor...*' raising the bar for quality and safety ever higher [25, 29].

Some preliminary suggestions for core standards of EI is appended in Table 27.3. It contains some samples of potential candidate standards for all EI programmes adapted from existing Standards for Early Psychosis Intervention, for example, Ministry of Health, Ontario, 2011, [19] and other sources, including the National Service Framework Standards [30], which provides evidence-based examples of the standards sought for early intervention, among other modules of mental health service. Both the original (1996) and the revised Australian National Standards for Mental Health Services [27] are useful, despite the regressive removal of a specific pre-existing early intervention standard and other specific intervention standards in the latter [29], as they also have an extensive standard on graduation from services when recovery is well advanced, including provision for orderly exit and re-entry if necessary. This may not apply to severe and persistent disorders, for example to some of the degenerative diseases of the elderly.

More specific standards could be developed for early intervention for each disorder, age-group and issue described in this volume.

Policy implementation guidelines and clinical practice guidelines

Policy implementation guidelines (PiGs) were introduced to mental health services in the United Kingdom in 2002 to support the consistent delivery of national mental health policy for all local service providers. Although certain service models are specified, there is also

Table 27.3   Potential candidate standards for all EI programmes: examples

1.   Facilitating access and early identification

1.1   EI programmes identify providers and organisations in their communities who are able to assist with early identification of the mental health disorder, help engage clients and make timely referrals for assessment, and be part of an effective early identification/rapid response system.

1.2   To promote early identification and referral of people with first-episode psychosis, EI programmes support providers and organisations in their communities by:

- providing initial and ongoing professional education on the relevant mental health disorder(s), including signs, symptoms and best practices in screening
- providing evidence-based screening tools as well as referral pathways for those organisations that do not have the skills to identify signs of psychosis
- working with members of the early identification (ID) system to ensure people with the relevant mental health disorder(s) access EI assessment services
- active urgent triage capability, not putting crisis assessment off on a waiting list, exercising a low threshold for expert assessment for any likely significant psychiatric disorder, getting to see a consultant psychiatrist within 1 week of referral, linking in to a clinically skilled care coordinator within 5 days of assessment.
- collateral accounts from family or other confidantes or trusted informants should be considered whenever possible
- encouraging the team to start the process of engaging the client in his/her own care
- encouraging schools and community mental health agencies to provide education for individuals with possible indications of the disorder and their families

2.   Comprehensive client assessment

2.1   Service-users referred for a comprehensive assessment are contacted by telephone within 72 hours of being referred, and a face-to-face meeting is offered to be held within 2 weeks. Service-users are made aware of crisis and other services such as crisis response teams, which they can use pending their first appointment or – if crisis response teams do not exist in the community – to the emergency department of the nearest hospital.

2.2   Comprehensive assessments are service-user centred. In keeping with a service-user and family centred approach, the programme strongly encourages service-user and family involvement in assessment and treatment. Families are involved in the assessment with the service-user's consent.

2.3   The programme follows established procedures for communicating with the service-user and family, which include providing a clear written description of the services the programme provides as well as the service-user's and family's role and responsibilities.

2.4   Engagement and assessment are continuous processes, not just restricted to the entry phase of service, but requiring repeated or continuing effort and commitment throughout the episode of care.

3.   Service-user interventions and service delivery systems

3.1   Provide an Interdisciplinary Team Approach, with a wide range and mix of clinical and functional skills, with 24-hour access for mobile crisis intervention [31, 32], individual care management and coordination and intensive/assertive community treatment if necessary.

3.2   To minimise disruption and anxiety for the service-user or family, treatment and support are actively provided in familiar and low-key community settings, including in the individual's home.

3.3   Treating symptoms that are affecting service-user function takes precedence over making a diagnosis. That is, developing our capacity to tolerate diagnostic ambiguity whilst addressing key problems by managing symptoms and addressing functional problems rather than definitive diagnosis.

Table 27.3 *(Continued)*

3.4	Service users receive regular physical and psychiatric re-assessment, and revision of physical and psychiatric treatments based on their changing needs and/or goals.
3.5	Emphasis is placed on providing evidence-based and service-user congenial psychosocial interventions, including cognitive strategies for medication adherence if needed. When clinically indicated, programmes use low dose, slow increment psychotropic medications only strictly as necessary.
3.6	Informed consent is required for all treatment, including treatment with medication. If service-users are clearly not capable of giving full informed consent, try to sustain the discourse and seek some level of understanding, agreement and cooperation, while also consulting substitute decisions makers (e.g., parents, partners, guardians) as set out in the relevant mental health legislation.
3.7	Service users taking prescribed psychotropic medications are monitored closely for side effects e.g., weight gain, cardiovascular abnormalities, changes in glucose or lipid metabolism, extra-pyramidal (Parkinsonian) or tardive dyskineticor sexual dysfunction (usually prolactin related) side effects and their treatment is adjusted as required. All service-users are taught to manage their medications and to self-monitor for adverse effects. A coaching approach is adopted while engaging both a health/sports physiologist and dietician in the interdisciplinary team.
3.8	Inpatient treatment is provided only when it is absolutely necessary. If inpatient care is required, it should be provided in age-appropriate locations (where available) that support the principles of EI, for example, voluntary care with no locked doors and no holding down, if possible. The EI team continues to provide support for the service-user in the inpatient setting (i.e., in-reach services) and advocates on behalf of the service-user to ensure he/she receives consistent treatment during the hospital stay.
3.9	Avoidance of compulsory treatment of all kinds, inpatient or community based, whenever possible, by applying systematically a repertoire of evidence-based alternative strategies including shared decision-making, advanced directives, negotiation of individual care/recovery/wellness plans including early warning signs and desirable responses to them, access to voluntary respite facilities [33].
3.10	Alternatives to inpatient care should be provided wherever possible, including home treatment or voluntary admission to 24-hour staffed age-specific community-based respite facilities.
4.	**Family education and support**
4.1	Programmes use an assertive community care mobile approach to provide support for the family and actively engage the family in the family member's ongoing care (with the service user's consent) and in the family home wherever possible.
4.2	To encourage the family's full engagement, programmes provide education about: the illness and symptoms and the role of treatment, including medications and side effects, including safety risks.
4.3	Specific communication and practical problem solving skills are imparted to and shared with the family.
4.4	At first and as necessary, family education and skills training are imparted in the family home, where feasible, but are also offered via ongoing multiple family groups
5.	**A welcoming age and phase-specific non-stigmatising therapeutic environment**
5.1	A normative and familiar community environmental setting (e.g. home visits or a community health centre in a familiar ordinary environment for that age-group) wherever possible rather than only having facilities and appointments in a hospital setting
5.2	The setting for care should be welcoming and friendly in the interaction offered by front-of-house and other staff

(continued)

Table 27.3   *(Continued)*

5.3	The décor and interaction should be respectful, welcoming, appropriate and sensitive to the age-group, condition and phase of care
5.4	A useful model is the 'headspace' programme (www.headspace.org.au/, accessed 3 June 2014), but for other age-groups and phases of care: that is, the community-based one-stop-shop, where the person can obtain general medical care and other primary health services, while also obtaining mental health, drug and alcohol, sexual health, advice re-health and disability benefits, vocational and housing support and linkage.
5.5	The setting for treatment support and care should be located on an ordinary domestic or shop or office setting in an ordinary streetscape in the person's familiar neighbourhood or often frequented mingling space, if possible.

6.   Relapse prevention strategies

6.1	Regular reviews if the condition persists. Consider possible need for prophylactic medication, behavioural activation and/or psychological therapy with continued support.
6.2	Individual care/wellness/recovery plan collaboratively devised.
6.3	Early warning signs elicited and noted jointly, and copies provided by service-user to nominated or caregiving family, and confidantes, with instructions to be built into 6.2 or 6.4.
6.4	Advanced directive or 'living will' collaboratively devised if acute episodes recur intermittently where judgement or 'capacity' can be lost temporarily.
6.5	Combined individual and family training in cognitive intervention strategies to prevent relapse.
6.6	Individuals with a slow or difficult or delayed recovery or frequent relapses may benefit from more intensive structured interventions, emphasising problem solving and communication skills and multiple family group techniques.

7.   Graduation from the programme: exit and re-entry [26]

7.1	When service-users graduate from the programme, they are linked to the least intensive, least intrusive level of care required to meet their ongoing treatment and support needs (e.g., primary/shared care, family health teams, tertiary care, such as ACT teams, and community mental health specialised programmes).
7.2	When a client graduates to another level of care, the team continues to be available to consult on his/her care.
7.3	The mental health service actively involve the service-user and their carer(s) in developing, when appropriate, an exit plan from the service, including providing a copy to the service-user, and with their permission, to the carers.
7.4	The mental health service provides ample information and ensures easy access for re-entry to the service if and when necessary.
7.5	Some sense of graduation and celebration should be marked and certificated once recovery, resilience, early warning response skills and stress-management skills are honed. This should occur when service-users are ready to leave mental health services with some confidence in their ability to self-manage in an ordinary community setting, with the support of primary health services and a clear pathway to re-entry if needed.
7.6	Not all service-users will be able to leave the mental health service, particularly if they have severe, persistent or recurrent, rapid cycling, or deteriorating disorders. However, recovery principles should be adapted and a sense of achievement, joint journeying and value of the experience, as well as developing unique personal recovery goals in the face of a persistent disorder, should be imparted in these circumstances wherever possible.

Adapted from Iris Guidelines 2012, Ministry of Health and Longterm Care: Early Psychosis Intervention Standards, Ontario, 2011 [19]; Australian Government: National Standards for Mental Health Services, 2010 [27].

emphasis placed on tailoring services to meet local needs. Engaging all local stakeholders in planning the change was designed into the process, recognising:

- The centrality of the service user and those who support them the diversity of need amongst those who use mental health services and of the mhs workforce, encompassing the statutory provider sector but also the voluntary and independent sectors, the service user movement, primary care, and, indeed all areas of the 'whole system'

- The need to value the lessons we learn from each other and the need wherever possible to avoid the blight of the 'not invented here syndrome'.

PiGs have been developed for many service delivery components (e.g. Crisis and Assertive Outreach Community Treatment teams, Inpatient Units and modules of intervention (e.g. dual AOD disorders and personality disorders).

The PiG on EI teams [34] specifies: Intervening early in the course of the disease can prevent initial problems and improve long-term outcomes. If treatment is given early in the course of the illness and services are in place to ensure long-term concordance (cooperation with treatment), the prospect for recovery is improved.

An EI service should be able to:

- reduce the stigma associated with psychosis and improve professional and lay awareness of the symptoms of psychosis and the need for early assessment.

- reduce the length of time young people remain undiagnosed and untreated

- develop meaningful engagement, provide evidence-based interventions and promote recovery during the early phase of illness

It then tabulates specific key components, elements and tasks associated with each component of service.

Clinical practice guidelines (CPGs) have been developed by professional bodies, often with government support, on the basis of expert committees and consensus, to encourage standardisation and consistency of practice of qualified members in line with scientific knowledge (e.g. RANZCP [35]). The aims appeared to be to lift the games of their professionals as a whole in line with evidence, and to ensure that their professional practices should not lie outside that of the majority of their peers. RANZCP CPGs are based on diagnostic categories such as Anorexia Nervosa; bipolar disorder; deliberate self-harm (youth and adult); depression; panic disorder and agoraphobia; and schizophrenia. They are published in versions for clinicians, consumers and carers (RANZCP, 2003 [35]). There have been similar advances in England and Wales with the National Institute for Health and Care Excellence (http://www.nice.org.uk/, accessed 3 June 2014). In achieving consensus guidelines, clinicians were joined by other disciplines, scientists, patients, carers, civil servants, nongovernmental organisations and sometimes the commercial sector.

CPGs were seen by some professionals at the time of development as an assault on their clinical autonomy and on individual innovation, but they have been seen widely as useful over time, as they are advisory only, not compulsory, and purport to leave room for justifiable variations in practice and clinical judgment in individual circumstances. The main problem is that they go stale: their development is too often a one-off project, whereas the need to update them regularly as evidence changes requires a standing body overseeing their continuous redevelopment, and an ongoing commitment of resources to do so.

The Australian Clinical Guidelines for Early Psychosis meets all these criteria, and encouragingly, came out in its 2nd edition in 2010. It also covers preventive phases including ultra-high risk states through to late problematic recovery and delayed discharge phases.

The IRIS Early Intervention in Psychosis Guidelines, originally published in the United Kingdom in 1998, were also revised in [36]. They are for service providers and commissioners of mental health services to help them to ensure high quality and cost effective delivery of care and support for people experiencing a first episode of psychosis. They emphasise the importance of dedicated leadership engendering a strong early-intervention culture, an interdisciplinary team structure dedicated to EI, low caseloads and need for Assertive Community Treatment (ACT) methodology, applied flexibly according to need.

Ripple effects of early intervention teams

It is becoming clear that early prevention and intervention methods and service delivery systems can fruitfully spread their influence to:

(a)   Other phases of care

(b)   Other age-groups

(c)   Other diagnostic categories of psychiatric disorder

(d)   Many intervention modalities and

(e)   All psychiatric workforce disciplines

We will now consider each of these in turn:

(a) Other phases of care   The practical components of early intervention mental health services for young people may well be a useful model of care for those individuals with severe disabilities continuing through all phases of care. For example, a team providing the intensity, home visiting, low-key biophysical, psychological, social and cultural interventions, including family and multiple family interventions. Consequently, it would be useful to be able to maintain the intensity and integrated components of largely community-based early intervention work for another 5–10 years, or more, if needed for selected clientele. For a small minority, this might need to be a relatively long term (e.g. 5–10 years) service commitment.

There is a dilemma, as it will be most unhelpful if managers decide that if we can apply EI calibre and range of interventions, even if in some diluted form, at every phase of care, then we might as well only have one generic team for all. This is not what is indicated by the evidence nor by the staging classification of conditions subject to EI, (see P McGorry in Afterword) and nor should it be implied by our approach.

A smallish subgroup will need intensive EI-type services on an ongoing intensive basis for a further 5–10 years, hopefully by a separate but linked team undertaking high-calibre services with a similar range of interventions, a EI with an ACT type of service delivery system [7]. If they are to avoid feeling alienated on entry, and feel comfortable with other service-users around them as a peer group, young people need a different team from 30–35 year olds with a more diagnostically established and still persistently buffeting condition. Generally, as concluded in the current NICE guidelines on Schizophrenia, generic CMHTs have not been supported in evidence in comparison to phase-specific modules of care [37].

(b) Other age-groups It has become increasingly clear via indications in the learned literature and with the most willing and enthusiastic input from the authors of this book project, that an early intervention approach to mental health services would be most useful throughout the life cycle from the antenatal to perinatal periods, infancy, childhood, adolescence, adulthood and in old age (see our series of different age-group chapters). Again, this does not imply that there is evidence to support a generic service covering all these age-groups in any urban/suburban environment, though small generic CMHC teams may have to prevail in rural/remote settings by necessity. These teams can be supported by regional EI specialty teams either or both by an interactive video telehealth link, or in person, on an itinerant outreach basis. Specific phase and age-related modules of treatment and care usually prove to be more effective, where they can be organised (e.g. in urban to regional centres), but should be set up with very permeable boundaries between teams, to enhance continuity of care [15, 28].

(c) Other diagnostic categories of psychiatric disorder Equally, it is becoming increasingly accepted that early intervention approaches have a crucial role in and should be applied to most disorders, including anxiety, mood, post-traumatic, psychotic, delirium, personality disorders, eating disorders, suicidal tendencies, and dual or comorbidity disorders including drug and alcohol, intellectual, autistic spectrum and learning disorders. We also considered community, hospital and forensic settings, and if there was only more space, we should have added early prevention and intervention in transcultural and indigenous mental health service settings.

(d) Many intervention modalities The implications of an EI framework for individuals, families and whole communities are drawn out in chapters and sections on psychotherapies, family interventions, social movement strategies, stigma and discrimination, including the influence of the media, for better or worse. This framework allows a full range (from psychosocial to biomedical) effective interventions to be applied as soon as they are needed, without leaving individuals, families or communities needlessly in states of distress. This can occur due to calamities which befall them all because a person with severe mental illness has been left untreated when timely intervention would have made a huge difference to their inner and outer turbulence and risk of harm to themselves or others. This is in accord with an integrated approach embracing complexity and incorporating the multimodal and holistic person-centred principles stated in the principles section above.

(e) All psychiatric workforce disciplines The relevance to all workforce disciplines of such a framework is considered for interdisciplinary teams (including consideration of generic CMHT versus specialised EI teams) sometimes combining or synergising the efforts of mental health professionals from the public, nongovernment and private fee-for-service sectors (e.g. 'headspace' type models), and consumer and family peer workers.

While at the same time.......

(f) Taking care not to unnecessarily intrude, over-diagnose or over-treat   We must continue to take care not to needlessly medicalise or pathologise ordinary problems of living or life crises where there is no definitive evidence of emerging or actual mental illness.

We should take care not to needlessly worry individuals or families by declaring them at 10% risk of developing schizophrenia early in life through screening programmes because of genetic heritage, where there is a 90% chance or more of NOT getting it, even with a first degree relative with the syndrome. False positives will still usually far outweigh true positives [38], unless rigorous steps are taken to ensure postponement of diagnostic and prognostic predictions until the clinical picture is compelling.

We should consider how *intrusive* or *invasive* the screening method is, both physiologically (e.g. blood tests) and psychologically (provoking anxiety in subjects by worrying them that they may have the disease-state in question). As pointed out by McGorry [39] and in Rosen [40], the concept of 'number needed to treat' (NNT) to prevent one negative outcome needs to be balanced by the 'number needed to inconvenience' (NNI), or moreover, the 'number needed to worry' (NNW) through screening, over-close preventive observation or pre-emptive intervention to prevent one negative outcome [40]. This has been scientifically codified more coarsely as Number Needed to Harm (NNH). There is also the danger of over-claiming the benefits of early prevention, so we should be cautious to balance early prevention and intervention strategies with such benefits, and be careful not to bother people too early, especially if they have only possible early stages of neurologically degenerative disorders, such as irreversible dementias, for which there may be no definitive treatments. This should be weighed against the possibility of referring early for investigation of possible reversible causes, and to assist with preparation, particularly with special relationships and interests, for inevitable decline.

So far, on the basis of Australian national survey data, iatrogenesis, misdiagnosis and unwarranted treatment has either not occurred, or if so, only very uncommonly, and to a slight degree [41]. Why is this over-treatment fear probably misplaced? Firstly, because EI services are generally so underprovided, the demand for EI services is so heavy, and the queues are so potentially long that EI services will only take on those with confirmed disorders or those individuals who are assessed as having a relatively high index of probability of an emerging disorder of clinical significance.

Secondly, clinicians working in early intervention teams tend to want to underplay clinical conclusions, and are wary of false positives and are reluctant to treat those without a confirmed disorder. They are usually reluctant to pathologise or clinically redefine issues that could be more usefully construed as problems of living, or as protracted life crises. They are often aware (although they may not yet have a term for it) that one of their important duties is the need to perform the 'undoing' [40] or 'undiagnosis' [42] of an inappropriate iatrogenic psychiatric diagnosis or over-treatment given during a transient period of stress or temporary life crisis by a previously consulted clinician or referring professional. Such iatrogenesis is now referred to increasingly as 'quaternary prevention' [43]. Quaternary prevention includes actions taken to identify patients who are at risk of over-treatment, and to protect them from unnecessary clinical interventions. Quaternary prevention is particularly relevant in the elderly, whose comorbidities are associated with increased fragility. Falls clinics across the world have identified over-treatment of hypertension, excessive prescription of painkillers and use of unnecessary sedation of older people (to name but three iatrogenic examples) as the main preventable causes of injury. Clinicians have ethical obligations to protect patients at risk of harm from excessive interventions [43].

Thirdly, mental health professionals working in EI teams or contexts usually try to work with a light touch, to avoid any undue trauma due to the intervention and to avoid adverse effects or unneeded hospital admissions that could impact on their engagement with the service-user. If in doubt, as with suspected prodromal symptoms, there is often an emphasis placed on psychosocial interventions from the very beginning, only resorting to medical interventions if absolutely necessary, and in very low doses if so.

Engagement here is not just the icing on the cake of EI: in many ways it IS the cake. If the person and the clinician make the transition to working alliance, the hard work of therapeutic assessment and building trusting relationships has already been done. Working actively on engagement must occur not just at the beginning, but throughout the therapeutic encounter, however long.

Can there be early prevention and intervention of chronicity?

Can we do EI of chronicity? Is this an oxymoron? Or should an EI approach replace chronicity thinking at every phase of care? Should not we replace the term 'maintenance stream' with the conviction that we can always create the conditions and provide assistance for a person with a long-term persistent and severe psychiatric condition to take the next constructive steps towards recovery and moving on in life?

This requires a conceptual map invoking the constructs of newsworthiness, readiness, therapeutic optimism and a life beyond 'woodshedding' [7].

Can we do EI of wellbeing and wellness?

Should not we speak about EI with wellbeing as well as with mental illness? Can we take a timely wellness approach to 'happiness' counselling or dealing with everyday 'home and garden' crises in the normalising context of general practice, or if necessary, at home or in a community mental health centre, to short-circuit the precipitation of significant anxiety and depression? (e.g. Improving Access to Psychological Therapies (IAPT) http://www.iapt.nhs.uk/). Can we take an EI and wellness approach to crises even when people are struggling with a longer-term mental illness, to prevent exacerbations and consequent life disruptions?

Finally, we should be taking preventive and EI approaches to physical disorders which may co-occur with psychiatric disorders (e.g. alcohol-related harm and obesity disorders co-occurring with psychiatric disorders), the excessive rates of smoking in psychiatric disorders and the unwanted neuromuscular, cardiovascular and metabolic consequences of taking psychiatric medications. Appropriate timely strategies include 'quit-smoking' programmes; dietary and activity programmes; sports physiology coaching and metabolic monitoring; using medications sparingly, in lower doses and for lesser periods, strictly as needed for acute treatment, follow-up and protective prophylaxis [44].

The overall benefits of an EI approach

So could EI be a fruitful approach across the range of clinical conditions, key mental health issues, stages of life and phases of care? Just consider the potential in terms of the following.

(a) The rational/logical benefit There is a high face validity to offering early rather than late intervention in most potentially severe and persistent clinical disorders. Cardiologists and oncologists will no longer tolerate late intervention in their fields, and their insistence on EI has paid off handsomely in terms of better clinical and functional outcomes, quality of life and survival rates. Gynaecologists soon saw the wisdom and moral arguments of the PapanicolaouTest ('Pap'/cervical smear), and provided proactive clinics with speedy colposcopies. It would be unthinkable if these programmes had failed to develop.

Until recently, the accepted norm for severe psychiatric conditions, many of which begin in teenage years, was to provide middling to late detection and intervention services. This has been challenged by the growing EI in psychosis international movement for young people and the Australian nationwide 'headspace' assessment and triage programme for young people with all psychosocial disorders.

However, most psychiatric systems for other age-groups are still predominantly late and slow intervention services. This is largely habitual and institutionalised within mental health services. Possibly this has been based on our professional upbringings, which have emphasized Kraepelinian therapeutic pessimism [7], and the false assumption that most of these disorders lead inexorably to deterioration. For whatever reason, this mindset has been habitually entrenched and largely institutionalized within mental health services. However, it may be also partly due to the stigma and personal sense of failure associated with seeking help with emerging psychiatric conditions, particularly in men. It is also due to the lack of community awareness about how disabling and lethal psychiatric disorders can be. Some people come to services late, sicker and with ingrained pessimism that they cannot be helped.

Rationally, the evidence favours EI [45], which decreases the duration of untreated psychosis, promotes early recovery, and decreases violence to self and others [46]. When users, carers, professionals, and the people who fund services agree to use their resources on services based on logical grounds and sound evidence, we glow in the bright warm haze of the Enlightenment.

(c) The clinical benefit Our co-authors have reviewed a wide array of promising to very high quality evidence to demonstrate the clinical benefit and to support the adoption of EI approaches in a wide range of disorders age-groups and settings, and with key mental health issues like self-harm and suicide prevention.

This should also include the benefit of timely crisis intervention or EI counselling to prevent stressful periods of life building up into major psychiatric disorders. Such stressful life events are often associated with losses of many kinds: by death, separation, or divorce, loss of accustomed occupation by redundancy or retirement, loss of limb or bodily function and so on. Occasionally, even positive life events like homecomings after prolonged absences, public recognition of achievements, birthdays, weddings and so on. can prompt mental illnesses in those who are vulnerable. Effective intervention entails dealing with stress and anxiety disorders associated with life events as a 'home and garden' crisis to be done in timely fashion, with competent counselling and involving the real people in your life. It should be dealt with in ordinary language rather than just providing a technical label. It should be addressed as soon as possible, rather than putting it on the back-burner or waiting list, or worse still, 'sitting on your hands' in a sedentary (do-nothing-much) service, or merely waiting until it becomes a full-blown clinical emergency [31].

(c) The economic cost-benefit   Earlier and more recent studies by health economists (e.g. [47–50]) strongly support the economic benefits of EI approaches. McCrone et al. [49, 50] demonstrated savings of at least 66% over 3 years with this approach, while Mihalopoulos et al. [47, 48] in Australia and Hastrup et al. [51] in Denmark show that short-term cost savings are maintained over an 8 year and 5-year follow-up period respectively, with the 10-year results also looking promising for the Danish group.

This evidence also applies to conditions where functional disability has already set in early.

In general, the overarching objective of EI is to incur some expenditure on a particular intervention today that, not only improves individual outcomes beyond that which would occur in the absence of the intervention, but also lowers the costs and impacts associated with the disability for individuals and the wider community over the longer term.

This is an objective that should apply to all care and support for people with disability. It should not be restricted to specific interventions just because they are usually performed at a certain time relative to (say) the identification or appearance of a disability.

The Productivity Commission of Australia [1] recommends that where there is strong evidence to support funding of an EI approach, this funding should be provided in addition to funding provided for ongoing care and support and not be able to be 'cashed out' by habitual clinical services or people with self-directed disability care packages.

Comprehensive EI treatment and care services are demonstrably an excellent 'buy' and begin to yield savings even in the first year of entry to care.

(d) The moral/equity/morale/ethical benefit   Individuals with psychiatric conditions and their families have a human right to the most timely access to the most effective interventions and service delivery systems, that is, congenial evidence-based care when it is most likely to be effective. Being given an appropriate differential diagnosis is often met with relief, though sometimes not so if the individual, family or community is more concerned with stigma than the illness. Such access should be available to all, regardless of their age, ethnicity, socio-economic class or ability to pay. Further, the earlier the person with an emerging or current psychiatric disability can be engaged in services which are seen by that person to be welcoming, congenial and of value, the less resort that will be necessary to involuntary or hospital inpatient care, which would compromise the person's life, liberty and human rights, and which could add an overlay of fear and trauma. The ethical dimension requires that the benefits of early screening, early assessment and treatment should be carefully weighed against preventing unwarranted alarm and worry [40].

(e) The cultural benefit   EI conveys benefits to the *micro-culture* of the extended kinship network, including immediate family, and if need be proxy families and friends [52]. This entails such families and/or confidantes, with permission of the service-user, being adequately informed, involved, consulted and supported at every stage of care. If the person's life is hardly or only briefly disrupted, afflicted individuals will not compromise or lose key relationships. Families and friends will feel relieved from worry, fear, trauma and anticipatory grief if the disorder is caught and effectively resolved early.

EI also includes benefits to and from the *macro-culture* of the service-user's community, society and national or cultural traditions [52]. The benefit from the culture should be respect and continued social inclusion, including if needed, community housing and employment, and freedom or relief from the blights of stigma and discrimination from that culture. The benefit to the culture is to have a productive and active citizen restored to full functioning within that culture.

With the example of homelessness: strictly, you cannot 'treat' homelessness. However, every roofless person on our streets tonight would have benefited from early, simple interventions (most especially in rehousing and preserving their mental and physical health, self-respect and dignity). Instead, worse in our cities, and worst of all in the United States, unacceptable levels of homelessness shame us all.

Strictly, you cannot 'treat' homelessness. However, every roofless person on our streets tonight would have benefited from early, simple interventions (most especially in preserving their mental and physical health, self-respect and dignity). Instead, worse in our cities, and worst of all in the United States, unacceptable levels of homelessness shame us all.

Conclusion

EI is not a new concept in medicine; the approach draws on lessons from improvements elsewhere in health care, most notably in cancer and cardiovascular disease, where intervening earlier, rather than later, with therapeutic strategies being chosen according to the stage of illness and on the basis of a careful risk/benefit assessment which is a standard practice. In psychiatry, EI provides a logical pathway, supported by strong evidence, towards achieving the reductions in mortality and morbidity seen in these other areas of medicine, yet which have remained elusive in mental health care. Furthermore, the EI paradigm provides a rationale and framework for developing and systematising evidence-based primary though to tertiary preventive efforts, as well as implementing more responsive and effective mental health services. It is an approach that can be offered across the lifespan, and the full diagnostic spectrum, to enable the timely provision of appropriate care to ensure better outcomes. The evidence has been building considerably for EI for young people experiencing an episode of mental ill-health that may represent the onset of a severe mental illness. Teams particularly serving these individuals and their families are increasingly supported by evidence of effectiveness in longer-term follow-up studies, and therefore they will continue to be needed with more of them being developed. However, there are also strong indications that systematised EI approaches may well be able to further alleviate suffering of those experiencing other significant psychiatric disorders, as well as their families.

So, discrete teams serving young people for EI in Psychosis should continue to be implemented, and, at the same time, we must ensure ample provision for active rehabilitation and recovery programmes for individuals with persistent disabilities. It is also timely for mental health services to develop and implement EI approaches across a much wider spectrum of conditions, age-groups and treatment settings, in line with advances in the contemporary management of many medical conditions.

References

1. Productivity Commission of Australia. (2011). Inquiry Report: Number 54: 31 July 2011: Disability Care and Support, Chapter 13 Disability Support: Early Intervention. http://www.pc.gov.au/projects/inquiry/disability-support/report (accessed 5 June 2014).
2. Haggerty R. and Mrazek PB. (eds). (1994). *Reducing Risks for Mental Disorders: Frontiers for Preventive Intervention Research*, pp. 53–71. Washington, DC: National Academy Press.
3. Caplan G. (1964). Principles of Preventive Psychiatry. New York: Basic Books.
4. Yung AR and McGorry PD. (1996). The prodromal phase of first-episode psychosis: past and current conceptualizations schizophrenia bulletin **22**(1): 353–370.
5. Falloon IRH and Fadden G. (1993). *Integrated Mental Health Care: A Comprehensive Community-Based Approach*. Cambridge: Cambridge University Press
6. Rosen A, Byrne P, Goldstone SD, and McGorry P. (2014). Early intervention approaches: for better mental health services, Chapter 99. In: A Tasman, J Lieberman, J Kay, M First and M Riba (eds), *Psychiatry*. New York: Wiley. In press.
7. Shiers D, Rosen A and Shiers A. (2009). Beyond early intervention: can we adopt alternative narratives like 'Woodshedding' as pathways to recovery in schizophrenia?. *Early Intervention in Psychiatry* **3**: 163–171.
8. Murray R, et al. (2012). The abandoned illness. A report by the Schizophrenia Commission, United Kingdom, http://www.schizophreniacommission.org.uk/the-report/ (accessed 8 May 2014).
9. Armando M, De Crescenzo F, Birchwood M. (2014). Early intervention services versus generic community mental health services: A paradigm shift, Chapter 15. In: P Byrne and A Rosen (eds), *Early Intervention in Psychiatry: EI of Nearly Everything*, pp. 167–184. Oxford: Wiley Blackwell.
10. Thornicroft G and Tansella M. (2002). Balancing community-based and hospital-based mental health care. *World Psychiatry* **1**(2): 84–90.
11. Rosen A. (2002). Integration is as essential as balance. *World Psychiatry* **1**(2): 91–93.
12. Rosen A, Gurr R and Fanning P. (2010). The future of community-centred health services in Australia: Lessons from the mental health sector. *Australian Health Review* **34**: 106–115.
13. Rosen A, Gurr R, Fanning P and Owen A. (2012). The future of community-centred health services in Australia: 'When too many beds are not enough.' *Australian Health Review* **36**: 239–243.
14. Thornicroft G, Alem A, Antunes R, et al. (2010). WPA guidance on steps, obstacles and mistakes to avoid in the implementation of community mental health care. *World Psychiatry* **9**: 67–77.
15. Rosen A, Killaspy H and Harvey C. (2013). Specialisation and marginalisation: How the world-wide experience with Assertive Community Treatment demonstrates the way interpretation of

evidence can impact adversely on investment for those with the most complex needs. *The Psychiatrist* **37**: 345–348.

16. Whiteford H, Harris M, Diminic S. (2013). Mental health service system improvement: Translating evidence into policy. *Australian and New Zealand Journal of Psychiatry.* doi:10.1177/000486741349486

17. Australian Healthcare and Hospitals Association. (2008). The Mental Health Services conference of Australia & New Zealand, Inc. Mental Health Funding Methodologies and Governance, National Roundtable discussion paper. Co-authors Eagar K, Rosen A, Gurr R, Gear C. Sydney: PriceWaterhouseCoopers. http://www.aushealthcare.com.au/publications/publication_details.asp?sr=0™pid=169 (accessed 1 March 2010).

18. Mezzich JE and Salloum IM. (2008). Clinical complexity and person-centered integrative diagnosis. *World Psychiatry* **7**(1): 1–2.

19. Ministry of Health and Long-Term Care, Ontario. (2011). Early Psychosis Intervention Program Standards, Ontario, Canada.

20. Rosen A and Teesson M. (2001). Does case management work? The evidence and the abuse of evidence-based medicine. *Australian and New Zealand Journal of Psychiatry* **35**: 731–746.

21. Teague GB, Bond GR and Drake RE. (1998). Program fidelity in assertive community treatment. Development and use of a measure. *American Journal of Orthopsychiatry* **68**: 216–232.

22. Brooker C. (2001). A decade of evidence-based training for work with people with serious mental health problems: progress in the development of psychosocial interventions. *Journal of Mental Health* **10**(1): 17–31.

23. Birchwood M, Lester H, McCarthy L, et al. (2014). The UK national evaluation of the development and impact of Early Intervention Services (the National EDEN studies): study rationale, design and baseline characteristics. *Early Intervention in Psychiatry* **8**(1): 59–67.

24. Australian Clinical Guidelines for Early Psychosis. (2010). *Early Psychosis Prevention & Intervention Centre*, 2nd edition. Orygen, Melbourne, Australia.

25. Rosen A, Miller V and Parker G. (1989). Standards of care for area mental health services. *Australian and New Zealand Journal of Psychiatry* **23**: 379–385.

26. Rosen A, Miller V and Parker GB, Area Integrated Mental Health Services (AIMHS) Standards. (1993). *Area Integrated Mental Health Services (AIMHS) Project.* Sydney: NSW Health.

27. Australian Government: National Standards for Mental Health Services. (1996), revised 2010, National Mental Health Strategy.

28. Rosen A, Stein L, Birchwood M, et al. (2013) Specialist community teams backed by years of research. *The Psychiatrist* **37**(1): 38–39.

29. Miller V, Rosen A, Gianfransesco P, et al. (2009). Australian National Standards for Mental Health Services: a blueprint for improvement. *International Journal of leadership in the Public Service* **5**(3): 25–42.

30. Department of Health: National Health Service. (1999). *National Service Framework for Mental Health: Modern Standards and Service Models*, Government of England.

31. Rosen A. (1997). Crisis management in the community. *Medical Journal of Australia* **167**(11/12): 633–638.

32. Rosen A. (2002). Crisis Intervention in Severe Mental Illness. Proceedings of The Working of Helplines Symposium. ARAFMI, Australia, 38–41.

33. Rosen A, Rosen T and McGorry P. (2012). The human rights of people with severe and persistent mental illness: Can conflicts between dominant and non-dominant paradigms be reconciled? In: M Dudley, D Silove and F Gale (eds), *Mental Health and Human Rights.* Oxford: Oxford University Press.

34. Department of Health: Mental Health Policy Implementation Guide. (2002). *Adult Mental Health Policy: National Health Service*, Government of England.

35. RANZCP. (2003). Clinical Practice Guidelines, Royal Australian & New Zealand College of Psychiatrists, Melbourne http://www.ranzcp.org/Publications/Clinical-Practice-Guidelines-2.aspx (accessed 8 May 2014).

36. IRIS Early Intervention in Psychosis Guidelines revised. (2012). http://www.iris-initiative.org.uk/ (accessed 8 May 2014).

37. Rosen A, Stein LI, McGorry P, et al. (2013). Specialist community teams backed by years of quality research. *The Psychiatric Bulletin* **37**: 38.

38. Jablensky A. (2000). Prevalence and incidence of schizophrenia spectrum disorders: implications for prevention. *Australian and New Zealand Journal of Psychiatry* **34**(Suppl.): S26–S34.

39. McGorry PD. (2000). The nature of schizophrenia: Signposts to prevention. *Australian and New Zealand Journal of Psychiatry* **34**(Suppl.): S14–S21.

40. Rosen A. (2000). Ethics of early prevention in schizophrenia. *Australian and New Zealand Journal of Psychiatry* **34**(Suppl): S208–S212.

41. Bobevski I, Rosen A and Meadows G. (2014). Mental health service use and need for care of Australians with and without diagnoses of mental disorders: Is there any "met un-need" in the findings from the National Survey of Mental Health and Wellbeing 2007. *BMC Psychiatry*. In press.

42. Patfield M. (2011). Undiagnosis: an important new role for psychiatry. *Australasian Psychiatry* **19**(2): 107–109.

43. Gérvas J, Starfield B and Heath I. (2008). Is clinical prevention better than cure? *The Lancet* **372**: 1997–1999.

44. HEAL Statement, Declaration & Campaign, Curtis J, Shiers D, et al. This international statement, called Healthy Active Lives (HeAL), aims to reverse the trend of people with severe mental illness dying early by tackling risks for future physical illnesses pro-actively and much earlier. http://www.iphys.org.au/what_is_HeAL.html (accessed 8 May 2014).

45. Schizophrenia Commission. (2012). The Abandoned Illness: A Report. Rethink Mental Illness.

46. Large MM, Nielssen O, Ryan CJ and Hayes R. (2008). Mental health laws that require dangerousness for involuntary admission may delay the initial treatment of schizophrenia. *Social Psychiatry & Psychiatric Epidemiology* **43**: 251–256.

47. Mihalopoulos C, Harris M, Henry L, et al. (2009). "Is early intervention in psychosis cost-effective over the long term?" *Schizophrenia Bulletin* **35**(5): 909–918.

48. Mihalopoulos C, McCrone P, Knapp M, et al. (2012). The costs of early intervention in psychosis: restoring the balance. *The Australian and New Zealand Journal of Psychiatry* **46**(9): 808–811.

49. McCrone P, Knapp M and Dhanasiri S. (2009). Economic impact of services for first-episode psychosis: a decision model approach. *Early Intervention Psychiatry* **3**(4): 266–273.

50. McCrone P, Craig TK, Power P and Garety PA. (2010). Cost-effectiveness of an early intervention service for people with psychosis. *British Journal of Psychiatry* **196**(5): 377–382.

51. Hastrup LH, Kronborg C, Bertelsen M, et al. (2013). Cost-effectiveness of early intervention in first-episode psychosis: economic evaluation of a randomised controlled trial (the OPUS study). *British Journal of Psychiatry* **202**(1): 35–41.

52. Rosen A. (2006). The community psychiatrist of the future. *Current Opinion in Psychiatry* **19**(4): 380–388.

Afterword for Early Intervention of Nearly Everything for Better Mental Health Services

Patrick McGorry

Orygen Youth Health Research Centre, University of Melbourne, Melbourne, Australia

The case for early intervention may seem so obvious, particularly when backed up by the sort of logic and evidence that this monograph has assembled, that one may be genuinely surprised to learn that it has been critiqued, often emotively and passionately, by a number of academic psychiatrists and other interests. How could anyone oppose early intervention? While some of this critique is certainly fuelled by a variety of sometimes undeclared vested interests [1, 2], all the same it is well worth considering when early intervention might *not* be justified.

I can think of two scenarios where caution is certainly required. First, even in the case of potentially serious conditions, such as Alzheimer's disease or motor neurone disease, which are inevitably deteriorating and ultimately fatal, if there is absolutely no effective treatment currently available to modify the impact and course of the disease, then it could be argued that early detection and intervention may be a waste of time or even harmful. However, even here, relief of suffering, the provision of personal and social support and especially care of the relatives may all be extremely worthwhile and may be much more helpful if offered early or in a timely fashion. The second scenario where the value of early intervention can be legitimately questioned is where the only available treatments are known to produce serious adverse effects, and to offer them in the early stages of illness may actually do more harm than good.

This latter scenario illustrates a broader principle, which has been at the very heart of ethical medical practice from the time of Hippocrates, namely the responsibility to "first,

Early Intervention in Psychiatry: EI of nearly everything for better mental health, First Edition.
Edited by Peter Byrne and Alan Rosen.
© 2014 John Wiley & Sons, Ltd. Published 2014 by John Wiley & Sons, Ltd.

do no harm". Prevention and treatment must be proportional to the risk and severity of the condition being treated. While early intervention strategies are designed to target treatment delay and under-treatment, there is a balancing responsibility to avoid over-treatment. This lesson has been learned in mainstream medicine, for example in the cancer field. David Sackett, the Eminent Canadian Clinical Epidemiologist, has emphasised that the earlier one ventures in prevention and early intervention, the greater importance must be attached to safety [3]. This principle has legitimately underpinned the critiques of early intervention in mental health, as well as in other branches of medicine.

A practical solution to this tension is clinical staging [4, 5], in which treatment in the earlier stages must not only be shown to be more effective than when offered later, but it must be demonstrably safer than no treatment and later forms of treatment. These features can be demonstrated in many cancers and other physical illnesses, where the consequences of over-treatment have also been demonstrated. Proportionality is the key to this enhanced approach to diagnosis and great sensitivity to risk/benefit balance is required. This is not exactly the same as "stepped care", where treatment non-responders graduate in a step-wise manner through sequential trials of treatment. With clinical staging, there is also an eye to the future. In addition to successful treatment of the current syndrome(s), an additional target is the prevention or the reduction of the risk of progression to the next and more advanced stage of illness and worsening disabilities.

In the mental health field, in addition to the specific adverse effects of treatments such as intensive and overly intrusive psychotherapies and medications (including over-medication and unbridled polypharmacy), the other potential source of harm flows from stigma and "labelling". Stigma may harm people at any stage of illness, yet which is of special concern when people are in the early stages prior to treatment and when there may be confusion as to whether the person has a need for care or is merely going through a troubling or distressing period of life. Stigma has also been a feature of many physical illnesses, yet has been dispelled by a combination of better education and community understanding, and decisively with the advent of highly effective treatments. Tuberculosis, epilepsy, cancer and even leprosy are excellent examples of this. These approaches will be essential in dispelling stigma in mental health and are well underway (see chapter by P. Corrigan). It is insufficient for effective treatments to exist. They must be delivered successfully in the real world, through translation and up-scaling mechanisms. An additional early anti-stigma intervention strategy in mental health, rarely achieved, is the delivery of care in positive, hopeful and welcoming environments and within positive cultures of care. We have seen this occur with the national roll-out of early prevention and intervention in psychosis (EPPIC) teams and "headspace" programmes, which provide easy access to youth-friendly one-stop shops for all their general medical and psychosocial concerns, located nearby communal youth mingling spaces in Australia [6, 7, www.headspace.org.au] and increasingly elsewhere (e.g. "headstrong" in Ireland). Ironically, *headspace* is the best antidote known to Allen Frances's stated concerns [8] of over-reliance on medication and "labelling". In fact, *headspace* has provided stigma-free access to care for the first time to now over 100,000 young Australians.

Early intervention and *headspace* services are led by people who are strongly committed to evidence-informed care and ensuring that these are carefully evaluated. With Early Intervention in Psychosis teams for young people, both short- and long-term outcomes are proving to be robustly positive, and the early data for *headspace* look very promising.

The introduction and concluding chapter of this volume promote the role of early intervention as a force for good in the rest of the system. The suggested further development of principles and standards exemplified in the tables of the concluding chapter begin to operationalise this approach. However, the concluding chapter also correctly identifies a dilemma and posits a caveat: taking an "early intervention" inspired approach in different age groups and in more phases of psychiatric illnesses should not be allowed to weaken the argument for stage-based care. If we were to say that people should stay long term in an early intervention service, managers will conclude that this could then become the whole service over time, in a merged generic sense. This would be a mistake, not supported by the evidence. As the editors state (Concluding chapter, Ripple Effects (a) and (b)): "Specific phase and age-related modules of treatment and care have usually proven to be more effective, wherever they can be organized (e.g., in urban to regional centres), but should be set up with very permeable boundaries between teams, to enhance continuity of care."

They also suggest: "A smallish subgroup will need intensive early intervention type services on an on-going intensive basis for a further 5–10 years, hopefully by a separate but linked team undertaking high calibre services with a similar range of interventions as early intervention with an ACT type of service delivery system". There has to be a tenure issue to make room for new referrals, but I also think 2 years is too short, and probably up to 5 years if required seems the best compromise. Also the later stage services can reform on-going services and be more responsive with an early intervention-type approach plus a recovery focus, without merging with early intervention services. There is also an age and developmental stage issue that fits with broadening early intervention by diagnosis. This is the reason we do not want to see 35 year olds with 10-year histories and with a less fluid, more definitive diagnosis mixed in with the early intervention youth-care zone.

A final challenge for proponents, and indeed the opponents, of early intervention in mental health is to acknowledge and embrace the ambiguity that characterises the onset stage of mental ill-health. The boundary between normal human experience and transient distress on the one hand and mental ill-health is not clear, yet is dynamic and contestable [5]. Positive mental health, resilience, coping repertoire and social support all mediate and moderate how people at risk for emerging mental ill-health navigate this boundary and whether they cross it. If we develop the right language and discourse, create fully permeable stigma-free portals to care and offer choice and evidence-based interventions, then I believe these problems and barriers to early intervention can be solved. Denial of the widespread and genuine need for early intervention and mental health care across the lifespan, but especially in young people, and conversely narrow medical reductionism and an unthinking defence of the status quo in psychiatry, pose the major threats to effective solutions.

If these issues are acknowledged, then early intervention in mental health will flourish and produce huge benefits in terms of both reduced human suffering and greater personal fulfilment and economic productivity. Facing and responding to key features of the early intervention critique will assist us in securing these social benefits and will expose the residual resistance for what it is: the familiar and expected defence of vested interests. Here this is spawned and fuelled by a misguided loyalty to the status quo in mental health care, which is so clearly deficient, or from the opposite side the more covert and denialist campaigns of extreme anti-psychiatry [9]. This volume sets out a comprehensive agenda for reform and progress based on the crucial early intervention paradigm. There is considerable potential utility of recommending and exemplifying the development of some core principles and standards which may underlie this approach. These necessarily lack specificity in this common-ground form, but will undoubtedly become more specific and elaborated as they are applied to different disorders, age groups and phases of care. The success or otherwise of this reform agenda will depend on the creation and translation of evidence, empowerment of consumers and families, giving voice to the wider society as a whole, and dauntless leadership from a phalanx of key professional, community and political leaders.

References

1. Oreskes N and Conway E. (2010). *Merchants of Doubt*. London: Bloomsbury Publishing.
2. Rosen A, Byrne P, Goldstone S and McGorry P. (2014). Early intervention for better mental health services, Chapter 99, In: A Tasman, J Kay, JA Lieberman, MB First, and MB Riba, *Psychiatry*. New York: Wiley. In press.
3. Sackett DL. (1995). Applying overviews and meta-analyses at the bedside. *Journal of Clinical Epidemiology* **48**(1): 61–66; discussion 67–70.
4. McGorry PD, Hickie IB, et al. (2006). Clinical staging of psychiatric disorders: a heuristic framework for choosing earlier, safer and more effective interventions. *Australian & New Zealand Journal of Psychiatry* **40**(8): 616–622.
5. McGorry P and van Os J. (2013). Redeeming diagnosis in psychiatry: timing versus specificity. *Lancet* **381**(9863): 343–345.
6. McGorry PD, Tanti C, et al. (2007). Headspace: Australia's National Youth Mental Health Foundation–where young minds come first. *Medical Journal of Australia* **187**(7 Suppl): S68–S70.
7. McGorry P, Bates T, et al. (2013). Designing youth mental health services for the 21st century: examples from Australia, Ireland and the UK. *British Journal of Psychiatry - Supplement* **54**: s30–s35.
8. McGorry P. (2011). The real questions in mental health reform. *Psychiatric Times*, http://www.psychiatrictimes.com/real-questions-mental-health-reform (accessed 20 June 2014).
9. McGorry P. (2013). Early clinical phenotypes and risk for serious mental disorders in young people: need for care precedes traditional diagnoses in mood and psychotic disorders. *Canadian Journal of Psychiatry* **58**(1): 19–21.

Index

Early Intervention in Psychiatry: EI of nearly everything for better mental health, First Edition.
Edited by Peter Byrne and Alan Rosen.
© 2014 John Wiley & Sons, Ltd. Published 2014 by John Wiley & Sons, Ltd.